Medicine, Health, and Healing in the Ancient Mediterranean (500 BCE–600 CE)

Medicine, Health, and Healing in the Ancient Mediterranean (500 BCE–600 CE)

A Sourcebook

KRISTI UPSON-SAIA, HEIDI MARX, AND JARED SECORD

UNIVERSITY OF CALIFORNIA PRESS

University of California Press
Oakland, California

Library of Congress Cataloging-in-Publication Data

Names: Upson-Saia, Kristi, author. | Marx-Wolf, Heidi, author. |
    Secord, Jared, author.
Title: Medicine, health, and healing in the ancient Mediterranean
    (500 BCE–600 CE) : a sourcebook / Kristi Upson-Saia, Heidi Marx,
    and Jared Secord.
Description: Oakland, California : University of California Press, [2023] |
    Includes bibliographical references and index.
Identifiers: LCCN 2022052882 (print) | LCCN 2022052883 (ebook) |
    ISBN 9780520299702 (hardback) | ISBN 9780520299726 (paperback) |
    ISBN 9780520971325 (ebook)
Subjects: LCSH: Medicine, Greek and Roman—Sources.
Classification: LCC R138 .U67 2023 (print) | LCC R138 (ebook) |
    DDC 610.938—dc23/eng/20230313
LC record available at https://lccn.loc.gov/2022052882
LC ebook record available at https://lccn.loc.gov/2022052883

Manufactured in the United States of America

32 31 30 29 28 27 26 25 24 23
10 9 8 7 6 5 4 3 2 1

CONTENTS

ILLUSTRATIONS

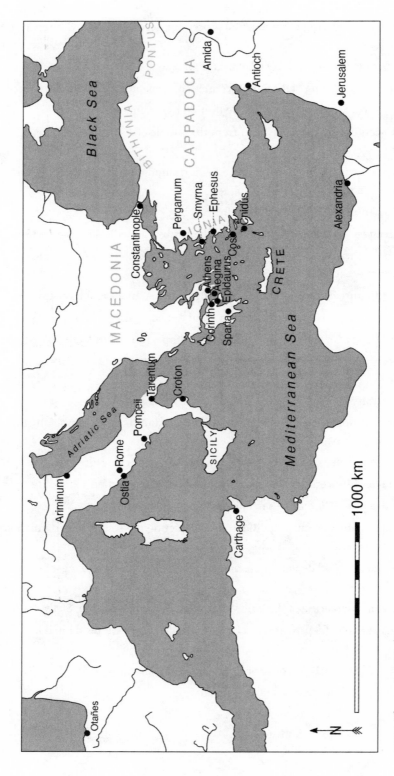

MAP 1 The ancient Mediterranean

ONE

Approaching the History of Medicine

WHY SHOULD WE STUDY THE HISTORY OF MEDICINE?

Students interested in health—especially those seeking careers in the medical professions—know they need to study anatomy, chemistry, and the biological systems of the human body. Many also know that they would benefit from courses beyond the sciences, including courses on the material and societal conditions that lead to health disparities across communities (epidemiology), on the economics of health-care systems (such as the US Affordable Care Act, Canada's Medicare system, and the UK's National Health Service), and on medical ethics. Yet, students may be less convinced that they should study the *history* of medicine. Why, they might ask, would it be important to study medical ideas and practices of the past, especially since we have long abandoned them as misguided and now obsolete? For example, medical theories based on the four humors (yellow bile, black bile, phlegm, and blood) are, to students' minds, wrongheaded, while practices such as bloodletting are even cruel. In short, what value is there in studying medicine, health, and healing of the past?

It is our conviction that studying history matters. Why? Because we can better understand where our own medical ideas, practices, and institutions came from, as well as how they have changed course over time. Moreover, we become better people when we cultivate new perspectives, intellectual sensitivities, and skills from our study of the past.

Let's explore the reasons to study the history of medicine in more detail. First, we can trace the origins and legacies of many medical approaches, values, and practices that we have in fact retained. For example, our modern medical values and ethics are rooted in the oaths that physicians have taken in the past, as well as in the principles that guided their conduct. Additionally, our diagnostic processes are indebted to the approaches ancient medical writers devised to detect what was happening inside the body in a noninvasive way, especially by reading signs or symptoms from the outside of the body. And the modern use of medical charts directly descended from ancient physicians' practice of taking careful clinical notes. Finally, our ideas about quality medical care derive from ancient physicians' discussions of "bedside manner." Although at first it may seem that our forms of medical care deviate starkly from medicine in the past, as it turns out we have inherited much from those who have gone before us. Thus, the first reason to study the history of medicine is to discern the ways in which the past continues to shape our approaches, practices, and values today.

Second, just as we can learn about *continuities* with the past, so too can we learn about *changes introduced over time*. Even when we retain medical ideas and practices from the past, they sometimes morph to better suit new historical moments and new social contexts. For example, one of the most famous legacies of the past comes from the Hippocratic *Oath* (Text 40), a vow made by physicians to follow certain guidelines in their medical practice. Among these guidelines is the vow of confidentiality, which remains important in most medical communities today. According to professional medical organizations of most countries (such as the Canadian and American Medical Associations), physicians pledge to keep medical information confidential in order to secure a patient's trust, in turn freeing the patient to divulge health information—especially sensitive information—that could help the physician arrive at a good diagnosis and treatment plan. Today, therefore, patient-physician confidentiality is primarily about both keeping health information secure and ensuring the best care for the patient. In the ancient Mediterranean, however, a physician's pledge of confidentiality related to something other than a patient's medical information. Ancient physicians made house calls, providing treatment in the private living quarters of patients' homes. In these spaces, physicians were afforded a glimpse into how the household was managed. They could see how orderly and well mannered (or not) the slaves and women of the household were, which was taken as evidence of the man of the house's ability to govern his household well and, when extended to the public sphere, as evidence of his potential for strong leadership within the community. Physicians might also overhear discussions of business affairs among slaves, family, and friends who were at the bedside of the sick. These kinds of information could be used to harm the household, whether undermining the man of the house's reputation or costing him clients. According to the ancient Hippocratic *Oath*, the physician pledged to keep all of this private household information strictly confidential: "Whatever I see or hear, which must never be divulged, I will keep silent and deem such things as not to be spoken" (Text 40). So, in contrast to the thrust of today's pledge, confidentiality in the ancient *Oath* was not limited to *health-care information* but included a wider range of information gleaned during treatment; nor was it motivated by the *health interests* of the patients, but rather by the social and economic interests of the household, and especially the men of households. Thus, studying the history of medicine enables us to see how ideas and practices we have retained have been reinvigorated with new meaning when situated in new contexts over time.

Third, studying the history of medicine complicates the narrative of progressive innovation: the notion that ideas and practices consistently improve over time, with modernity representing the pinnacle of scientific achievement. We very quickly learn that our predecessors had medical insights long before we did. For instance, physicians in the ancient Mediterranean discovered that foxglove could be used to regulate heart rate; they knew the antimalarial properties of sweet wormwood; they used galantamine as a treatment for dementia; and they devised effective techniques to treat hip dysplasia. Study of the past reveals the longevity of a wide swath of remedies still in use today. Scientists today still look to the past to guide innovative new treatments. For example, scientists are studying ancient stool samples—which reveal much richer and more diverse microbiomes than ours today (since ours have been compromised by antibiotics and processed foods)—searching for ways to improve gut health.

In addition to remedies, we also have much to learn from the past about "soft skills," such as those in the clinical context. As modern researchers are beginning to unpack how the quality of a patient's experience when engaging with their physician augments the effectiveness of medical treatments and enhances health outcomes, they can turn to ancient discussions on these topics. Sources from ancient Greece and Rome note the importance of a physician's tone, confidence, warmth, touch, and time spent with patients, all features of the patient-physician relationship that remain significant in modern studies. Moreover, ancient sources draw our attention to other aspects of the clinical encounter that are not receiving adequate scholarly attention, such as ancient medical writers' focus on how physicians' dress, comportment, movements, and handling of instruments contributed to patients' confidence in their physician and optimism about a successful treatment, in turn boosting actual health outcomes. Thus, the history of medicine is a resource we can mine to learn about ancient ideas and practices that can enhance current scholarly investigations and clinical conduct.

Fourth, studying the past can unstick us from the routine, unquestioned ways we tend to think about medicine and health care, and inspire new perspectives. Seeing the medical questions, interests, and priorities of people in a different context attunes us to aspects of health and medicine that are not always at the front of our minds. In other words, studying medicine in a time period and context other than our own can have a productively reorienting and refocusing effect. For instance, many students who have their sights set on careers in the health professions tend to be attuned to certain features of medicine: they focus on anatomy, the nature of disease (pathology), treatments and remedies (such as pharmacology, physical therapy, etc.), and the technological tools used to measure health and illness (such as lab tests and machines that take measurements of the body, such as blood tests or heart rate monitors) or technology used to treat ailments (such as laparoscopic instruments). When students study health care in a different period, especially in the ancient Mediterranean, they see that ancient people cared about a myriad of things beyond the *science* of medicine, including the *human* elements of health care. For example, students encounter patients' fears, worries, anxieties, and priorities. Students see that patients did not always trust their physicians and often refused to follow physicians' orders. Students notice how sick and suffering people turned to family, friends, temples, magicians, community healers, and tradespeople, in addition to physicians, for help. Finally, students perceive physicians themselves fretting about the myriad challenges they face: from the difficulty of sorting all the symptoms they observed to determine which were most significant for their diagnosis, to negotiating with patients (and their families and friends) about a treatment plan, to making financial ends meet. In short, studying the past attunes us to a broader range of issues in the humanistic and social spheres of health and medicine—to patient-centered concerns, preferences, and agency; to communities of care; to nonmedical domains of healing; and to patients and physicians as whole people—and we become sensitized to a wider array of aspects, features, and elements of medicine in our own moment that may have escaped our notice. Thus students entering the health professions who have studied the history of medicine will necessarily be better at their jobs because of their more capacious perspective on the field.

Fifth, when we study the past, it can be easier for us to discern how society's medical ideas and practices are tethered to their specific material and cultural context. For example, a large proportion of medical sources from the ancient Mediterranean address reproduction, which we can understand as a direct response to a historical context constantly in the throes of demographic instability (people dying at a higher rate than being born). Thus the priorities of ancient Greek and Roman medicine were clearly informed by the material conditions and societal interests of its context. Additionally, we see how social and cultural norms infiltrate medical reasoning. For instance, ancient medical gynecology was infused with pervasive gender stereotypes. For example, when discussing an ailment called the "wandering womb," ancient physicians described the womb with misogynistic characteristics commonly attributed to ancient women, characteristics used to deem women the inferior gender: the womb was mercurial, driven by emotions rather than reason, and in need of male pacification and control to be whole and healthy.

As students of history become attuned to how ancient medical priorities and ideas were informed by their context, we become better able to perceive such influence in our own time and context. The study of the past prompts us to question our own modern medical priorities and investments. We are primed to ask questions like the following: What individual and societal problems are motivating medical research? Which research projects are most funded, and which least funded? Whose interests are being served by such research, and whose problems and interests are being ignored? How does our own culture creep into modern medicine (for example, descriptions of the body's defense against disease agents in terms of military metaphors; culturally gendered ways describing the activities of sperm and egg in the fertilization process; culturally racialized and gendered ways of explaining the pain threshold of people of color and women)? When standing in the middle of our own context, it can be difficult to discern how our own societal interests and cultural norms inform our medical priorities and reasoning, but as we become practiced at identifying such sociocultural influence by studying other historical contexts, we cultivate the impulse and capacity to do so.

Sixth and finally, by studying the history of medicine we cultivate an impulse to be empathetic, to discern different points of view, and to respect people who are different from ourselves. Studying the past puts us in contact with a wide range of worldviews, practices, preferences, and values—put simply, students of history encounter a plurality of people. And we are also asked to cultivate the historian's instinct to strive to understand and to respect people who are unfamiliar and unlike ourselves, attempting to discern the reasonableness of their views and practices within their context. In short, the study of the past becomes an occasion in which we practice becoming comfortable with diversity and difference and in which we cultivate the habit of charitable engagement with others. These skills and impulses, in turn, make all of us better able to navigate our own diverse world. And, in particular, these skills and impulses make those entering the health professions better clinicians. As medical ethicists explain, physicians who build stronger relationships with their patients devise treatment plans with which patients are more willing to comply, and the result is better health outcomes overall. In fact, medical schools are recognizing the importance of being able to work with patients from a range of sociocultural backgrounds, something they test for in the Multiple Mini-Interview (MMI) questions that many medical schools now use in the Admissions process.

For all of these reasons and more we are convinced of the importance of studying ancient medicine.[1] An understanding of the past is vital for aspiring health-care professionals, but also for anyone seeking to engage thoughtfully with humans' ongoing—and unending—desire to be healthy.

HOW DO WE STUDY THE HISTORY OF MEDICINE?

Now that we understand *why* studying history is important, the next question to ask is, *how* do historians of ancient medicine do their work? In terms of method, historians of medicine take a multilayered approach. We study important developments in the science of medicine, and the people who had the greatest impact on the history of health and health care, while we also study more commonplace materials that give us glimpses into everyday people's experiences of health and sickness, their views and values regarding health, the kinds of health care available to them, and how their social, religious, economic, political, environmental, and material contexts informed their health and health care. By studying both the big picture and the little picture, we glean an expansive view of ancient medicine, health, and healing. And as we engage these different levels of perspective, we let the myriad and varied details of the ancient world wash over us until it becomes second nature to occupy the position of people in antiquity, and until it becomes second nature to think like someone living in that context. In short, the historian's approach is an immersive, humanistic practice.

Our approach impels us to study as many types of extant evidence as possible, including different kinds of written records (such as formal treatises, letters, and inscriptions), artistic

---

1. Aspiring health-care professionals also benefit from learning the origins and conceptual development of medical terminology, much of which is rooted in or is even a direct transliteration of Greek and Latin terms.

records (such as paintings and statues), and physical remains (such as archaeological sites, artifacts, and human remains). Let's examine the wealth of sources available to us in greater detail. We possess various genres of medical texts, including treatises that articulate general theories of illness; detailed studies on the anatomy, physiology, and pathologies of specific parts of the body (such as gynecological or ophthalmological texts); detailed studies of particular ailments (such as wounds); guides for medical techniques (such as surgery and joint relocations); collections of medicinal recipes (such as pharmacological texts, and recipes for food); and ethical texts and oaths (see fig. 59). These texts help us understand how health-care providers envisioned the problems they were trying to address, and the different steps they took to treat the sick and suffering. Historians also possess extant medical instruments and devices, including scalpels, knives, probes, anal and vaginal specula, forceps, hooks, catheters, drains, cupping vessels, and spatulas (see figs. 22, 24, 26, 48). We possess the botanical remains of medical remedies that survive as residues in the bowls in which drugs were crushed and mixed, and in the containers in which they were stored (see fig. 43). From the archaeological record, we can also see how patient rooms were set up in physicians' clinics or private homes (see fig. 70), as well as the layout of military infirmaries (see fig. 72), healing temples and chapels, and other curative sites. Taken together, these sources provide a textured picture of medicine in ancient Greece and Rome, enabling us to envision medical ideas and treatments concretely and viscerally.

While the sources described above paint a picture of healing professionals, other ancient sources give us a glimpse into sick and suffering people's experiences. In letters exchanged between friends, individuals described their ailments and the symptoms they were feeling, the impact their ailments had on their livelihood as well as how it affected their loved ones, how they explained the cause or source of their ailments, and their reasoning about when and what kind of medical care to seek out. Other letters provide insight into the founding of the first hospitals: how the institutions were organized and staffed, the social services provided, and what the public thought of them. In literary sources, such as poems and plays (sometimes satire), we hear criticisms of medicine and physicians, alerting us to patients' fears, anxieties, and worries, and explaining why some chose nonmedical remedies when they became sick. For those who sought aid at healing sites, we possess votive offerings—clay or stone objects shaped to resemble body parts affected by illness or injury—which were offered to the gods along with prayers/petitions for healing (see figs. 21, 32). We also possess inscriptions and graffiti from healing sites, where the sick and suffering scribbled their petitions for help or their gratitude for healing (see Text 39). Finally, from epitaphs on tombstones, we learn the causes of deaths, especially the most common causes (such as war injuries, childbirth, or occupational hazards).

In the past few decades, historians have made use of an even wider set of sources and scientific techniques to illuminate our understanding of ancient health. For instance, the study of human remains—known as bioarchaeology or osteoarchaeology—provides information about people's diets, bodily injuries, and diseases, information that complements our textual records. For example, scholars conduct carbon and nitrogen isotope analysis of bones in order to detect an individual's diet in the last few years before death, and they also analyze the microscopic structures of teeth to glean information about nutritional deficiencies. When enough individual data is amassed, researchers can reach conclusions about how much access ancient communities had to nutrient-rich foods, as well as about nutritional disparities across regions and social classes. Because malnutrition is linked to injuries (less dense bones make people more susceptible to fractures and breaks) and to illness (malnutrition compromises the immune system), this scholarship on the prevalence and patterns of malnutrition affords us a sharper picture of the daily life conditions that influenced health and illness in the ancient Mediterranean.

The study of human remains also provides information about the specific kinds of bodily trauma and diseases ancient people experienced. For example, bioarchaeologists and osteoarchaeologists estimate the prevalence of rheumatic ailments from lesions and eburnations they find in the joints of human remains. And paleogeneticists can construct a picture of the disease ecology of the ancient Mediterranean by analyzing pathogen DNA extracted from human dental pulp (see fig. 37). Finally, paleoparasitologists can identify the prevalence and kind of parasitic infections within a city or region by harvesting evidence of parasites—whether adult parasites, parasite eggs, their DNA, or their protein byproducts—from latrine soil or calcified human feces at ancient sites (see fig. 25). This range of scientific findings provides us with a sense of the kinds and prevalence of injuries and illnesses, further nuancing our understanding of the routine forms of suffering people in the ancient Mediterranean endured.

Scientific approaches also provide us with information about how ancient people dealt with certain health issues. For example, bioarchaeologists' study of human remains reveals medical interventions, such as the surgical technique of cranial trepanation: boring a hole into the skull to relieve pressure on the brain (see fig. 47). And scientists can also assess ancient physicians' degree of success in these interventions. For instance, some scholars remark on the advanced techniques of setting bones that make some fractures and breaks nearly imperceptible to modern scientists, healing that reveals the patient survived the surgery.

Finally, historians of medicine study the epidemiological conditions that would have influenced health and illness. We learn about the health disparities that must have resulted from different environmental conditions, such as those in cities and in the countryside. For instance, people in cities that were trading centers often would have had access to a wider variety of foods, while people in the countryside often would have had access to cleaner water sources. Moreover, in Rome, we surmise that lower-class people living in marshy, low-lying areas of the city experienced health risks due to standing water and regular flooding that, in turn, spread more mosquito-borne illnesses. They were also susceptible to the more highly concentrated air pollution that settled in the pockets between the city's hills. These were health risks that elite people living in the higher elevations of Rome's seven hills avoided. We also make use of newly available scientific evidence from ice cores bored from the Greenland ice sheet that helps us understand the levels and dispersion of air pollution generated by ancient, especially Roman, mining and smelting operations. When we pair this atmospheric pollution with ancient people's practices of drinking water that had passed through lead pipes, eating food from lead cooking and serving bowls, and even ingesting lead as food additives (*defrutum* or *sapa*), it explains the high levels of Pb toxicity bioarchaeologists are finding in human remains from the period. By studying these kinds of exposure to environmental pathogens and toxins, historians can reach conclusions about the symptoms and health maladies people living in the ancient Mediterranean likely experienced. For example, lead poisoning causes chronic ailments (such as hypertension, kidney issues, and immunotoxicity) and reproductive impairments (such as reduced and abnormal sperm, miscarriages, and stillbirths). Lead poisoning also impairs the brain and central nervous system, resulting in coma, convulsions, and even death.

Taken together, all of these sources and scholarly methods provide historians of medicine with a rich sense of the conditions, experiences, ideas, practices, and approaches toward illness, health, and healing in the ancient Mediterranean. The best histories of ancient medicine are interdisciplinary projects, coordinating various kinds of evidence and using an array of humanistic, social scientific, and scientific methods.

SCOPE AND APPROACH

The materials in this volume encompass medicine, health, and healing in the ancient Mediterranean from approximately 500 BCE to 600 CE (from the emergence of Greek science and medical profession through its development across the Roman Empire).[2] As we selected the topics and sources to cover, we were motivated by two guiding principles. First, we endeavored to paint a representative picture of medicine, health, and healing in ancient Greek and Roman territories. We have included sources from a range of medical authors, traditions, and schools in order to give readers a sense of what ideas and practices garnered consensus and had staying power over time, as well as to reveal minority opinions and changes over time. We also aimed to include a range of genres of medical sources, including medical lectures and treatises, case histories, medical reference works, and medical compendia. Yet, to avoid giving a distorted impression that physicians and professional medicine were the only form of health care in ancient Greece and Rome, we widened our gaze to include materials on health and healing beyond professional medicine, including discussions of religious and so-called magical healing. We discuss philosophical and metaphysical texts, natural histories, collections of herbal remedies, spells and magical recipes, healing at religious sites, miracle stories, personal letters, and inscriptions. When studied alongside professional medical sources, these materials reveal the range of options that sick and suffering people had when seeking healing, and illuminate the fluid boundaries between medicine, philosophy, religion, and "magic" in the ancient Mediterranean. And by highlighting

---

2. We shop at the time when Islamic medicine was on the rise, introducing developments beyond the scope of this volume.

the overlap of healing domains we aim to disrupt the tendency to project into the past a modern notion that medicine was the only or the superior form of health care.

Our second goal was to incorporate an array of nontextual evidence and an array of methodological approaches. When possible, we discuss physical remains, including artistic evidence (such as statues of famous healers and frescoes depicting medical procedures), artifacts (such as anatomical votives, surgical instruments, and drug paraphernalia), and archaeological evidence (such as military hospitals, surgeons' houses, and incubation chapels). And we discuss scientific scholarship that nuances our understanding of the conditions and health of people in the ancient Mediterranean (for example, paleoparasitology and bioarchaeology). We include this wide variety of evidence in order to demonstrate the different kinds of information we can glean from different kinds of sources, which, when taken together, paint a rich and layered picture of ancient health and medicine. After readers have finished this volume, we hope they will have gained a good sense of the landscape of ancient Greek and Roman medicine, health, and healing, understanding the ideas of health and illness, health-care practices, healing institutions and spaces, and experiences of suffering and healing, while also becoming familiar with the scholarly approaches utilized by historians and scientists.

Although we tried to create a comprehensive picture of health and healing in the ancient Mediterranean, we were forced to exclude many topics and materials simply because of space limitations. For example, readers will notice that most of our materials relate to ancient Greek and Roman communities. We made the decision to exclude a wider breadth of communities (represented in Babylonian, Mesopotamian, Egyptian, Syrian, Persian, and Islamic sources) in order to provide greater depth. Even so, we still could not include every aspect of Greek and Roman medicine. We chose to highlight the humanistic side of medicine—for example, materials that give us a glimpse into the experiences, practices, decisions, challenges, and complications faced by health-care professionals and by sick and suffering people—at the expense of diving more deeply into more technical aspects of medical theories and knowledge. Finally, we must acknowledge that some choices have been made for us in terms of what kinds of information were recorded and what ancient sources have been preserved. Most extant sources from antiquity come to us from literate, wealthy men who lived in urban centers. Thus, the perspectives of others—namely, less prominent healers, people in rural areas, and marginalized groups, such as slaves, women, and lower-class people—are not as well documented. Moreover, the survival of sources has depended on accidents of history; for example, sources kept in dry climates tend to survive better than in moist climates, and some medical sources have been lost in disasters, like the fire at the Temple of Peace in Rome. We must remain cognizant of how these lacunae and losses in the historical record have necessarily created distortions in our picture of ancient medicine, health, and healing.

In chapter 2 we provide a chronological overview of the key developments and figures of Greek and Roman medicine, health, and healing from approximately 500 BCE to 600 CE, and in chapter 3 we describe the material conditions that gave rise to sickness, injury, and death, prompting the need for health care. These introductory chapters attempt to set the stage so that readers can engage with the primary sources and evidence in the remainder of the volume.

The subsequent chapters are arranged according to thematic focus.

Chapter 4 discusses ancient theories about the connections between humans and the cosmos: how human bodies were thought to share the same material and ordering as the cosmos, as well as how human health was linked to environmental factors.

Chapter 5 describes the emergence of a professional field of medicine, and ancient people's initial skepticism and criticism of the new science.

Chapter 6 provides an overview of the ways ancient thinkers defined health and illness, their range of theories about what caused illness, and their range of principles about how to avoid illness and how to restore health.

Chapter 7 explains the diagnostic protocols followed by ancient physicians, including the bodily signs they looked for when giving a physical examination, the questions they would ask patients, and how they sifted this evidence to reach a diagnosis and prognosis.

Chapter 8 discusses the case notes and case histories taken to track the progress of individual illnesses, and the kinds of information we glean about the clinical context from these records.

Chapter 9 provides an overview of common complaints: the ailments that show up most frequently in ancient sources and thus either were the most prevalent or caused the most distress.

Chapter 10 provides an overview of common treatments or therapeutic approaches that were taken to combat illness or maintain health.

Chapter 11 discusses the training, education, and status of physicians and other kinds of health-care providers.

Chapter 12 focuses on the sick and suffering person's perspective: their experiences of being sick, their use of home health care, their fears and worries about medicine, and their resistance to and disobedience of physicians' instructions.

Chapter 13 discusses the vows and ethical principles that governed physicians' practice, as well as their professional clinical conduct.

Chapter 14 describes medical views of salient life stages: pregnancy and obstetric care; childhood ailments and pediatric care; and end of life and geriatric care.

Chapter 15 discusses a variety of healing sites in the ancient Mediterranean and considers the role of place and space in healing.

Each of these chapters includes headnotes that orient readers to the topic, explaining how the sources in the chapter fit within a wider range of extant evidence and highlighting important issues. Text introductions for each primary source provide contextual information about the text, along with its date and the original language in which it was written.

TRANSLATIONS, TERMINOLOGY, AND CONVENTIONS

Many decisions went into the translations we include, the terminology we favor, and the conventions we employ in this volume. We aimed for the translations, whether newly commissioned for this volume or reprinted from recent publications, to be the most up-to-date. New translations matter because we are better able to render the ideas of ancient Greek and Latin medical thinkers as our understanding of texts improves, whether through the reexamination of existing manuscripts or the discovery of new manuscripts. Although new discoveries are rare, they do happen periodically. In the 1970s a new manuscript of *On Medicine* by the Roman author Celsus was found, which contained material missing from other manuscripts we already had of this text. And in 2005 a manuscript containing texts by the physician Galen was discovered, including a text that we previously did not have, called *On the Avoidance of Grief.* New translations are important because they take into account knowledge we glean from these new manuscripts and new texts.

New translations also matter because they keep up with changing medical and anatomical terminology. For example, the only existing English translations of some of the texts in this volume were made in the nineteenth or early twentieth century. These older translations tend to use medical terminology that will seem strange to modern readers—for instance, the word "epistaxis" rather than "nosebleed." Older translations are also sometimes coy in translating medical discussions or anatomical terms that past translators considered lewd. In these cases, translators sometimes actively censored the text, refusing to translate it into English—for example, a translator of Theophrastus refused to translate the words for a prolapsed anus and instead gave the Latin: "And, if he is cutting the root at the time, he gets *prolapsus ani*." Or translators used more oblique words like "fundament" rather than "buttocks" or "anus." Furthermore, because language is always evolving, new translations are essential to convey meaning more effectively through words, phrases, and style that contemporary readers will best understand.

Finally, new translators fix mistakes and avoid the pitfalls made by past translators and scholars. For example, new translators are more careful about identifying ailments mentioned in ancient medical texts and avoiding the conflation of ancient and modern conditions that share the same name. Translating some ancient terms is challenging because so many medical terms in English are drawn directly from Greek or Latin words. One illustrative example is the use of the term *cholera*. This Latin word also exists in English, referring to an infectious disease, transmitted by contaminated food or water, that typically causes vomiting and diarrhea. But the disease that most of us now associate with the word "cholera" seems not to have existed in the Mediterranean in antiquity.[3] Both the ancient and modern illnesses called "cholera" get their names from Greek words that refer to one of the principal symptoms—the "flow" (*rhoea*) of excretions filled with "bile" (*cholē*)—but the causes of the

3. Occasionally, modern people will call the cholera mentioned in ancient Greek and Latin texts European, sporadic, or summer cholera as a way to distinguish it from the modern form of cholera, which has also sometimes been called Asiatic cholera.

ancient and modern illnesses are different. When European physicians in the nineteenth century first encountered the disease, they simply borrowed the word *cholera* from older medical sources, wrongly concluding that what is now familiarly known as cholera was the same as the condition mentioned by Hippocrates, Celsus, and other ancient authors. Another example is the English word "cancer," which derives from the Greek word *karkinos* and the Latin word *cancer.* The basic meaning of these words in their respective languages was "crab," but they also came to be associated with a range of sores, tumors, and weeping ulcers, evidently because the sores' shape resembled a crab's body and the sores were as hard as a crab's shell. Some of the conditions that ancient medical writers described as *karkinos* in Greek or *cancer* in Latin may have actually been what modern physicians now define as cancer, but other times the ancient term referred to sores that do not fit our modern classification of cancer. In our translations we have sought to be very clear when ancient ailments are in fact different from modern conditions with the same or similar names.[4]

Furthermore, our translations also avoid another misstep of older translators: retrospective diagnosis, which involves diagnosing ancient illnesses based on the symptoms described in ancient sources and using modern disease names or classifications. It is often tempting for modern readers to diagnose ancient people with modern illnesses or conditions based on vague or ambiguous descriptions of symptoms in ancient literature (descriptions that oftentimes were not intended to be used for this purpose). This tendency creeps into translations and interpretations of ancient texts. See, for example, the suggestion that Favorinus, a famous orator of the second century CE, was born with an intersex condition called Reifenstein's syndrome because he is described by ancient authors as being an androgynous "man-woman" with no beard or testicles, a conjecture that assumes (wrongly, we think) that the information in our sources is sufficiently detailed, reliable, and objective to allow modern readers to use our knowledge of medical science to arrive at a reliable diagnosis. Many similar examples of this sort exist, including how to translate "leprosy" (Greek *lepra*, Latin *lepra*), a term that was applied to skin conditions of all sorts in the ancient world, few of which had anything to do with the condition that physicians today call Hansen's disease. In order to avoid using categories of illness that would be illegible to people in antiquity, and to avoid the potential for misdiagnosis, our translations resist the temptation of retrospective diagnosis as much as possible.

Finally, our translations aim to be readable, literal, and consistent. These three features of translation, however, are not always compatible, so we periodically sacrifice literalness and consistency in the interest of readability and conveying meaning that makes sense for both ancient authors and modern readers.[5]

4. For the same reason that we cannot conflate ancient and modern terms, we have also chosen not to offer firm identifications of the various plants and animals in the translations.

5. Regarding consistency, in the reprinted translations we were sometimes granted permission to make minor changes (such as changing British spellings to American and standardizing spellings of Greek names), but in some cases we were not allowed to make edits, leading to some inconsistencies across translations in this volume. In some of the reprinted translations, we have made changes to the footnotes.

While our overarching goal was to make the ancient texts comprehensible for readers who do not read Greek and Latin, we also did not want to give the misleading impression that ancient medical writers and physicians operated with the same assumptions and ideas and thought-world as people today. So, at times we have allowed the strangeness of our sources to stand in the translation, and then used footnotes to provide further explanation or clarity.

There were occasions when we had a choice of English words to use in our translations. For example, there were a number of Greek and Latin terms that we could have translated as "illness," "sickness," "ailment," "injury," or "disease." We chose to avoid translating the Greek term *nosos* and the Latin term *morbus* as "disease," since the modern notions of disease as a long-term illnesses with a specific set of features (for example, obstructive pulmonary disease, Lou Gehrig's disease, heart disease) would not have made sense to ancient medical thinkers. They, on the contrary, had different ways of categorizing some illnesses (such as acute or chronic) or did not formally categorize illnesses at all.

Our translations follow standard numbering conventions: including book, chapter, and paragraph numbers for texts written in prose, and book (where applicable) and line numbers for texts written in verse. Readers can use these conventions to track down references cited in footnotes. For instance, a footnote that points to Homer, *Iliad* 11.833 refers to line 833 of the eleventh book of the *Iliad,* Homer's epic poem. Similarly, a reference that reads Pliny the Elder, *Natural History* 7.13–15 refers to chapters thirteen through fifteen of the seventh book of Pliny's encyclopedic text written in prose. References to texts written by medical authors follow similar principles, though there is some additional complexity in standard references to texts by Galen and those attributed to Hippocrates; these typically include references to volume and page numbers in standard editions of their Greek text edited respectively by Kühn and Littré.

Readers should be aware that the numbering systems, and sometimes even the titles, used in English translations were not originally part of the ancient texts. Later editors often added the text divisions and created titles taken from words in the opening lines of the text. A text by Rufus of Ephesus, which in this volume we title *On The Importance of Questioning the Sick Person,* illustrates such a case. The numbering that appears in this text derives from the first printed edition of the Greek text, and was assigned by its editor in the nineteenth century, nearly 1,800 years after Rufus wrote the text. A subsequent edition of the Greek text published in the 1960s further divided up the text into chapters to reflect the editor's sense of the logical segments of the text. Following the suggestion of our translator Melinda Letts, we have not included these chapter numbers, on the grounds that they limit how readers may interpret Rufus's structure. Furthermore, while the traditional title assigned to this text is *Medical Questions* (typically given in Latin: *Quaestiones Medicinales*), Letts argues that the longer form of the title is a more accurate reflection of the text's content, and also remains faithful to the text's opening phrase: "You must ask the sick person questions." Readers should consequently use caution when seeking to understand a text based on its conventional title and chapter divisions that appear to organize it, since, in many cases, neither has any relation to how the text was originally written and published in antiquity.

In the translations we use three asterisks (*) to indicate places where we are choosing to omit part of a text and jump ahead. When portions of a paragraph or sentence are missing in the original text itself, we use square brackets. When the original text contains a corrupt section that the editor has attempted to restore but cannot be confident in its accuracy, we indicate this with a symbol called an obelus (†) at the beginning and end of the restored section. And when a text (or inscription) has been damaged and words are missing or break off, though we know there was more to follow, we use square brackets and ellipses [. . .] to indicate a missing portion of the text. When editors are relatively confident about what letters or words are missing—because, for instance, they are words that are commonly used in inscriptions or deduced through the context of the surrounding words—the restored text will be placed inside square brackets.

Throughout the volume, we often provide dates in centuries. The second century CE refers to the period from 100 CE to 199 CE, the third century CE to the period from 200 to 299 CE, and so on. For the centuries Before the Common Era (BCE), remember that dates progress counting downward (rather than upward as in the Common Era)—for example, the fourth century BCE refers to the period 399–300. Also note the use of the following abbreviations:

c.   circa. This indicates that the date or dates given are approximate.

BCE   Before the Common Era. (BCE is equivalent to BC, which stands for "Before Christ.")

CE   Common Era. (CE is equivalent to AD, the abbreviation for the Latin phrase *Anno Domini,* which means "In the year of the Lord.")

As for reading aids, at the end of the volume you will find a glossary of subjects that defines words that have a distinct meaning or significance in the context of ancient medicine. We have not defined every technical term; we have left out terms whose meaning has not changed since antiquity and whose definition readers can easily find in a standard dictionary or by way of an internet search. By this rationale, we have not included a glossary entry for a word like "lientery," the correct meaning of which readers could easily discover on their own and that meant something similar in antiquity to its meaning today. We have, however, included entries for seemingly familiar words that refer to ancient concepts or practices but have different meanings in our context. For example, we have a glossary entry for "fumigate" that explains how fumigation was used as a therapeutic tool by some ancient physicians, a process rarely, if ever, used in medical treatment today. Finally, we have also included in the glossary some ancient units of weights and measures that may be unfamiliar to modern readers.

Throughout the volume, terms are bolded (the first time they appear in chapter headnotes and in translations) to indicate when there is a corresponding entry in the glossary of subjects. Readers will also find the names of physicians and philosophers in bold font (the first time they appear in chapter headnotes and in translations). These figures have short biographical entries in the glossary of people. To help readers situate these figures with their contemporaries and in their context, the more significant of these people also appear in the timeline at the end of this volume.

We consulted hundreds of primary and secondary sources in the production of this volume. Although we cannot adequately recognize them all in an itemized list, we wish to signal our indebtedness to the scholars on whose shoulders we stand. At the end of the volume we have included a section titled "Further Reading" to help readers navigate the available primary sources and identify some of the foundational recent scholarship.

TWO

Greek and Roman Medicine: A Chronological Overview

In the preface to his text *On Medicine*, **Celsus** (first centuries BCE and CE) wrote that "nowhere is medicine absent, since even the most uncivilized peoples are familiar with herbs and other things brought forth for aiding wounds and illnesses" (Text 4, Preface 1). Although, as Celsus notes, people in all times and places have developed ingenious and effective ways of dealing with suffering and illness, in this chapter we trace important developments in the history of ancient Greek and Roman medicine from roughly 500 BCE to 600 CE. We begin with the Hippocratic school in Greece in the fifth to fourth century BCE, which marked a notably more systematic, theoretical approach to health, as well as new professional identities for healers. And we trace the development of the early science and profession as they spread throughout the Mediterranean. We will see that the field of medicine encompassed a diverse set of ideas, practices, and personnel.

As we learn about some of the most important medical thinkers and innovations of this period, it is important to keep in mind that many other people—beyond physicians—were involved in providing health care to the sick and suffering. Physicians sometimes competed, and sometimes collaborated, with root cutters (Greek *rhizotomos,* sometimes used as a synonym for "sorcerer"); **drug** traders, sellers, and makers (i.e., pharmacists); **obstetricians;** massage therapists; gymnastic trainers; bone setters; surgeons; lithotomists (surgeons who specialized in the removal of bladder stones); ritual or shamanic healers of various sorts, including exorcists; temple priests; and the gods and other immortal spirits. From this range of healing domains—often referred to as the ancient "medical marketplace"—we understand that the sick and suffering had many options available to them, and we seek to learn when and why they chose one over the other.

We must also keep in mind that, before the Greek science and profession of medicine developed, communities across the Mediterranean had established healing practices and traditions, some of which influenced Greek and Roman medicine. For example, the Egyptians and Babylonians developed sophisticated and fascinating approaches to healing. Studying papyri documents from Egypt, such as the Edwin Smith Papyrus (c. 1600 BCE) and the Ebers Papyrus (c. 1550 BCE), we find elaborate descriptions of procedures used to staunch bleeding and suture wounds, recipes for drugs to treat intestinal complaints and eye infections, and descriptions of the heart and the vessels attached to it for conveying blood to the entire body. Readers interested in ancient medicine will find much to discover in textual and archaeological records from these earlier civilizations.

Before we start our chronological overview of Greek and Roman medicine with a discussion of the scientific approach to health introduced by early Greek natural philosophers, we need to first consider the prevailing religious explanations of illness from which they broke.

RELIGIOUS EXPLANATIONS OF SUFFERING AND ILLNESS ACROSS ANTIQUITY

When scientific views of the world were developing, most people—both educated and uneducated, from all socioeconomic classes—believed that human suffering of all kinds was caused by immortal beings who were expressing displeasure with humans. They reasoned that individuals or communities had failed to show proper reverence or worship to the gods, or they had failed to uphold their moral responsibilities, so the gods sent misfortune as a punishment. Take, for example, the collective suffering the gods sent upon the Greek army in Homer's *Iliad,* and the seven plagues the Judean God sent to induce the Egyptians to free the Jewish people from captivity. Moreover, individual illnesses, injuries, and death were explained as retribution for broken vows to the gods or for immoral conduct.

Although most of the time humans' relationships with the gods followed a straightforward theory of reciprocity—rewards for good behavior and punishments for bad behavior—religion could be complicated. For example, the mercurial goddess Tuche (sometimes spelled Tyche) or Fortuna was believed to dole out prosperity and suffering, fortune and misfortune, somewhat indiscriminately. She was often depicted holding the wheel of fortune, which she spun to determine someone's fate. And Greeks and Romans needed to pacify a wide range of immortal beings who were in charge of many important aspects of life, such as planting and growing food (for instance, the Greek goddess Demeter and the personified Roman gods Blight and Rust, who could cause crop failure), and the fraught and dangerous process of carrying a child to term and giving birth to it (the Greek goddess Hera, for example). Still more, the gods were not the only immortals who could bring suffering. Jews and Christians told stories of malign daemons who caused illness and injury, as well as mental distress when they possessed individual bodies. The Gospel of Mark, for instance, reports

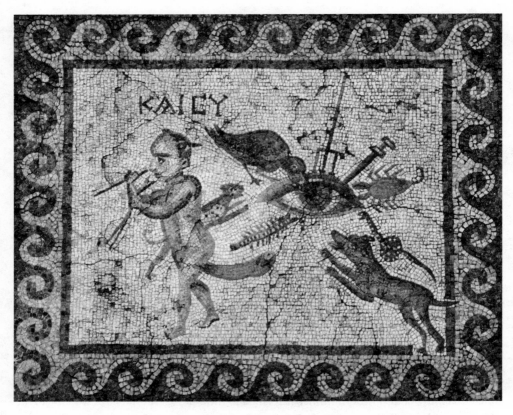

FIGURE 1 Second-century CE Roman mosaic depicting the evil eye—a symbol of misfortune—being attacked by a centipede, cat, bird, trident, sword, scorpion, snake, and dog. The figure on the left, represented with an enlarged phallus (also a symbol of power, sometimes used apotropaically to ward off evil), may be either a harmful spirit allied with the evil eye, or a good spirit helping to subdue the evil eye. The Greek KAI SU—which translates as "and you too"—wishes for the viewers of the mosaic a similar protection against evil. Hatay Archaeology Museum, Antioch (inv. no. 1024). Photo credit: Tahsin Firuz Soyuer.

that the Jewish holy man Jesus cast out an "unclean spirit" from a boy experiencing seizures that caused him to fall down and foam at the mouth.

Many people also believed that the good things in life—such as health, children, and comfort afforded by wealth—were in limited supply. If one person had more of any one of these it was because someone else had less (what we today call "zero-sum thinking"). Moreover, they believed these limited goods and evils could be redistributed or preserved through ritual means. For example, it was thought that an envious glance could lead to the drying up of vital fluids, the loss of health, illness in one's children, and so forth. Thus, the evil eye was a representation of what people believed were the withering effects of envy (see fig. 1). And many people sought to protect themselves and their health through apotropaic objects that could repel evil powers, such as amulets worn like jewelry or stationed in or around one's house (see fig. 2).

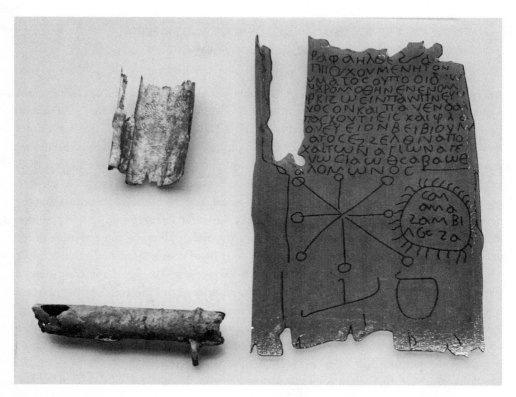

FIGURE 2 Fourth- to fifth-century CE curative amulet. Fourteen lines of script were inscribed on thin silver lamina (*top left*), then rolled up and placed inside a cylindrical bronze container with two suspension rings (*bottom left*). The inscription (enlarged, *right*) is an invocation to the angels, the Holy Spirit, and the Lord followed by a formula imploring that Bibius Mamas, the owner of the amulet, "who suffers from headaches and ictus" might be delivered from evil spirits and from the demon responsible for gingivitis that prevents him from speaking. A set of symbols is engraved under the text, including a star with eight rays. This symbol—which is associated with Helios, the Greek god and personification of the Sun—is also found at the Asclepian temple in Epidaurus, Greece, alongside inscriptions asking Helios for healing. Naples Archaeological Museum. Photo credit: Kristi Upson-Saia.

Finally, misfortune—including illness and death—could be caused by curses inscribed on metal, rolled up, and tucked away near the intended victims. For example, a tablet found at a temple and bath complex in Aquae Sulis (modern-day Bath in England) records a curse against an unknown thief or anyone who has knowledge of the theft of a ring: "Anyone, whether slave or free, who knows anything about the theft and keeps silent, he may be accursed in (his) blood, and eyes and every limb and even have all (his) intestines quite eaten away if he has stolen the ring or if he is withholding information (about the theft)" (*Tabellae Sulis* 97). These ideas about suffering and illness persisted throughout the period we are exploring, but around the sixth century BCE they began to be challenged by both philosophers and medical writers.

EARLY GREEK NATURAL PHILOSOPHERS AND MATERIAL EXPLANATIONS OF THE WORLD (SIXTH–FIFTH CENTURY BCE: GREEK ARCHAIC PERIOD)

Against the backdrop of such religious views, alternate explanations of the causes of illness began to develop among philosophers in the Greek colonies of ancient Ionia (on the west coast of modern-day Türkiye) and southern Italy. These thinkers—who are sometimes known collectively as the pre-Socratic or Ionian philosophers but who are more accurately referred to as early Greek natural philosophers—sought to replace religious or supernatural explanations with explanations that were based on principles of nature itself. They undertook the task of carefully observing the material world, and then devised theories about the laws and principles that governed the operations of the world. For example, instead of understanding weather events as signs of the gods' pleasure and displeasure, some of these thinkers observed cycles of seasons. This paradigm shift freed people from understanding the gods alone to be in control, and allowed them to engage with the world and contribute to their own well-being. For example, once they could understand the cycles of the seasons, humans could make agricultural decisions in concert with weather patterns and, in turn, maximize their harvest. Thus, the natural philosophers introduced a new way of viewing the operations of the world, one that gave a degree of agency to humans. Similar modes of thinking are evident in the ideas of early Greek medical writers from roughly the same period about the nature of the human body and the phenomena of health and illness.

Beyond this general orientation, the early Greek natural philosophers also developed a number of specific ideas that contributed to early medical thinking. First and foremost, the observations of certain philosophers about the makeup and functioning of the natural world would come to influence views about the makeup and functioning of the human body. For example, **Empedocles of Acragas** (fifth century BCE), who was likely a healer himself, was the first to posit the four elements—earth, water, air, and fire—as the building blocks of matter. He called them "roots," and he taught that all things in the cosmos were made up of the mingling of these elements, in different ratios and different states of mixing. These ideas would form the basis of later humoral theories that the human body was composed of the four **humors**—black bile, phlegm, blood, and yellow bile—and that health and illness related to their ratios and mixing in the body. The "atomists," **Democritus of Abdera** (c. 460–380 BCE) and Leucippus (Ionia, fifth century BCE), held a different view about the makeup of the world; they proposed that "atoms" were the building blocks of all things. Atoms—indestructible particles that were in constant motion—combined and separated in patterns that caused things to exist and then disintegrate. According to this atomic theory, health in human beings was explained to be the result of atoms combining and remaining together in specific patterns, whereas people became ill upon the dissolution of these atomic patterns. Despite their disagreement, the views of both Empedocles and Democritus about the material components of the cosmos would inspire later medical writers to generate systematic explanations of the material components of human bodies.

Some of the early Greek natural philosophers also initiated discussions about human anatomy and physiology that would influence later medical discussions. **Alcmaeon of Croton** (early fifth century BCE) seems to have made some of the earliest anatomical observations of the optic nerves and of the passages between the nasal and ear cavities, perhaps as a result of dissection. **Anaxagoras of Clazomenae** (fifth century BCE) devised a theory that all things were made up of an infinite number of kinds of invisible "seeds" in order to explain how food could be transformed into other things, such as hair and fingernails: the seeds of these kinds of matter were digested and reconstituted in new forms. Alcmaeon, followed by Diogenes of Apollonia (fifth century BCE), also theorized about the body's *pneuma*—which could mean anything from air, wind, or breath to enlivening spirit—understanding it to be the medium that transmitted sensations from the brain to other parts of the body. Later medical writers would continue to chart anatomical structures, discuss physiological processes like digestion, and debate the qualities and role of *pneuma* in the body's operation and health.

Finally, these natural philosophers advised their audiences to adopt certain bodily practices in order to heighten their well-being. For instance, Alcmaeon followed his teacher, **Pythagoras** (c. 570–495 BCE), in believing that the soul was divinity trapped in the body and that the soul could escape cycles of reincarnation only through practices that enhanced one's spiritual and physical purity. Such practices seem to have taken the form of dietary restrictions, such as vegetarianism and a prohibition against eating beans. In addition to regimen, later accounts of Pythagoras depict him healing his students using music therapy. This link between bodily practices and well-being would be developed in detail by later medical thinkers.

In short, the early Greek natural philosophers introduced a new way of making sense of the world, understanding natural phenomena in terms of logical principles and the order of the natural world (not solely in terms of the powers of the gods). Additionally, they provided a reservoir of discrete ideas that would be developed by subsequent thinkers, not only in the domains of natural science and philosophy, but also in the field of medicine. In conversation with these philosophical thinkers, the field of professional medicine could develop not just as a craft or a profession, but also as a science: a coherent system of knowledge and practice grounded in empirical research.

THE HIPPOCRATIC SCHOOL (FIFTH CENTURY BCE: GREEK CLASSICAL PERIOD)

A seminal moment in early attempts to think about medicine, health, and healing in a systematic fashion and as a professional pursuit is associated with **Hippocrates** and the Hippocratic school (fig. 3). According to a biography written centuries after his life, Hippocrates was born in 460 BCE on Cos, an island off the west coast of modern-day Türkiye where he later founded his medical school. He was reputed to have drawn his lineage from the family of Asclepiads, healers who traced their origins back to the healing god **Asclepius** (discussed in more detail below). Growing up in Cos and in close proximity to the nearby coastal

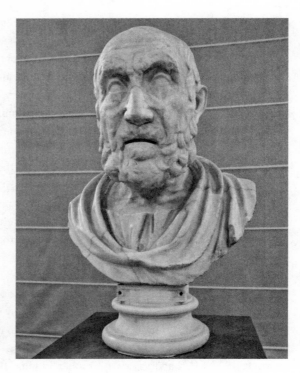

FIGURE 3 First-century CE marble bust of Greek physician Hippocrates of Cos. Naples Archaeological Museum (inv. no. 6131). Photo credit: Kristi Upson-Saia.

city of Cnidus—both places known for their healers—Hippocrates must have been steeped in the healing traditions not only of his family but also of the region. After some time leading the group of healers on Cos, Hippocrates is reported to have left the island to work as a physician in Thessaly (a region in northern Greece) and in Athens. As his fame spread, Hippocrates was invited to practice in the court of the Persian ruler, Artaxerxes.

Unfortunately, we have few ancient testimonies as to what Hippocrates actually thought or taught. Contemporary witnesses tell us when and where Hippocrates was born and that he would teach medicine to anyone who could pay his fee. **Plato** (428–348/7 BCE) cryptically said that Hippocrates believed one could not treat illness without knowledge of the whole, though whether that meant knowledge of nature as a whole, of the body as a whole, or just of the patient's environment as a whole, we cannot know for certain. Writing a generation later, Meno (Greece, late fourth century BCE) attributed to Hippocrates a view on the origins of illness that is very similar to that held by earlier Egyptian medical writers: that illness arises from the gases that emanate from undigested food residues putrefying in the body. These gases then overwhelm or displace health-giving *pneuma* in the body.

We are fortunate, however, to possess a large set of texts—approximately sixty Greek medical texts called "the Hippocratic corpus"—that give us a strong sense of early Greek medical thought. The Hippocratic corpus is a treasure trove of information on almost every aspect of medicine. It includes texts that discuss anatomy, physiology, pathology, diagnosis, prognosis, case studies, regimen, therapy, surgery, pharmacology, medical ethics, "bedside manner" or etiquette, and also subspecialties such as pediatrics, gynecology, obstetrics, and even psychology. Given that some texts represent views developed decades and even centuries after Hippocrates's lifetime, it is clear that the corpus includes texts written by a range of authors over time. It is possible that some of these texts were written by Hippocrates himself, but we cannot know for certain which ones. (The puzzle of whether any of these texts, and which texts, were written by Hippocrates is called "the Hippocratic question.") Some of the earliest texts could have been written by students of Hippocrates or by those subscribing to his medical approach, who co-opted Hippocrates's name as a way of showing their indebtedness to their teacher or honoring him. And it is probable that some texts might represent the curriculum—possibly even lecture notes—from a Hippocratic school on Cos. Some texts in the Hippocratic corpus, however, offered contradictory views, suggesting either that Hippocratic views changed over time or that some texts were written by a range of authors. The latter could have been authors who wanted to capitalize on Hippocrates's fame, using his name in order to find a readership for their ideas. Or Hippocratic authorship could have been attributed to certain books by readers and editors who thought the ideas therein resembled those of the iconic physician, or by traders trying to sell books.

Despite some differences of opinion, the texts in the Hippocratic corpus participate in the scientific project launched by the early Greek natural philosophers: making sense of the body, health, and illness in terms, not of religion, but of material elements in the world that could be observed, studied, and thus predicted. This came to be characterized as the Rationalist approach or school of thought. Moreover, we can trace a set of consistent threads that run through many of the texts in the Hippocratic corpus, perhaps suggesting some of Hippocrates's core approaches and ideas. First, texts in the Hippocratic corpus understood the human body to be made up of humors and tended to define health in terms of balance and illness in terms of imbalance of the humors. That said, across Hippocratic texts we find different views about what is supposed to be in balance, whether elements (earth, water, air, fire), qualities (hot, cold, wet, dry), or humors (blood, phlegm, yellow and black bile) of the body. And, in the case of the humors, we also find various opinions across Hippocratic texts about how many primary humors there are. In some Hippocratic texts, for instance, black bile was understood not to be a core humor, but rather a corrupted form of yellow bile; whereas *On the Nature of Humans* is the only text to assert that there were four humors, a view that would become canonical in later medical theorizing.

Authors in the Hippocratic corpus also focused a good deal of attention on the internal structures and workings of the human body (anatomy and physiology, as we would call them). Given that the Hippocratic corpus represented a greater understanding of these matters than earlier texts, we can surmise that the authors gained their knowledge through careful study and observations, possibly animal dissections and opportune examinations of wounded bodies. Hippocratic authors, like their philosophical counterparts, shared a propensity for thinking about bodily processes as analogous to processes they observed in the world around them: for example, the processes of digestion were likened to cooking, baking, or grinding food; the process of organs drawing in substances was likened to the principle of a vacuum; the phenomenon of cold and warm fluids meeting suddenly in the body was likened to the clashing of cold and warm currents of water. In other words, Hippocratic writers used mechanical or natural processes in the world to think about what might be happening inside the hidden recesses of the body.

Perhaps most importantly, the Hippocratic corpus reveals a development in the professionalization of medicine. We see a move to create a field of medicine that is distinct from and more specialized than philosophy, despite significant overlap in epistemology and subject matter. And we see a move to privilege one kind of healer—the physician who employs a Rationalist approach—as superior to all other options in the medical marketplace. Finally, we see a move for Hippocratic physicians to understand their medical practice as far more expansive than healing practices had previously been conceived. Physicians were to make comprehensive, holistic recommendations on healthy lifestyles for clients related to diet, sleep, sexual activity, exercise, massage and bathing treatments, and entertainment and education. They offered guidance to patients who were ill in order to restore health, but they also began to market themselves as purveyors of regimens that would maintain health. This elevation of a specialized set of knowledge, their Rationalist approach, and their comprehensive scope set them apart from other kinds of healers.

HEALING IN TEMPLES OF ASCLEPIUS (FIFTH CENTURY BCE: GREEK CLASSICAL PERIOD)

At the same time as the Hippocratic texts were being written and compiled and Greek physicians were developing medical theories and professional identities, another healing-related trend was underway: the burgeoning of the cult of Asclepius.

Recall that people in antiquity thought that many gods and goddesses could and did cause illness, and that these same gods and goddesses healed. For instance, people petitioned the god **Apollo,** who was well known for his healing activities, when they needed help with illness, but they sought his help for a myriad of other issues as well. None of the gods specialized exclusively in healing like the god Asclepius and his goddess daughter **Hygieia** (from whose name the terms "hygiene" and "hygienic" are derived).

According to the numerous legends about the life and deification of Asclepius that were circulating in the fifth century BCE, Asclepius was the son of Apollo and a mortal woman. When Asclepius's mother abandoned her child, Apollo raised his son, handing him over to the centaur Chiron for instruction in the healing arts and the medicinal properties of plants. Under Chiron's tutelage, Asclepius was purported to have become very skilled and famous as a healer, so much so that some legends reported he was even able to bring the dead back to life. Worried about humans overstepping the powers of the gods, Zeus struck Asclepius down with a thunderbolt, killing him. Upon his death, Asclepius was deified and joined the pantheon of gods from whom mortals could seek help.

The cult of Asclepius spread rapidly and widely in the fifth and fourth centuries BCE, with many cities setting up shrines to Asclepius, often as a response to the outbreak of an

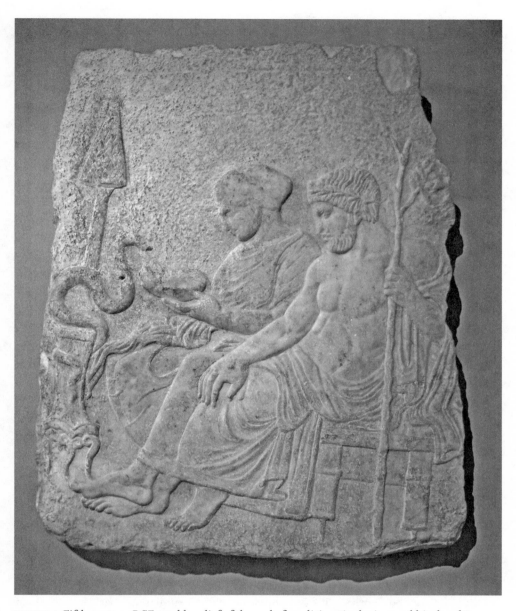

FIGURE 4 Fifth-century BCE marble relief of the god of medicine, Asclepius, and his daughter, the goddess of health, Hygieia, from the Therme of Thessaloniki, Greece. Asclepius is pictured with his characteristic staff, and Hygieia presents an offering to a snake, an animal whose periodic shedding of its skin symbolized the shedding of illness and the recovery of health. Istanbul Archaeological Museum (inv. no. 109 T). Wikimedia Commons, Creative Commons Attribution 3.0.

epidemic. For example, a temple to Asclepius was set up in Athens circa 420 BCE in the wake of a devastating plague. In total, we know of hundreds of Asclepian temples throughout the Mediterranean, with the best-known and largest complexes in Epidaurus (in mainland Greece), Cos (the Greek island homeland of Hippocrates), and Pergamum (in modern-day Türkiye) (see fig. 49).

We hear reports of sick and suffering people traveling for days to seek healing at these religio-medical centers. Upon arrival, they often presented the god with offerings of anatomical votives, objects fashioned in the form of body parts (such as arms, hands, legs, feet, ears, eyes, genitals, and viscera such as intestines, wombs, liver, and heart) they hoped the god would heal. The votives that survive from antiquity were made of clay and stone, but we know that others were made from more ephemeral materials, such as wood and wax.

Asclepian temples were best known for a healing ritual called "incubation": sick individuals slept in a special sanctuary where they would either experience the god healing them within a dream or receive a dream in which the god would prescribe a regimen or remedy they should follow upon waking in order to be cured. For the latter, they would work with the priest who interpreted the dreams and oversaw the administration of the prescribed remedy at the therapeutic sites in or near the temple: bathing in the bathhouse, engaging in exercise at the on-site gymnasium, ingesting drugs prepared by the priests or local pharmacologists, or receiving surgical treatment (archaeologists have found medical instruments on the temple grounds). (For a more detailed discussion of incubation, see chapter 10.)

Inscriptions found at Asclepian shrines report stories of the healings enacted there, describing individuals' ailments and the remedies pursued, touting the god's power, and expressing gratitude for the healings performed. These inscriptions were displayed prominently on-site for new arrivals to see, enhancing the god's reputation and instilling optimism in visitors. Artistic representations of Asclepius—statues and paintings alike—depict him holding a staff with a snake wound around it (see fig. 4). The snake, and particularly the snake's practice of shedding its skin, served as a symbol of those who underwent the process of shedding their illness when under the care of the god-physician Asclepius.

Given modern distinctions between religious healing and medical healing, we might be tempted to think of the Asclepian healing cult as an alternative to professional medicine. But, as indicated above, priests at these temples employed similar approaches in terms of regimen, drugs, and surgery, and cooperated with local physicians and pharmacologists in carrying out the god's dream therapies. Moreover, Asclepius became a patron deity for many physicians, as sources such as the Hippocratic *Oath* (Text 40), sworn in the name of Asclepius and Hygieia, attest. Some physicians supported temples to the god with offerings of medical instruments and money, and some physicians eventually became priests of Asclepius. This overlap should not be surprising, inasmuch as, according to legend, Asclepius was himself a physician during his mortal life.

THE INFLUENCE OF PLATO AND ARISTOTLE ON MEDICAL THOUGHT
(FIFTH–FOURTH CENTURY BCE: GREEK CLASSICAL PERIOD)

Although not physicians themselves, the philosophers Plato (427–348/7 BCE) and **Aristotle** (c. 384–322 BCE) made a number of important contributions to the history of ancient Greek medicine. First and foremost, Plato theorized that the human body was deliberately and purposefully created by a cosmic divinity called "the demiurge," a divine craftsman we might think of as consonant with Nature. (See Text 1 for selections from Plato's *Timaeus* discussing the demiurge.) With other ancient philosophers and scientists who held the view that "Nature does nothing in vain," Plato explained in detail how the parts of the body were designed with specific purposes or for certain "ends" (Greek *telos*; this kind of thinking is called "teleological")—namely, for the body's optimal functioning. For instance, Plato suggested that the intestines were intentionally made long (and ingeniously coiled to fit in the body) so it took a long time for food to be digested and people would feel satiated longer, giving them time to focus on their philosophical pursuits rather than spending their time eating. Plato also explained that the body was designed with temperature-modulating mechanisms built in. For example, the body's moisture—in the form of sweat—helped to keep the body cool in the summer heat. This kind of logic impelled philosophers and physicians to detect signs of rational, well-ordered design in the anatomy and physiology of the human body.

Plato laid the foundation for later discussions of bodily humors and pathological theories. Following Empedocles, Plato understood the body to be made up of the four elements: earth, water, air, and fire. Plato combined this elemental system with Pythagorean thought, ascribing geometric shapes to each of the elements. For instance, Plato explained that fire burned and caused pain when touched because it was made up of triangular shapes with sharp edges. Plato also suggested a few pathological theories that later medical writers would develop. Illness could be the result of an excess or deficiency of elements within the body, the decomposition of parts of the body into these elements, or changes in *pneuma*, bile, and phlegm in the body.

Finally, Plato's reflections on the relationship between the body and soul would be of utmost importance to later medical theory. In both his *Republic* and *Timaeus*, Plato advanced the view that the soul was divided into three parts: the rational or reasoning part, the spirited or emotional part, and the appetitive or nutritive part. Each of these mapped onto a different internal organ: the rational was associated with the brain, the spirited with the heart, and the appetitive with the liver. This division influenced later writers, including **Galen** (c. 129–c. 216 CE), who imagined health and medicine as encompassing not only the body, but also the soul.

Aristotle was Plato's most famous student at the Academy in Athens. He was the son of a physician, which explains his avid interest in biology, zoology, botany, and natural science more generally. Aristotle followed Plato in his commitment to teleological explanations of human and animal anatomy and physiology. Yet his methodology differed significantly from his teacher's in that he emphasized empirical observation as a starting point for philosophical reflection. In this regard, Aristotle's contributions to the history of medicine are considerable. He was committed to dissecting as many animal specimens as he could and seems to have succeeded in the case of over fifty species, including rare marine life, birds, and insects. Aristotle wrote on a wide variety of topics, including the generation (i.e., reproduction) of animals, and even the details of the sex lives of crustaceans.

Aristotle should also be credited with teaching a number of students who went on to become physicians or to write on medical topics, including Meno (Greece, late fourth century BCE), who wrote something like an early history of medicine; **Theophrastus** (c. 372/1–287/6 BCE), who wrote some of the first treatises we have on the medicinal properties of plants; and **Diocles of Carystus** (fourth or third century BCE), who wrote treatises on physiology, pharmacology, and regimen. Aristotle's most famous student, however, was the Macedonian ruler, Alexander the Great (356–323 BCE), to whom we now turn.

MEDICAL DEVELOPMENTS IN PTOLEMAIC ALEXANDRIA (FOURTH–SECOND CENTURY BCE: HELLENISTIC PERIOD)

Carrying out the imperialistic ambitions of his father, Alexander first conquered the Greek city-states and then extended his domination further abroad. By the time Alexander died at the young age of thirty-two, he had expanded his rule throughout the Levant, Persia, Babylonia, Mesopotamia, Egypt, and all the way to the western parts of modern-day India. As Alexander conquered new territories, he disseminated Greek culture, including customs, law, and science, to the lands and peoples he conquered—a process scholars now call "Hellenization," during a time (323–31 BCE) known as the Hellenistic period. The spread of medicine, both as a scientific pursuit and as a professional practice, was part of this process.

The Ptolemaic kingdom in Egypt, one of the regions to undergo Hellenization, was especially enthusiastic about promoting Greek culture and knowledge. The state sponsored the proliferation of Greek natural sciences and medicine by establishing a museum (more precisely, a Hall of the Muses) and a library in its capital city of Alexandria. The two institutions became a place for scholars—drawn from all parts of the Greek-speaking world—to congregate, read books, give lectures, and discuss intellectual matters. Alexandria during this time was an especially fruitful place for medical research.

Of particular importance, Alexandria became a hub for anatomical study, where scientists engaged in the dissection of animal and human cadavers. At public dissections scientists walked viewers through the anatomical structures and parts they were exposing. Although dissection was taboo in other parts of the Mediterranean, it may have been more palatable to the Egyptians, who had a custom of opening up and removing internal organs from dead bodies in their funerary practice of mummification. Moreover, Greek scientists and physicians who traveled to Alexandria to learn from public dissections might have been more willing to treat the corpses of colonized subjects and especially criminals (the bodies most likely used for dissection and anatomical studies) with little dignity. Given aversion to the practice, however, human dissections in Alexandria did not last long.

During the time in which human dissection was practiced a number of remarkable strides were made by two leading figures in Alexandria. The first was **Herophilus of Chalcedon** (c. 330–c. 260 BCE), whose most important discoveries related to the anatomy of the eye, brain, and liver and vascular, reproductive, and nervous systems. It was Herophilus who discovered the Fallopian tubes and ovaries, and also the various coverings and ventricles of the brain. Herophilus also developed a diagnostic procedure using the pulse, a technique that would be elaborated in subsequent centuries.

Where Herophilus excelled at anatomical study, **Erasistratus of Ceos** (fourth and third centuries BCE) came to be known as the "Father of Physiology." Erasistratus focused his studies on the nervous system, experimenting on live brains in order to determine how damage to different parts affected motor function. Erasistratus explained bodily processes in mechanical terms. For example, he explained blood being drawn into arteries using the model of a vacuum; and he likened the stomach to a grinder, the heart to a pump, and the kidneys to a filter. He also earned a reputation for being a highly competent surgeon, helping to establish surgery as a subspecialty in medicine and Alexandria as a center for its practice.

Whereas the combined discoveries of Herophilus and Erasistratus moved anatomical and physiological knowledge forward in unprecedented ways, other scientists and medical thinkers in Alexandria (including successors of Herophilus) made discoveries in the field of pharmacology. A city such as Alexandria was a rich environment for the development of new drugs: with robust trade networks across sea and land, and in a region with indigenous botanical variety, it was well positioned to experiment with new mixtures and compounds of medicinal plants.

Another important development that began in the Hellenistic period was the creation of new schools or sects of medicine. Because the term "schools" can be somewhat misleading, we should clarify that the ancient "schools" of medicine were closer to "schools of thought"— differing approaches to the science and the practice of medicine—rather than institutions or buildings where medical students were trained. In fact, many physicians-in-training did not learn their craft in the kind of formal educational setting we think of when we use the term "school"; rather their training often took the form of apprenticeships (for a more detailed discussion, see chapter 11). Since some methods (or "schools") became popular in certain cities or regions, physicians' approaches were often shaped by where they were trained. Finally, we should also acknowledge that the approaches within each school were not monolithic but changed over time, so any introduction to ancient medical schools should be regarded merely as a rough sketch, and the situation, in reality, was much more complex. (See Text 4, from Celsus, *On Medicine*, for the defining features of each school.)

All of the medical writers and theorists we have discussed thus far, despite the significant differences between them, can be grouped together under the heading Rationalists (sometimes also called "Dogmatists"). Even though physicians might affiliate themselves with one of these thinkers—for example, identifying as Hippocratics, Herophilians, or Erasistrateans—all of these Rationalist thinkers shared a similar approach. They attempted to devise general *theories* that could guide their clinical practice. Specifically, they sought to theorize what characterized an unhealthy body, and to theorize how forces outside and within the body put someone in such a state. Rationalists also devised theories of treatment—for example, the "principle of opposites" or "principle of contraries"—that could combat the cause of illness. Armed with these general principles, Rationalists understood themselves to have the ability to diagnose and treat all individual cases, no matter how different they were from one another.

In the Hellenistic period, a new school arose, called "Empiricism," that provided an alternative to the Rationalist approach. The approach was popularized by **Heraclides of Tarentum** (first century BCE), though adherents claimed a much longer intellectual heritage. While Rationalists based their work in theory, Empiricists relied primarily on experience: trial and error. In other words, for Empiricists, the art of medicine was characterized by experiments that revealed which remedies worked for which specific ailments. They focused on documenting and collecting case histories and past successes. When physicians encountered a new case, therefore, they could reference similar cases in the past and devise a similar treatment plan. In general, Empiricists agreed with Rationalists that bodies, illnesses, and remedies worked in terms of a consistent set of principles, but Empiricists were pessimistic about humans' ability to understand what those principles were (especially given the number of contingent factors they took into account, such as region, season, age, gender, and so forth). Empiricists argued that the time of scientists and physicians was better spent on the experimentation necessary to test effective remedies than on theoretical speculation.

MEDICINE IN THE ROMAN EMPIRE (FIRST CENTURY BCE–THIRD CENTURY CE: ROMAN IMPERIAL PERIOD)

When Alexander the Great's successors ruled in the eastern Mediterranean (roughly the late fourth to first century BCE), the city-state of Rome began expanding its power and scope in the western Mediterranean. At first Rome gained control of the Italian peninsula and then expanded its territories beyond Italy to create a vast empire. By the second century CE, the Roman Empire included Spain, Gaul, Britain, North Africa, and regions in the east formerly governed by the Greeks.

Romans had their own healing customs and practices that could be referred to as a kind of "agrarian self-help." As we learn from writers such as **Cato the Elder** (234–149 BCE), Varro (116–27 BCE), and **Pliny the Elder** (c. 23 or 24–79 CE), health care was the responsibility of individual households and was based largely on herbal remedies and basic wound care, along with petitions to the gods and the use of charms and incantations. When Greek physicians arrived in the west, most of them brought to Rome as slaves acquired through conquest, they were treated with suspicion and their art was maligned as butchery and poisoning. Such negative assessments stemmed from Romans' sense of ethnic superiority, from the low status of Greek physicians, and from the treatments advised by Greek medicine, which seemed more violent and painful than Roman therapies.

This suspicion and denigration notwithstanding, Romans slowly began incorporating Greek forms of medicine into their households and institutions. For example, recognizing the financial incentive to keep slaves on large Roman estates healthy enough to work, estates trained one or more of their slaves in Greek medicine so they could treat their sick and injured peers, providing such care in the slave quarters (*valetudinaria*), and sometimes treating the freepersons in the household too.

Greek medicine made further gains among Romans when emperors who understood the need to keep Roman troops healthy enough to fight employed physicians as part of army personnel. Emperors also sought to cultivate loyalty among their troops, by creating the impression that the emperor cared about their well-being (unlike in earlier periods when Rome was expanding within the Italian Peninsula and the protocol was to patch up soldiers in the field and then return the seriously wounded to their homes or to station them temporarily in the homes of allies in friendly towns nearby). When campaigns took place outside of Italy, hundreds of miles from home and where the locals were decidedly unfriendly, the Roman military set up medical tents in temporary encampments, and they built infirmary buildings (also called *valetudinaria*) at the fortified bases at their outposts. These infirmaries were staffed by professional physicians and specialists (such as surgeons), along with other military personnel who were less extensively trained (such as "wound dressers" and "caretakers"). Although there is scant information about the treatments performed in military infirmaries, the conditions of war and a few daily rosters listing the ailments that made soldiers unfit for service suggest that the most commonplace treatments involved the patching up of injuries incurred on the battlefield (such as mending bodies wounded in combat or extracting arrows or projectiles), and dealing with intestinal distress or eye troubles.

As Greek healing practices became more prevalent in Roman society, they gained a more positive reputation, and the status of physicians also rose considerably. Eventually, some physicians came to be employed exclusively by wealthy senatorial and imperial families as their private physicians. But while Romans eventually came to accept Greek medicine as a preferred form of health care, elite Romans rarely became physicians themselves; instead our most important medical figures of the Roman Empire, such as Galen (c. 129–c. 216 CE), **Soranus** (second century CE), and **Aretaeus** (second century CE), were Greeks from the eastern parts of the empire who traveled to practice medicine in the west.

In the first centuries BCE and CE, a new approach to medical thinking was on the rise: the Methodist school of medicine. Methodists were like the Rationalists in that they attempted to generate general theories that they could employ when confronted with various individual cases. Yet, unlike the Rationalists, their theories were not concerned with the *causes* behind an illness, because, they asserted, knowledge of the causes had no bearing on the course of treatment. Rather, Methodists focused exclusively on the *properties* of illness. More specifically, they understood the body to be made up of atoms, and noted that all illness stemmed from the inability of these atoms to move properly through what they called the pores or channels in the body because of either too much constriction or too much loose-ness. When Methodists analyzed the properties—also called "indications"—of various ill-nesses, they recognized three general categories or kinds of illness: those characterized by flux, laxity, or looseness (*status laxus*), those characterized by constriction, tightness, or ten-sion (*status strictus*), and those that involved both flux and constriction (*status mixtus*).

Their treatments aimed to counteract the nature of the problem they observed, recom-mending remedies to relax parts of the body that were overly constricted or tense, and con-stricting or styptic remedies to parts of the body that were overly relaxed. For example, if one observed that the bowels were constricted, the treatment should be to relax the bowels; and conversely if one observed diarrhea, the treatment should be to encourage constriction. Again, although they agreed with Rationalists regarding the treatment principle of oppo-sites/contraries, Methodists targeted not the cause (that which was hidden behind the ill-ness) but rather addressed the manifest properties of the illness itself.

Methodists were also innovative in their categorization of illnesses into chronic and acute, a distinction first proposed by the physician **Themison** (first century BCE), whose ideas influenced the subsequent development of the Methodist school. No previous medical school or thinker had focused as much attention on chronic conditions like arthritis and asthma, a fact that helps to explain the popularity that the Methodists enjoyed.

In the early centuries of the Common Era, there was an impulse to create practical medi-cal guides. For example, Aretaeus and another physician now called the **Anonymus Parisi-nus** (late first century CE?) authored comprehensive volumes cataloging the causes and treatments of acute and chronic illnesses. A handful of pharmacological handbooks were likewise produced: **Scribonius Largus** (first centuries BCE and CE) amassed 271 different drug recipes, and **Dioscorides of Anazarbus** (second half of first century CE; fig. 5) authored an immense pharmacopeia recording mostly herbal remedies, but also remedies derived from animal and human products, minerals, and metals. These reference works had lasting clinical value, as is evidenced by the fact that Dioscorides's volumes were copied and recop-ied not only in their original Greek, but also in Latin and Arabic translation for fifteen cen-turies after his lifetime.

Finally, one of the most famous physicians and medical writers of antiquity lived and practiced during the early imperial period of the Roman Empire: Galen of Pergamum (c. 129–c. 216 CE; fig. 5). Born to a wealthy family, Galen was afforded a top-notch education, studying medicine in Pergamum (his hometown), Smyrna, and eventually at Alexandria (see Text 34, *On Anatomical Procedures,* for details of this training). Galen's training was enhanced by the wealth of knowledge and experience he gained as a gladiator physician in Pergamum. Stitching up wounds, treating injuries, and also keeping the gladiators in good condition through regimen and diet provided Galen with ample opportunity to enhance his study of anatomy and physiology, and improve his skills in surgery. When he moved to Rome (162 CE), he established a reputation for himself through a series of public lectures involv-ing anatomical demonstrations on animals. These spectacles—intended to impress elite audiences in the highly competitive medical marketplace of the imperial capital—won him

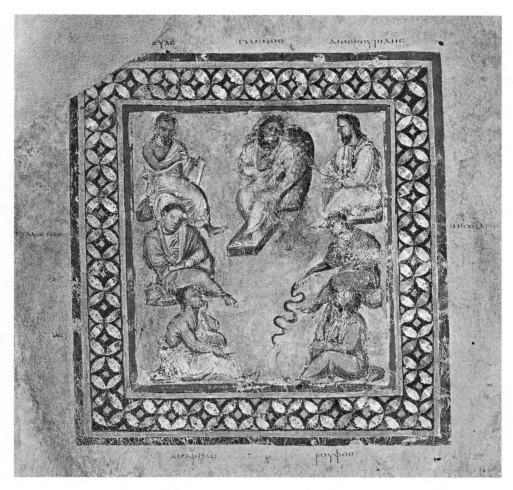

FIGURE 5 Illustration in the sixth-century CE Vienna Dioscorides codex depicting a collection of famous medical writers in conversation with each other (though they lived at different times and in different places). From the labels in the margins, we can identify the physicians: Galen sits at the top center, then moving clockwise, Dioscorides (the author of the pharmacological work in which this illustration is found), Nicander (pictured with a snake, referencing his writings on poisonous substances, such as venom, and their antidotes), Rufus of Ephesus (who had wide-ranging expertise in anatomy, physiology, and human emotions, and was known for his advocacy of questioning patients as part of the diagnostic process), Andreas of Carystus (personal physician of Ptolemy IV Philopator), Apollonius (who could be one of several medical figures who share the same name), and Crateuas (a botanist). Vienna Dioscorides, folio 3v, Austrian National Library, Vienna. Wikimedia Commons.

a collection of wealthy supporters among the Roman elite. Eventually, as his reputation continued to bloom, he was hired to serve as physician to the emperors Marcus Aurelius, Lucius Verus, Commodus, and Septimius Severus.

Because of his high status and important patrons, Galen was afforded the time to compose over 350 medical treatises, and his medical ideas carried a good deal of weight. Marshaling his education, experience, and success, Galen wrote on a wide variety of topics in medicine, as well as philosophy, logic, and etymology. He held the view that good physicians were philosophically trained, and his texts regularly reveal his indebtedness to the ideas of previous philosophers (such as Plato and Aristotle).

Given his voluminous writings, Galen's voice threatens to drown out many others from this period in ancient medicine. Moreover, Galen was thoroughly convinced of his own superiority, and he was not shy about denigrating his many competitors at Rome, especially those from the Empiricist and Methodist schools. But we must resist the urge to think of Galen as the undisputed authority of his time; rather, we get the sense that Galen would not have had to protest so vociferously against competing views if everyone agreed with him. And we certainly should not think of all physicians of his time as cast in his mold, since the vast majority would have had far less training, expertise, and imperial patronage.

MEDICAL DEVELOPMENTS IN LATE ANTIQUITY (FOURTH–SIXTH CENTURY CE)

The most important medical innovation of late antiquity was the development of institutions that many scholars consider predecessors to the hospital as we know it. This development can be traced to a cultural change taking place in the third and fourth centuries CE: the gradual and uneven Christianization of the Roman Empire. Christians, who preserved earlier Jewish moral principles, believed in the importance of providing care for the vulnerable, especially those without familial support, such as orphans, widows, and foreigners. Christians were guided by biblical commandments to provide hospitality and charity, and—because they considered all members of Christian communities, or all of God's creation, as "brothers" and "sisters"—they extended care to those they considered part of their "family." Their charity took the form of alms and food doles, and by the fourth century CE was institutionalized in full-blown "hospitality" centers that were founded by wealthy Christians or were outgrowths of Christian monasteries (where male and female monks lived in community and vowed to make the world better through prayer, work, and charity).

For example, the fourth-century Christian noblewoman Fabiola spent her wealth on the creation of a sick house outside the city of Rome, the first institution of this kind, according to a contemporary. She was reported to have "gathered sufferers out of the streets," caring for people with ghastly ailments—such as "having their noses slit, eyes put out, feet half burnt, hands covered with sores, limbs dropsical and atrophied, and **flesh** alive with worms" (Jerome, *Letter* 77). At her sick house she provided them with nursing care, washing the discharge from their wounds, hand-feeding them, and moistening their parched lips with sips

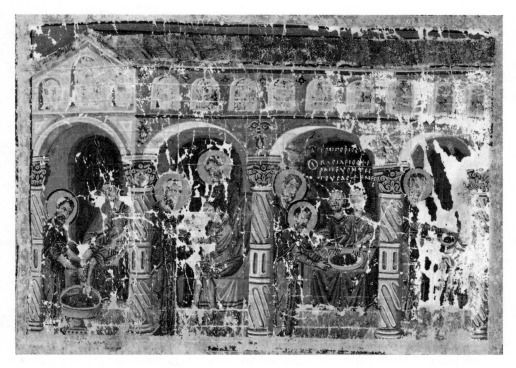

FIGURE 6 Illustration from a ninth-century manuscript that depicts the types of care provided at Basil of Caesarea's hospital complex, including bathing, preparing food, and hand-feeding patients. Gregory of Nyssa, *Homilies*, BnF MS Gr. 510, folio 149r. Permission: Bibliothèque Nationale de France.

of liquid. As new institutions like Fabiola's developed, they grew in complexity. The fourth-century complex of Basil of Caesarea—known as the "Basiliad"—included separate spaces for the poor, the dying (hospices), orphans, lepers, and the sick (see fig. 6).

The introduction of Christian hospitals was a revolution in the organization of medical care in that, for the first time, the public had access to free, in-patient health care under the supervision of medical professionals. Support staff provided basic nursing care, while some monks (including Basil himself) were formally trained in medicine. These institutions were also revolutionary in that they provided care for a class of people physicians often refused to treat: the chronically ill and dying. For this innovation, Christians earned the devotion of their communities, and also induced the jealousy of the emperor Julian, who worried that non-Christians who benefited from Christian health care might shift their political loyalties from him to the religious community. The introduction of Christian hospitals spurred a burst of philanthropic one-upmanship among Christian and non-Christian leaders in the late ancient Mediterranean, the latter wanting either to imitate Christians' good works or to shore up the good will of the people.

The other important trend in late antiquity was a shift from specialized medical treatises (such as a text on head wounds or gynecology) to increased production of medical digests, compilations, and handbooks. For example, **Oribasius** (c. 325–400 CE) and **Aëtius of Amida** (sixth century CE) wrote compilations and handbooks for diverse audiences, sometimes for other physicians and sometimes for learned friends who had an interest in and knowledge of medicine. Many historians of medicine value compilations and handbooks only because they preserve earlier medical texts that no longer exist on their own, assuming that late antiquity was a time when medicine remained largely stagnant, merely recirculating ideas from past generations. More recent scholarship, however, has begun to discern the many innovations, revisions, and adaptations compilers made of earlier medical ideas and practices and how compilations were themselves new forms of medical thinking. Moreover, compilations give us a sense of medical education in late antiquity, as some contain the medical treatises, and commentaries on those treatises, of a medical curriculum in the order in which students should progress through them.

The consensus represented by late ancient handbooks was the outcome of the thousand-year history discussed in this chapter. Medical handbooks and compilations drew heavily on the texts of the Hippocratic corpus as filtered through the writings of Galen and others. Despite this accumulation of knowledge, professional physicians in late antiquity still had to compete with other healers (both human and divine) just as they had to in the fifth century BCE. Even if people were no longer incubating in temples of Asclepius by the fifth century CE, they were sleeping in shrines of Christians martyrs and saints, awaiting dreams of healing and using oil, water, dust, and textiles that had come into contact with the relics of these holy persons, in order to recover health and alleviate suffering.

THREE

Living Conditions in the Ancient Mediterranean

Sickness, suffering, and premature death were commonplace in the ancient Mediterranean. The average life expectancy was approximately 25–30 years old. (Compare this with life expectancy figures from 2021: 77.1 in China, 78.9 in the US, 81.6 in Germany, and 82.7 in Canada.) This does not mean that most people lived to the age of 25–30. Rather, many died early, from complications in childbirth or from childhood illness. We estimate that approximately one-third of all infants died in their first year and up to one-half of all children died before they reached the age of five. If someone survived childhood, their chances of living into old age increased dramatically (see fig. 7).

Yet even those who escaped an early death could expect to endure a life filled with sickness, injuries, physical impairments, and pain. Although they sought health, it seems that ancient people understood sickness and suffering to be the normal, default state of being, with health being a respite they only occasionally and fleetingly experienced. Compare this to contemporary views of health as the steady state, with sickness being something we experience only occasionally and temporarily. For example, while we might bemoan an especially bad illness that lasts a long time, the second-century CE Roman orator **Fronto** celebrated when he enjoyed a "lengthier period of health than usual" (*Letter to Antoninus Pius* 8.2).

In this chapter, we examine the conditions of the Greco-Roman world that made Fronto's view understandable: given the vulnerabilities, hazards, and disasters people in the ancient Mediterranean faced on a daily basis, life and health were precarious. Understanding the conditions in which ancient people lived helps to contextualize their desire for health care, which could prevent or provide relief from sickness and suffering.

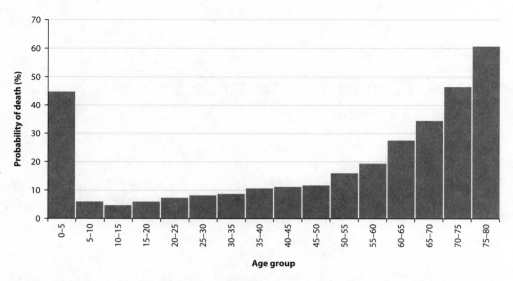

FIGURE 7 Probability of death in the ancient Mediterranean across age groups (using data from Coale and Demeny Model West). Created by Cassandra Gutiérrez.

HOUSING

The housing conditions of the poor lower classes and the wealthy elite varied widely, resulting in disparities of health risks. The poorest people who lived in cities erected shanties and huts wherever they could find a little space, or sought shelter under porticoes or in enclosed tombs in cemeteries. Lower-class families may have been able to rent space in a tenement building, but to save money a multigenerational family might need to crowd into a single room (see fig. 8). In these cases, people lived in very close proximity to one another: archaeologists calculate approximately 302 people per acre in ancient Rome and 195 people per acre in ancient Antioch (for a sense of scale, compare these figures with approximately 122 and 100 people per acre today in Calcutta and Manhattan, respectively). This population density created ideal conditions for the rapid spread of illness, especially highly contagious diseases, such as tuberculosis, and especially when a city was under siege and the residents were forced to remain within the city walls.

Still other dangers lurked in such living quarters. In the colder months, when people covered their windows with cloth to keep in the heat, they routinely inhaled air polluted by oil lamps, fecal matter that collected in chamber pots, and smoke from fires to cook food and heat the room. So polluted was the air in these residences that scholars who have examined human remains from the ancient Mediterranean have found inflammation of the lung lining and even anthracosis (carbon accumulation in the lungs, an ailment that affects many coal miners today). In the heat of the summer months, when people left their windows uncovered to let in cooling winds, strong gusts could blow over their cooking braziers, resulting in fires. These fires not only burned the buildings in which they lived, but

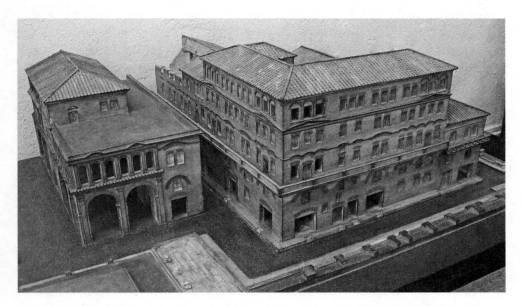

FIGURE 8 Model of a Roman tenement building (*insula*), pictured on the right. Tenement buildings were typically six to seven stories high. The bottom floor consisted of shops that opened onto the streets, and sometimes a cesspit toilet for the residents. The rest of the building was made up of residential apartments. These apartments averaged approximately 1,000 square feet, though those closest to the ground floor that housed middle-class families tended to be larger, and those on the uppermost floors that housed lower-class people tended to be smaller. Museum of Roman Civilization, Rome. Photo: Bent Christensen.

because of the close proximity of buildings (the broadest streets in Rome, for example, the Via Appia and Via Latina, were only fifteen–twenty feet wide) spread rapidly across a neighborhood or city.

The poorest people, residing in the least-appealing parts of unsafe buildings, suffered the most from their housing situations. Landlords charged the cheapest rent for the top floors because these residents had to take so many stairs to their rooms—the Roman poet Martial reports that there could be up to 200 steps!—and because they were exposed to the cold and moisture from leaking roofs, as well as the droppings of birds and vermin that lived in the eaves. When poor people crowded into these upper-floor rooms, they made the buildings top-heavy, at times causing whole buildings to collapse. Yet this was not the only reason buildings collapsed. Landlords who wished to maximize their profits ignored legal codes that set a maximum height for buildings, constructing up to ten stories (an apartment complex still standing in Ostia, the port city of Rome, for example, measures seventy feet tall). Building to such heights was precarious, given uneven foundations (sometimes built on the rotting trash that piled up on city streets, as we will see in the next section) and cheap and shoddy construction (such as walls with rubble cores, or constructed with sun-dried—rather than fired—clay bricks), in addition to the top-heavy crowding of the upper floors. As a

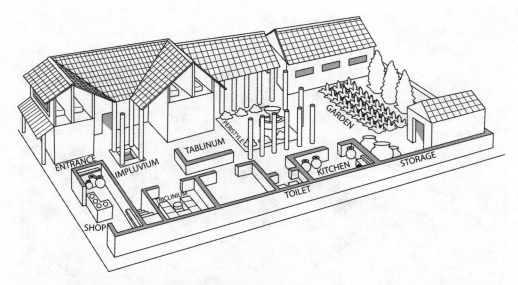

FIGURE 9 Illustrator's rendering of a two-story Roman home (*domus*). Wealthy families who lived in such residences had access to more space—thus slowing the spread of contagious illnesses and allowing sick people to isolate and recuperate in a quiet room of their own. These families might also have grown plants used as medicinal remedies in their courtyard or backyard gardens. Created by Gina Tibbott.

result, we hear reports of buildings collapsing, and sometimes toppling over neighboring buildings, causing dozens of deaths in an instant.

Because they could avoid these housing conditions, wealthy families escaped many of these perils. They lived in single- or double-story houses with several rooms and often a courtyard(s) (see fig. 9). Houses contained separate rooms with dedicated purposes: rooms facing the street could be used as shops, and other rooms could be used to receive guests and business associates. Still other rooms served as sleeping quarters, dining spaces, and kitchens. Other spaces included animal stalls and courtyards or a backyard where plants for cooking and household medicine could be grown. Although houses might contain an extended family—including multiple generations, slaves, and animals—the occupants had room to spread out, and the sick might be able to isolate in a room of their own (which, we now know, inhibits the spread of disease). Additionally, in times of epidemics, the wealthy must have fared better than those who lived in closer proximity to neighbors, since—when conditions proved unbearable in the city—many of the wealthy could escape to second homes they owned in the countryside.

WASTE AND WATER

Some health risks were unavoidable, regardless of a person's status. The sanitary conditions of Greek and Roman cities were ideal for pathogens to flourish and included multiple vec-

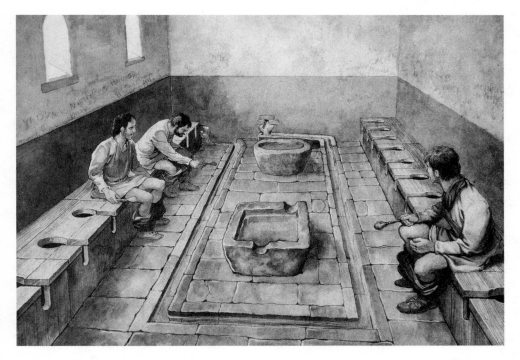

FIGURE 10 Illustrator's rendering of communal toilets at the Roman fort, Vercovicium (modern-day Great Britain). Photo credit: Carole Raddato (CC BY-SA 2.0).

tors by which disease could spread, so that even the wealthy were susceptible to the spread of germs and parasites. To illustrate, let us look first at sewage systems.

Most cities across the ancient Mediterranean had public, communal toilets, often set up as a horseshoe-shaped row of seats, with a pool in the middle to diffuse the smell (see fig. 10). These were social spaces in which people chatted while they relieved themselves. In place of toilet paper, Greeks and Romans used leaves, moss, or a sponge tied to the end of a stick, the latter of which was shared communally in the toilet rooms. Users would rinse off the anal sponge in a channel of water flowing through the toilet room. People also rinsed their hands in this channel or in a wash basin in the room. Without a robust germ theory to explain the spread of illness, these practices seem to have been largely about keeping people's bodies clean from filth, rather than preventing the spread of illness. Although these cleansing practices likely reduced the rate of cross-contamination, they would not have effectively curtailed the spread of illness owing to contact with others' feces.

These public toilets incorporated ingenious systems for flushing and evacuating sewage: collecting rainwater on roofs that was periodically released so that the sewage was carried away by gravity, channeling runoff from nearby hills or mountains, or piping in the waters of adjacent bathhouses. These dynamic systems would have forestalled the thriving of pathogens in standing sewage, but when sewage was flushed with force, we can imagine the aerosolization of microbes up through the toilet seats.

When we follow the pipes to investigate where the sewage went after it left the toilet rooms, an array of additional health hazards become clear. Sewage was usually piped under city streets, until it was eventually dumped into a nearby sea or river. Disposed in this way, sewage contaminated the water people collected to drink, the water in which they washed their clothes and dishes, and the water in which they might bathe. Additionally, the fish and animals who lived in or drank from these water sources likewise became contaminated, in turn striking ill the humans who ate them. Although ancient thinkers did not devise detailed theories about the relationship between raw sewage and illness, medical writers intuited that there was something unhealthy about these conditions. For example, **Galen** observed that "the worst fish live at the outlets of rivers which clean out the sewers, the tavern, and the baths," and advised against consuming such fish (*On the Properties of Foods* 3.29 [6.721K]). Finally, these sewage systems were vulnerable in times of war, as it was a common siege tactic to block up pipes leading out of a city, causing a backflow of sewage and filth into the closed-off city.

Some people had access to private, single toilets, such as the wealthy who installed them in their private homes and some lower-class families who were lucky enough to live in a tenement that had a single toilet (usually located on the ground floor) shared by the residents of the building. Although private toilets were convenient, this seeming luxury had health risks. Some of these toilets in private households were connected to pipe and flushing systems similar to public toilets, but most of these single toilets simply emptied into a pit latrine. When vermin and insects trod through these cesspits, they picked up germs that they then transferred throughout the rest of the living quarters, including to food they walked or crawled over.

When unable to visit the public toilets or if a private toilet was unavailable, most people were forced to evacuate their waste into chamber pots. The wealthy might isolate their chamber pots in a remote part of the house or task slaves with emptying the pots, but these were options tenement-dwellers did not have. Rather they were forced to trudge up and down their steps to dispose of their own waste or to endure the concentrated odors of human waste in their cramped living quarters (heightening the spread of fecal-borne illnesses). Perhaps it is not surprising, then, that we hear reports of people dumping the contents of their chamber pots out their windows. From the numerous laws forbidding such a practice, we surmise that this was a regular occurrence.

Finally, with respect to illness spread through sewage, our agricultural sources report that "professional waste removers" collected human and animal waste (from cesspits in private homes or pits where chamber pots were emptied), composted it, and used the compost to fertilize crops. Although this practice enhanced crop yields, if the feces of people infected with parasites was not composted long enough to break down parasite eggs, the fertilizer could spread parasites to the crops, and in turn (re)infect humans who consumed the food.

Illnesses spread not only from sewage, but also from trash. Some cities, like Rome, occasionally organized workers to collect trash and to cart it outside of the city, but we do not have evidence of a regular waste-removal system, and even when such measures were in place, they did not clear out all of the trash. Rather, building owners were responsible for cleaning the sidewalks in front of their properties, and individuals were expected to haul their own trash to garbage heaps. And despite regulations against and fines imposed for dumping one's trash in the streets, especially near public fountains, it seems these regulations were routinely ignored or surreptitiously violated especially in the dark of night. The first-century CE Roman poet Juvenal warns those out on the streets at night to look out for trash being thrown out of windows: he warns that tossed ceramics could crack open one's head, leftovers from cooking pots could scald a passerby, and one doesn't even wish to think about being doused with the contents of a chamber pot! We hear reports of trash piling up in the streets and alleyways of cities to the extent that streets became clogged and difficult to traverse. In such cases, one solution was to put stepping stones over the trash so that one could navigate a way through.

Trash piles included discarded rubbish and even animal and human remains: animal remains from butcher shops and tanners, and the bodies of feral animals; as well as the bodies of the homeless or those who did not have family or friends with sufficient means for a proper burial or the ability to carry their loved ones to the mass burial pits outside the city. As the trash rotted and bodies decomposed, insects that transmitted disease—such as flies, mosquitoes, roaches, lice, and fleas—flourished. Animals that scavenged through the trash for food—dogs, birds, and rats—were also vectors for infection and illness. For example, when we hear reports such as those from the ancient Roman biographer Suetonius about instances when a street dog carried partially eaten body parts into the middle of a meeting in the Forum and into the banquet hall where the emperor Vespasian was dining, we can surmise how toxic substances arising from decomposing bodies spread. Furthermore, rotting trash heaps that leached into the earth could contaminate groundwater, while trash (including animal and human remains) thrown into nearby waterways could likewise contribute to water pollution.

Water technologies developed by Greeks, and especially Romans, addressed some of the unsanitary conditions by helping to flush sewage and waste. Aqueducts, which used gravitational force to channel water from higher elevations into lower-lying cities, were connected to sewage pipes, leveraging natural water pressure to push waste through the system. Aqueducts also supplied higher-quality drinking water to cities, since the water was purified as it moved through settlement ponds or channels built into the aqueducts. Moreover, some cities had access to high-quality freshwater sources. Although ancient medical writers did not have a concept of waterborne bacteria, they intuited that some water sources were more healthful than others, preferring the running water of rivers and waters that bubbled up from springs to the stagnant waters of marshes and lakes (see Text 2, *Airs, Waters, Places* 1).

Yet even as water sources and systems curbed some forms of illness, they were also a cause of other illnesses. Water directed into the city for drinking was collected in open-air or underground cisterns before being piped to public fountains (see fig. 11). In the time that

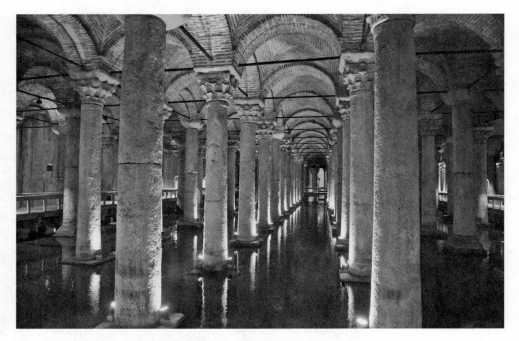

FIGURE 11 Underground cistern that collected and disseminated water throughout the capital city of Constantinople. This massive cistern was built in the sixth century CE by approximately 7,000 slaves, many of whom died during its construction. It is 105,000 square feet in size (9,800 square meters) and could hold up to 2,800,000 cubic feet of water (80,000 cubic meters). Photo credit: © Dick Osseman, Wikimedia Commons, Creative Commons Attribution 4.0.

the water lay stagnant in the cisterns, it could accumulate organisms that caused illness when ingested (for instance, standing water provided the ideal conditions for mosquitoes that carried illnesses like malaria). Additionally, water was piped through clay and stone pipes, but sometimes also lead pipes, resulting in low-level lead poisoning across a person's lifetime (see fig. 12).

Finally, although bathing was a societal custom intended to enhance cleanliness (as well as create community), the public bathhouses—especially the rooms with hot baths—were spaces that incubated microbes and thus were a source of sickness (see fig. 40)—even more so since physicians recommended that their sick patients go to the baths to treat illnesses we now know to be communicable. For example, Fronto reports that his physician sent him to the baths when he was experiencing cramps and diarrhea (see Text 37, *Letters* 5.69). Yet even ancient medical sources recognized that baths could exacerbate some problems: **Celsus** notes that open wounds tended to fester after exposure to water in public baths.

Taken together, we can see how the epidemiological conditions of ancient Mediterranean cities were ideal for the flourishing of pathogens, which need warmth, moisture, and food

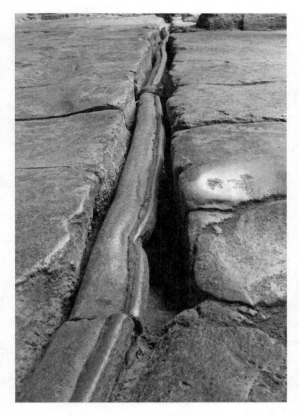

FIGURE 12 Lead pipe that supplied water to the Roman bath complex in Bath, England (constructed in the first century CE). Pipes that carried water for bathing, washing, and drinking could be made from various materials, but lead pipes were preferred because of their superior durability. Water that ran through ancient lead pipes is estimated to have had 100 times more lead than local spring waters. Ingested lead is a significant health hazard, causing neurological and nervous system disorders, and is especially harmful for children. (The association between pipes and lead has remained so synonymous that the English word "plumbing" derives from the Latin *plumbeus*, meaning "made of lead.") Photo credit: © Andrew Dunn, Wikimedia Commons, Creative Commons Attribution 4.0.

on which to live and breed. Moreover, a city possessed numerous vectors by which those pathogens could be spread. Insects and vermin—which likewise flourished in these conditions, the former breeding in standing water and the latter finding plenty to eat in rubbish heaps—were highly mobile creatures that transferred germs from feces and decomposing matter. People ingested food contaminated by feces from unwashed hands, fertilizer, or contaminated soil; they drank water riddled with bacteria or pollutants; and they breathed in noxious air. For those living in high-density residences, the dangers of these conditions were amplified as germs spread more quickly from person to person through coughing, sneezing, and shared surfaces.

Considering these conditions, and the ailments on which ancient medical sources focused the most attention, we get a sense of the kinds of illnesses that were most prevalent and that were regarded as the most distressing by people living in the ancient Mediterranean (see chapter 9). For example, the spread of germs and parasites from unsanitary conditions led to widespread gastrointestinal ailments. The vomiting and diarrhea associated with these ailments would have left victims dehydrated, unable to absorb nutrients from food, which could be deadly especially among children. Respiratory illnesses, whether from inhaling smoke (including burnt dung) from fires used to cook food and to keep warm or derived from the toxicity of mining and smelting operations, were common. And fevers, stemming from a range of illnesses, were a persistent worry. Thus, regardless of the specific ailments any individual might have experienced, we can be quite confident that chronic health problems and pain were a constant presence in the lives of nearly everyone living in the ancient Mediterranean.

NATURAL DISASTERS

In addition to the unhygienic conditions of cities, people in the ancient Mediterranean also faced threats posed by their natural environment. Most readers will be familiar with some well-known disasters, such as the volcanic eruption of Mt. Vesuvius in Italy. Many lives were lost to this eruption from the ash, pumice, and cinders, as well as the heat surges, that spread across the bay of Naples. Yet readers may not understand that volcanic eruptions also triggered earthquakes and landslides that caused destruction in nearby cities. Moreover, the ash and cinders strewn from the volcano ignited fires among wood structures. We have a report of people living near Vesuvius debating whether to stay indoors to avoid the heat and seek shelter from volcanic projectiles, or to take their chances in the open to avoid becoming trapped in a building that collapsed from the earth's tremors and shocks. Scholars estimate that in the nearby city of Pompeii, approximately 1,500 people (out of a population of approximately 20,000) perished from some element of the Vesuvian eruption.

Because the Mediterranean region is riddled with faults, seismic activity—great or small—was common (see fig. 13). Our sources describe earthquakes that hit several major cities in Asia Minor (modern-day Türkiye) in 17 CE and the city of Antioch in 526 CE, describing injuries and deaths caused by collapsing buildings or by the fires that erupted in the earthquake's wake. Theophanes writes that Antioch "became a tomb for its inhabitants" (*Chronicle* 172). **Procopius** adds that the whole city was "reduced to ruins, with most buildings immediately razed to the ground," estimating 300,000 people dead (*History of the Wars* 2.14.6). The devastation did not end when the earth stopped shaking. Survivors fought one another over the possessions they could scavenge; food production and trade were disrupted, triggering food shortages; and clean water became scarce.

Regular flooding created additional challenges for the health of people across the ancient Mediterranean world. Most communities were located near waterways—such as seas, rivers, and lakes—that provided them with an abundant supply of water for drinking, bathing, and cleaning. These locations also afforded easy access to goods moved along waterway trade routes. And their natural floodplains provided irrigation and nutrient-rich soil for agriculture. These water-proximate locations, however, made cities susceptible to the dangers of flooding. We estimate, for example, that the Tiber River flooded the city of Rome about once every twenty years, with high waters lasting on average five days. In the case of major floods, waters were sometimes powerful enough to collapse cheaply constructed buildings immediately or to weaken the foundations of even sturdy structures such that they collapsed at

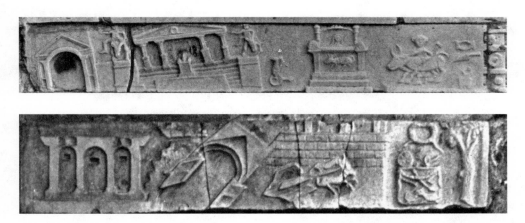

FIGURE 13 Carved stone reliefs from the House of Caecilius Iucundus, Pompeii, depicting the 5–6 magnitude earthquake that hit the region in 62/63 CE. The earthquake—a precursor of the eruption of Mt. Vesuvius in 79 CE—caused severe damage to the city's buildings, as illustrated in the reliefs. Photo credit: Ernest Nash. Permission: HEIR Project, Institute of Archaeology, University of Oxford.

some point thereafter. Thus people died not only by drowning or from injuries sustained while being swept away in the floodwaters, but also by being hurt or trapped in collapsed buildings.

Floods also triggered food shortages. Because food warehouses, especially grain storage, were located near waterways (to expedite the loading and unloading of goods traded to/from other cities), floods could waterlog a city's food supply, causing it to rot and become inedible. And because major flooding made roads impassable (although several of our ancient sources mention that people traveled through the streets in boats), it could be hard for people to secure food from marketplaces during a flood. The stagnant waters left behind by flooding bred insects, such as mosquitoes, that transmitted diseases. Likewise, disease spread when floodwaters backed up underground sewage systems, so that the streets filled with waste; when sewage combined with trash, and with the (human and animal) corpses of flood victims, the waste, in turn, contaminated the city's water supplies.

In addition to the food shortages caused by the natural disasters described above, bad weather—whether too much or not enough rain—and pestilence could likewise cause crop failure. Additionally, in times of war, enemies laying siege to a city might intentionally raze its fields (lighting them on fire) or harvest the crops to feed their own troops, either way limiting a city's food supply in order to weaken its defenses. Whatever the cause, food shortages made people more susceptible to injury and to the diseases that permeated their environments (see fig. 14). When coupled with nutrient deficiencies experienced by those communities without robust trade networks and thus with limited access to a range of kinds of foods, and with the foodborne illnesses resulting from food handling and preparation customs (such as fermenting foods, smoking meats, lack of refrigeration), food shortages

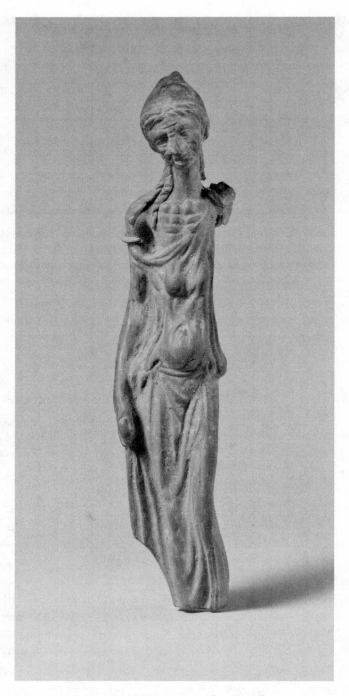

FIGURE 14 First-century BCE terracotta figurine of emaciated woman, perhaps suffering from lack of food, malnutrition, or a debilitating illness. Found near Ephesus. Metropolitan Museum of Art (89.2.2141).

merely exacerbated existing health vulnerabilities. Finally, during food shortages, we hear of desperate people consuming grasses, bulbs, and plants (such as darnel, a toxic weed that was ordinarily sifted from the wheat before harvest), and food normally served to animals (such as raw acorns), which could have serious side effects, including digestive ailments and liver damage.

It must have been common for people who lived in the ancient Mediterranean to have experienced a natural disaster themselves or to have known someone killed, injured, or sickened by such catastrophes. So terrifying were these disasters, and so serious were the health risks they posed, that it is not surprising to find depictions of these calamities—such as fire spewing from the ground, earthquakes shaking and toppling structures, floods engulfing vast regions, and famine striking down whole communities—in ancient dystopian literature and apocalyptic visions of Hades or Hell.

HAZARDS OF DAILY LIFE

Our sources likewise alert us to the myriad hazards people faced in merely going about their daily routines. For example, **Hippocratic** collections of case histories report on a range of injuries workers incurred on the job: we hear of a skipper whose hand was crushed by an anchor, a carpenter who suffered a fractured skull, a vineyard worker who suffered from paralysis in the arm he used to tie up grapevines, and a cobbler who stabbed his thigh with an awl while repairing a shoe. We also hear of farmers who were injured using the tools of their trade, such as sickles, and we have numerous reports of others working outdoors who were bitten by wild animals (Galen tells us, for example, about a vineyard worker who cut off his finger to minimize the effect of a snake bite).

Across occupations, we hear reports of bodies worn out by heavy labor. These reports— and the prevalence of work-related stress on the body—are confirmed by scientists' analysis of human remains from the period. For example, archaeologists who studied the remains of those killed during the Vesuvian eruption found that 41.3 percent of men showed signs of extreme physical stress in the bones of the head, shoulders, upper limbs, and spine that likely derived from heavy lifting, construction work, hand-plowing, and rowing. And scientists who studied the bodies of the Casal Bertone cemetery in Italy found an even higher rate of skeletal abnormalities among those who worked in the local tannery: 90 percent of the adult bodies examined showed signs of bodily trauma.

Researchers have also found more work-related injuries in children than we might expect. The majority of children would have finished with rudimentary schooling at a very young age and then would have been expected to engage in some sort of work (for example, in the family business, working on a farm, or minding smaller children). Our medical case histories are peppered with incidents in which children were injured on the job (see, for example, the report of a child kicked by work animals in Text 8, *On Epidemics* 5.16). And archaeologists have unearthed human remains—from children as young as five years old at Herculaneum—whose eroded shoulder bones show evidence of prolonged,

SCENE XXIV

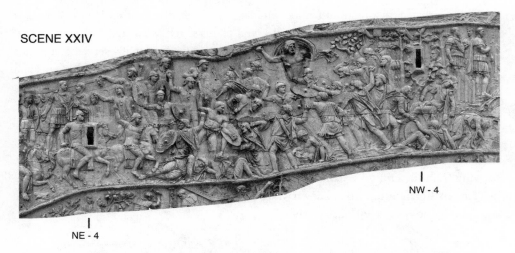

NE - 4

NW - 4

FIGURE 15 Plaster cast of a battle scene from the First Dacian War (scene 24) from Trajan's column (completed in 113 CE). The middle of the panel depicts the serious injuries that could be sustained in battle, such as being wounded by swords and projectiles, as well as being trampled by horses. The right side of the panel shows soldiers providing assistance to injured or fallen comrades. In other scenes of Trajan's column, army medics are depicted bandaging and hauling away wounded soldiers. From the Museo della Civiltà Romana, Rome. © Rome, Capitoline Superintendency of Cultural Heritage. Photo credit: trajans-column.org, used with permission of Roger B. Ulrich.

heavy activity of the muscles. When bones were broken or fractured while children were still growing and developing, we can assume this would have led to lifelong pain and impairments.

So common were hazards of everyday life that we get the impression that nearly everyone was marked by some sign of a past illness or injury. In fact, contracts from the time—which included physical descriptions of the people signing the documents (in lieu of surnames)— suggest that many people were identified by their bodily disfigurements or scars. For example, in a first-century CE will from Egypt, a testator bequeathed property to his son, Phibis, who had "a scar on the right elbow," and among the six witnesses to the will, two were identified by their own scars: "Pathoutes, about 35 years old, of medium stature, of honey-colored complexion, long-faced, with a straight nose, and a scar on his left shin," and "Paesis son of Chenamounis, about 45 years old, with a scar on his right shin." Bodily deformities resulting from illness and injury were so common that one of the other witnesses was notable precisely because he was "without scars" (*CPR* VI 72).

One of the leading causes of death among women was childbirth gone wrong (see fig. 61). We hear of difficulties in delivery (such as when young girls' pelvic bones were not yet sufficiently developed to allow passage of the fetus, when the baby was breech or sideways, or when complications arose in surgical interventions during delivery), as well as after birth (such as postpartum infections and hemorrhaging). Even if a woman escaped death after giving birth to her first child, the fact that she was expected to have many children (in order to counteract the high death rates) increased the likelihood that she would die from childbirth at some point. Infant and childhood mortality was also high. For the young, digestive issues, especially those that resulted in diarrhea, were regarded as the most dangerous. Celsus explains that children under the age of ten regularly succumbed to such ailments. And even things as seemingly mundane as teething, with the potential for ulcers and infections of the gums, could endanger an infant's life. For men, a leading cause of death was injuries sustained in battle, whether a fatal blow or infections from war wounds (see fig. 15). Finally, we know of mass casualties from epidemics. For example, scholars estimate that 75,000–100,000 lives were lost in the plague of Athens (25–35 percent of the city's population), in 430–427 BCE; and a witness to the Justinianic plague, of 541–543 CE, claimed that up to 10,000–16,000 people died each day for four months.

CONCLUSION

In sum, the daily life of people in the ancient Mediterranean was precarious. Illness and injuries were pervasive and could result in painful, chronic ailments. Moreover, death could strike at any moment. In such a world, philosophers urged people to focus on the things under their control—namely, the manner in which they responded to crises with bravery, wisdom, and dignity. A life well lived was one characterized by an individual's proper orientation to suffering more than a life free from suffering. As we consider the experiences of people living in such an environment, we gain a clear picture of the ubiquity of sickness and suffering, as well as the ailments they regarded as most distressing. Moreover, we better understand their desperate desire for relief and appreciate the refuge from illness and pain that they sought from health-care providers.

FOUR

The Cosmos and the Body as a (Micro)cosm

In the ancient world, the human body was understood to be a mirror of the cosmos and to be interconnected with the environment in inextricable ways. In other words, ancient cosmology—ideas about the nature, systems, and movements of the universe—served as a basis for thinking about the nature, systems, and movements of the human body. The body was literally a "micro"-cosm, a small-scale version of the cosmos. Once we see how people in antiquity conceived of the similarities and overlap between the cosmos and human bodies, we better understand how they approached bodily health and medical treatment.

Ideas about the natural world were developed by early Greek philosophers who carefully studied their surroundings and attempted to explain natural phenomena in terms of materiality rather than with reference to the gods (for an in-depth discussion, see chapter 2). From patterns they observed in nature, they devised unified principles and laws of nature in a range of fields: physics, astronomy, biology, what we might call "rudimentary chemistry," and medicine. Medical thinkers also participated in these kinds of unified and systematic ways of thinking, understanding the human body likewise to participate in a set of coherent patterns, rules, and principles.

Although the cosmologies of the natural philosophers and medical writers were based on material explanations instead of mythological accounts, most still believed in the existence of the gods and in a divine creation of the cosmos. Thinkers like **Plato** believed in a single, highest god who was all good and all intelligent. This god organized the preexisting matter of the cosmos, which was originally in a state of chaos, into a good, beautiful, whole, and rationally ordered world (similar to the Jewish God's creation of the world in Genesis). And the principles and laws of nature—its order and regularity—were regarded as an imprint of the divine on creation. As we see in the selections below from Plato's *Timaeus*

(Text 1), the main character in the dialogue presents a likely story about the origins of the cosmos (a kind of scientific myth) that starts with the creation of a World Soul to inhabit what will become the body of the universe. This ensoulment of the cosmos involves the divine infusion of what Plato calls Reason into preexisting matter, bringing it into the perfect symmetry of a sphere, and characterized by equal, regularized movements (such as the revolution of heavenly bodies and cycle of the seasons).

The *Timaeus* also expounded on the composition of the world from four elements—earth, water, air, and fire—a view that would become widespread in subsequent generations. According to the *Timaeus* the human body was made up of the same materials as the cosmos, and souls were likewise imparted to human bodies. Yet, if the divine creator was good and the process of divine ensoulment was characterized by order, how to explain the disorder and irregularities of human bodies? The *Timaeus* explained that humans were formed in a second-tier creation not by the highest god who created the cosmos but by lower immortal beings (called "young gods"). Thus their creation was less perfect. The bonds between the elements in human bodies were not as indissoluble as those that bound the elements of the cosmos, resulting in the body's vulnerability to decay and ultimately to death. Moreover, the irregular shape of human bodies and the irregular movements of humors within human bodies deviated from the more perfect form and movements that characterized the celestial bodies of the planets and stars. Finally, human bodies were thought to be vulnerable to the disturbances of environmental factors, such as winds, high and low temperatures, and diet.

Many of the ideas found in the *Timaeus* also can be found in medical thinking about the makeup and workings of the human body. First and foremost, each element came to be defined by its qualities on two scales: the degree to which it was hot or cold, and the degree to which it was wet or dry. Earth was regarded as cold and dry, water as cold and wet, air as hot and wet, and fire as hot and dry. Over time, there would also be widespread consensus that the human body was made up of bodily substances called "humors" that were likewise characterized on the same scales that defined the elements: hot/cold and wet/dry. As we see in figure 16, black bile was the humor like earth because it was cold and dry; phlegm was the humor like water because it was cold and wet; blood was the humor like air because it was hot and wet; and yellow bile was the humor like fire because it was hot and dry. And these qualities also became central to discussions of how to diagnose illness and prescribe treatments.

Plato's principle that the cosmos was an ordered and rational place was mirrored in medical ideas about health and illness of the body. An ordered body was assumed to be most healthy. Health, for many medical thinkers, was defined as an appropriate balance of the four humors. Yet as in Plato's *Timaeus,* most medical thinkers recognized that human bodies were rarely in a state of perfect equilibrium and balance. Rather, all four humors were present in different amounts for different individuals. This was evident in the temperaments people exhibited, temperaments associated with the predominance of one of the humors in the body: **bilious/choleric** (after yellow bile or *choler*), **phlegmatic** (after phlegm), **melancholic** (after black bile), and **sanguine** (after blood). Thus the humors characterized an individual both physically and psychologically.

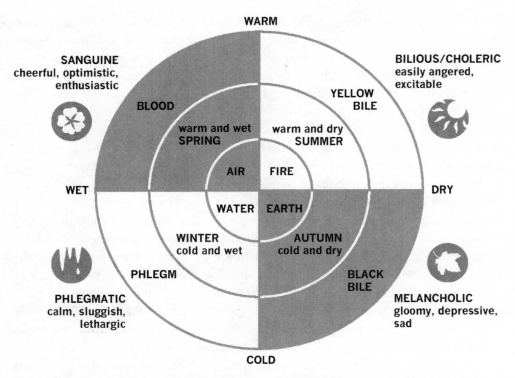

FIGURE 16 Diagram of ancient humoral theory. According to this theory, each of the four humors was characterized by its unique qualities (warm/cold and wet/dry). Each of the four humors was associated with one of the four elements and one of the four seasons that shared the same qualities. A person with a preponderance of one of the humors was associated with a particular temperament. Created by Monica Hellström.

Finally, the *Timaeus* laid a foundation for understanding the sympathetic connections woven into the very fabric of the cosmos: because they derived from a common creation and because of the principle of like things attracting to like, all parts were connected to and interacted with each other. Philosophers, natural scientists, and medical thinkers came to understand that the four elements were ordered in terms of density, with earth as the densest element, followed by water, air, and finally fire, the finest element. This ordering of the elements according to density explained, for instance, why heavy objects fall to the ground: because the earth in them "desires" to join its predominant element where it is most concentrated. Air bubbles rise in water and fire rises in air for the same reason. In the realm of human health, medical writers understood human bodies to be affected by their environment (see Text 2, *Airs, Waters, Places* and Text 5, *On the Nature of Humans;* see fig. 16). For example, the cold and wet climate of winter would trigger a production of the cold and wet humor, producing an excess of phlegm. Or a hot and wet wind would trigger a production of the hot and wet humor, an excess of blood. So, too, astronomical events such as the movements of the stars and planets altered the body, the position of the moon in its cycle influenced the best time for picking a medicinal plant, and so forth.

When observing these interactions between health and the environment, ancient thinkers also acknowledged that the elements were rarely, if ever, in their pure state; rather, they were always mixed to some degree with each other. For example, water from a spring or river was never purely water, but was always mixed with other elements, such as earth. For this reason, different kinds of water from different sources varied in quality, and also interacted with the human body in different ways, some causing sickness and some improving health. We see this logic at work when the author of *Airs, Waters, Places* stated a preference for waters that come from springs that face the rising sun because these waters are imbued with the first light of the sun, with particles of fire, which make it sparkly and more refined. The author also preferred rain water because it is made up of particles of the finest part of water found on earth, drawn up by the refined fire of the sun, like drawn to like.

Situating medical views within conversations about the cosmos helps us understand how people in the ancient Mediterranean conceived of themselves—their bodies and their health—as embedded within and interrelated with their world. It enables us to discern the logic of medical treatments, and the field of medicine more broadly, as modeled on restoring order and balance to the body, order and balance that characterized the goodness and beauty of the divinely created cosmos.

TEXT 1. PLATO, *TIMAEUS* SELECTIONS (27C–34B, 42D–44C)

Plato (427–348/7 BCE) was an Athenian philosopher and a student of **Socrates**. *His texts were written in the form of dialogues, most featuring Socrates in conversation with other people about important philosophical topics. Although Plato's* Timaeus *is technically a dialogue between Socrates and Timaeus, a philosopher of the Pythagorean school, Timaeus does most of the talking. The passages below center on the creation and nature of the universe (or cosmos). In the first selection, Timaeus explains how a divine craftsman, called the Demiurge, created the universe from a proportional balance of the four elements of earth, water, air, and fire. In the second selection, Timaeus explains how human beings were created from a mixture of the same four elements and given souls that governed them; he also discusses why they contain imperfections despite being patterned after the perfect form of the cosmos.*

SOURCE: Translation by Donald J. Zeyl based on the Greek text from J. Burnet, *Platonis Opera*, vol. 4 (Oxford: Clarendon Press, 1902). First published in *Timaeus* (Indianapolis: Hackett, 2000). Reprinted with permission of Hackett Publishing Company, Inc. All rights reserved.

27C. Timaeus: Surely anyone with any sense at all will always call upon a god before setting out on any venture, whatever its importance. In our case, we are about to make speeches about the universe—whether it has an origin or even if it does not—and so if we're not to go completely astray we have no choice but to call upon the gods and goddesses, and pray that they above all will approve of all we have to say, and that in consequence we will, too. 27d. Let this, then, be our appeal to the gods; to ourselves we must appeal to make sure that you learn as easily as possible, and that I instruct you in the subject matter before us in the way that best conveys my intent.

As I see it, then, we must begin by making the following distinction: 28a. What is *that which always is* and has no becoming, and what is *that which becomes* but never is? The former is grasped by understanding, which involves a reasoned account. It is unchanging. The latter is grasped by opinion, which involves unreasoning sense perception. It comes to be and passes away but never really is. Now everything that comes to be[1] must of necessity come to be by the agency of some cause, for it is impossible for anything to come to be without a cause. So whenever the craftsman[2] looks at what is always changeless and, using a thing of that kind as his model, reproduces its form and character, then, of necessity, all that he so completes is beautiful. 28b. But were he to look at a thing that has come to be and use as his model something that has been begotten, his work will lack beauty.

Now as to the whole heaven [*ouranos*], or world order [*kosmos*]—let's just call it by whatever name is most acceptable in a given context[3]—there is a question we need to consider first. This is the sort of question one should begin with in inquiring into any subject. Has it always been? Was there no origin [*archē*] from which it came to be? Or did it come to be and take its start from some origin? It has come to be. For it is both visible and tangible and it has a body—and all things of that kind are perceptible. 28c. And, as we have shown, perceptible things are grasped by opinion, which involves sense perception. As such, they are things that come to be, things that are begotten. Further, we maintain that, necessarily, that which comes to be must come to be by the agency of some cause. Now to find the maker and father of this universe [*to pan*] is hard enough, and even if I succeeded, to declare him to everyone is impossible. And so we must go back and raise this question about the universe: Which of the two models did the maker use when he fashioned it? 29a. Was it the one that does not change and stays the same, or the one that has come to be? Well, if this world of ours is beautiful and its craftsman good, then clearly he looked at the eternal model. But if what it's blasphemous to even say is the case, then he looked at one that has come to be. Now surely it's clear to all that it was the eternal model he looked at, for, of all the things that have

---

1. "Becoming" and "coming to be" here as elsewhere translate the same Greek word, *genesis*, and its cognates. The Greek word does not say, as English "comes to be" does, that once a thing has come to be, it now *is*, or has *being*.

2. "Craftsman" is a translation of the Greek *dēmiourgos*, whence the divine "demiurge" one reads about in accounts of the *Timaeus*.

3. The three primary terms Plato uses to refer to the universe are *ouranos* ("heaven" or "heavens"), *kosmos* ("world" or "world order"), and *to pan* ("universe"—literally "the whole"). The first of these is properly the designation of the realm of the fixed stars but is also used to designate the universe as a whole. The second refers to the world as an orderly system, while the third considers it in its totality.

come to be, our world is the most beautiful, and of causes the craftsman is the most excellent. This, then, is how it has come to be: it is a work of craft, modeled after that which is changeless and is grasped by a rational account, that is, by wisdom.

29b. Since these things are so, it follows by unquestionable necessity that this world is an image of something. Now in every subject it is of utmost importance to begin at the natural beginning, and so, on the subject of an image and its model, we must make the following specifications: the accounts we give of things have the same character as the subjects they set forth. So accounts of what is stable and fixed and transparent to understanding are themselves stable and unshifting. We must do our very best to make these accounts as irrefutable and invincible as any account may be. 29c. On the other hand, accounts we give of that which has been formed to be like that reality, since they are accounts of what is a likeness, are themselves likely, and stand in proportion to the previous accounts, that is, what being is to becoming, truth is to convincingness. Don't be surprised then, Socrates, if it turns out repeatedly that we won't be able to produce accounts on a great many subjects—on gods or the coming to be of the universe—that are completely and perfectly consistent and accurate. Instead, if we can come up with accounts no less likely than any, we ought to be content, keeping in mind that both I, the speaker, and you, the judges, are only human. 29d. So we should accept the likely tale on these matters. It behooves us not to look for anything beyond this.

Socrates: Bravo, Timaeus! By all means! We must accept it as you say we should. This overture of yours was marvelous. Go on now and let us have the work itself.

29e. Timaeus: Very well, then. Now why did he who framed this whole universe of becoming frame it? Let us state the reason why: He was good, and one who is good can never become jealous of anything. And so, being free of jealousy, he wanted everything to become as much like himself as was possible. In fact, men of wisdom will tell you (and you couldn't do better than to accept their claim) that this, more than anything else, was the most preeminent reason for the origin of the world's coming to be. 30a. The god wanted everything to be good and nothing to be bad so far as that was possible, and so he took over all that was visible—not at rest but in discordant and disorderly motion—and brought it from a state of disorder to one of order, because he believed that order was in every way better than disorder. Now it wasn't permitted (nor is it now) that one who is supremely good should do anything but what is best. 30b. Accordingly the god reasoned and concluded that in the realm of things naturally visible no unintelligent thing could as a whole be better than anything that does possess intelligence as a whole, and he further concluded that it is impossible for anything to come to possess intelligence apart from soul. Guided by this reasoning, he put intelligence in soul, and soul in body, and so he constructed the universe. He wanted to produce a piece of work that would be as excellent and supreme as its nature would allow. This, then, in keeping with our likely account, is how we must say divine providence brought our world into being as a truly living thing, endowed with soul and intelligence.

30c. This being so, we have to go on to speak about what comes next. When the maker made our world, what living thing did he make it resemble? Let us not stoop to think that it was any of those that have the natural character of a part, for nothing that is a likeness of anything incomplete could ever turn out beautiful. Rather, let us lay it down that the world resembles more closely than anything else that Living Thing of which all other living things are parts, both individually and by kinds. For that Living Thing comprehends within itself all intelligible living things, just as our world is made up of us and all the other visible creatures. 30d. Since the god wanted nothing more than to make the world like the best of the intelligible things, complete in every way, he made it a single visible living thing, which contains within itself all the living things whose nature it is to share its kind.

31a. Have we been correct in speaking of *one* heaven, or would it have been more correct to say that there are many, in fact infinitely many? There is but one, if it is to have been crafted after its model. For that which contains all of the intelligible living things couldn't ever be one of a pair, since that would require there to be yet another Living Thing, the one that contained those two, of which they then would be parts, and then it would be more correct to speak of our heaven as made in the likeness, now not of those two, but of that other, the one that contains them. 31b. So, in order that this living thing should be like the complete Living Thing in respect of uniqueness, the maker made neither two, nor yet an infinite number of worlds. On the contrary, our heaven came to be as the one and only thing of its kind, is so now, and will continue to be so in the future.

Now that which comes to be must have bodily form, and be both visible and tangible, but nothing could ever become visible apart from fire, nor tangible without something solid, nor solid without earth. That is why, as he began to put the body of the universe together, the god came to make it out of fire and earth. 31c. But it isn't possible to combine two things well all by themselves, without a third; there has to be some bond between the two that unites them. Now the best bond is the one that really and truly makes a unity of itself together with the things bonded by it, and this in the nature of things is best accomplished by proportion. 32a. For whenever of three numbers (or bulks or powers) the middle term between any two of them is such that what the first term is to it, it is to the last, and, conversely, what the last term is to the middle, it is to the first, then, since the middle term turns out to be both first and last, and the last and the first likewise both turn out to be middle terms, they will all of necessity turn out to have the same relationship to each other, and, given this, will all be unified.

32b. So if the body of the universe were to have come to be as a two-dimensional plane, a single middle term would have sufficed to bind together its conjoining terms with itself. As it was, however, the universe was to be a solid, and solids are never joined together by just one middle term but always by two. Hence the god set water and air between fire and earth, and made them as proportionate to one another as was possible, so that what fire is to air, air is to water, and what air is to water, water is to earth. He then bound them together and thus he constructed the visible and tangible heavens. 32c. This is the reason why these four particular constituents were used to beget the body of the world, making it a symphony of proportion. They bestowed friendship upon it, so that, having come together into a unity with itself, it could not be undone by anyone but the one who had bound it together.

Now each one of the four constituents was entirely used up in the process of building the world. The builder built it from all the fire, water, air, and earth there was, and left no part or power of any of them out. 32d. His intentions in so doing were these: First, that as a living thing it should be as whole and complete as possible and made up of complete parts. 33a. Second, that it should be just one world, in that nothing would be left over from which another one just like it could be made. Third, that it should not get old and diseased. He realized that when hot or cold things or anything else that possesses strong powers surrounds a composite body from outside and attacks it, it destroys that body prematurely, brings disease and old age upon it and so causes it to waste away. That is why he concluded that he should fashion the world as a single whole, composed of all wholes, complete and free of old age and disease, and why he fashioned it that way. 33b. And he gave it a shape appropriate to the kind of thing it was. The appropriate shape for that living thing that is to contain within itself all the living things would be one which embraces within itself all the shapes there are. Hence he gave it a round shape, the form of a sphere, with its center equidistant from its extremes in all directions. This of all shapes is the most complete and most like itself, which he gave to it because he believed that likeness is incalculably more excellent than unlikeness. 33c. And he gave it a smooth, round finish all over on the outside, for many reasons. It needed no eyes, since there was nothing visible left outside it; nor did it need ears, since there was nothing audible there, either. There was no air [**pneuma**] enveloping it that it might need for breathing, nor did it need any organ by which to take in food or, again, expel it when it had been digested. For since there wasn't anything else, there would be nothing to leave it or come to it from anywhere. It supplied its own waste for its food. Anything that it did or experienced it was designed to do or experience within itself and by itself. 33d. For the builder thought that if it were self-sufficient, it would be a better thing than if it required other things.

And since it had no need to catch hold of or fend off anything, the god thought that it would be pointless to attach hands to it. 34a. Nor would it need feet or any support to stand on. In fact, he awarded it the movement suited to its body—that one of the seven motions which is especially associated with understanding and intelligence. And so he set it turning continuously in the same place, spinning around upon itself. All the other six motions he took away, and made its movement free of their wanderings. And since it didn't need feet to follow this circular path, he begat it without legs or feet.

34b. Applying this entire train of reasoning to the god that was yet to be, the eternal god made it smooth and even all over, equal from the center, a whole and complete body itself, but also made up of composite bodies. In its center he set a soul, which he extended throughout the whole body and with which he then covered the body outside. And he set it to turn in a circle, a single solitary heaven, whose very excellence enables it to keep its own company without requiring anything else. For its knowledge of and friendship with itself is enough. All this, then, explains why this world which he begat for himself is a blessed god.

. . .

42d.[4] And he would have no rest from these toilsome transformations until he had dragged that massive accretion of fire-water-air-earth into conformity with the revolution of the Same and uniform within him, and so subdued that turbulent, irrational mass by means of reason. This would return him to his original condition of excellence.

Having set out all these ordinances to them—which he did to exempt himself from responsibility for any evil they might afterward do—the god proceeded to sow some of them into the Earth, some into the Moon, and others into the various other instruments of time. After the sowing, he handed over to the young gods the task of weaving mortal bodies. He had them make whatever else remained that the human soul still needed to have, plus whatever goes with those things. 42e. He gave them the task of ruling over these mortal living things and of giving them the finest, the best possible guidance they could give, without being responsible for any evils these creatures might bring upon themselves.

When he had finished assigning all these tasks, he proceeded to abide at rest in his own customary nature. His children immediately began to attend to and obey their father's assignment. Now that they had received the immortal principle of the mortal living thing, they began to imitate the craftsman who had made them. 43a. They borrowed parts of fire, earth, water, and air from the world, intending to pay them back again, and bonded together into a unity the parts they had taken, but not with those indissoluble bonds by which they themselves were held together. Instead, they proceeded to fuse them together with copious rivets so small as to be invisible, thereby making each body a unit made up of all the components. And they went on to invest this body—into and out of which things were to flow—with the orbits of the immortal soul. These orbits, now bound within a mighty river, neither mastered that river nor were mastered by it, but tossed it violently and were violently tossed by it. 43b. Consequently the living thing as a whole did indeed move, but it would proceed in a disorderly, random, and irrational way that involved all six of the motions.[5] It would go forward and backward, then back and forth to the right and the left, and upward and downward, wandering every which way in these six directions. For mighty as the nourishment-bearing billow was in its ebb and flow, mightier still was the turbulence produced by the disturbances caused by the things that struck against the living things. 43c. Such disturbances would occur when the body encountered and collided with external fire (i.e., fire other than the body's own) or for that matter with a hard lump of earth or with the flow of gliding waters, or when it was caught up by a surge of air [*pneuma*]-driven winds. The motions produced by all these encounters would then be conducted through the body to the soul, and strike against it. (That is no doubt why these motions as a group came afterward to be called "sensations,"

4. At this point in the dialogue, Timaeus has finished describing the process whereby the Demiurge creates souls for all of the heavenly bodies and next proceeds to make souls of lower orders (including human souls). He assigns the task of making bodies for these lower souls to what are called the "young gods," who are also called his "children" in 42e.

5. Timaeus is here describing the uncontrolled movement of a newborn infant. He goes on to describe the confusion produced in its soul by its first sensations.

as they are still called today.[6]) It was just then, at that very instant, that they produced a very long and intense commotion. 43d. They cooperated with the continually flowing channel to stir and violently shake the orbits of the soul. They completely bound that of the Same by flowing against it in the opposite direction, and held it fast just as it was beginning to go its way. And they further shook the orbit of the Different right through, with the result that they twisted every which way the three intervals of the double and the three of the triple, as well as the middle terms of the ratios of 3/2, 4/3, and 9/8 that connect them. [These agitations did not undo them, however,] because they cannot be completely undone except by the one who had bound them together. 43e. They mutilated and disfigured the circles in every possible way so that the circles barely held together and though they remained in motion, they moved without rhyme or reason, sometimes in the opposite direction, sometimes sideways and sometimes upside down—like a man upside down, head propped against the ground and holding his feet up against something. In that position his right side will present itself both to him and to those looking at him as left, and his left side as right. It is this very thing—and others like it—that had such a dramatic effect upon the revolutions of the soul. 44a. Whenever they encounter something outside of them characterizable as *same* or *different,* they will speak of it as "the same as" something, or as "different from" something else when the truth is just the opposite, so proving themselves to be misled and unintelligent. Also, at this stage souls do not have a ruling orbit taking the lead. And so when certain sensations come in from outside and attack them, they sweep the soul's entire vessel along with them. It is then that these revolutions, however much in control they seem to be, are actually under their control. All these disturbances are no doubt the reason why even today and not only at the beginning, whenever a soul is bound within a mortal body, it at first lacks intelligence. 44b. But as the stream that brings growth and nourishment diminishes and the soul's orbits regain their composure, resume their proper courses, and establish themselves more and more with the passage of time, their revolutions are set straight, to conform to the configuration each of the circles takes in its natural course. They then correctly identify what is the same and what is different, and render intelligent the person who possesses them. 44c. And to be sure, if such a person also gets proper nurture to supplement his education, he'll turn out perfectly whole and healthy, and will have escaped the most grievous of illnesses. But if he neglects this, he'll limp his way through life and return to Hades uninitiated and unintelligent.

TEXT 2. HIPPOCRATIC CORPUS, *AIRS, WATERS, PLACES*

Airs, Waters, Places *was attributed to* **Hippocrates,** *but as with all the texts in the Hippocratic corpus, the authorship is uncertain. Scholars have identified some similarities between it and other texts in the Hippocratic corpus, especially* On the Sacred Illness *(Text 17), and believe the text was likely written in the mid- to late fifth century BCE. The author was clearly a physician*

6. It is not clear what etymological point involving the word *aesthēseis* (sensations) Plato wants to make here. He may think (incorrectly) that *aesthesis* is etymologically related to *aïssein,* "to shake."

writing for other physicians, especially those who traveled from place to place, within and beyond the Greek world. The author explains how different features of geography and environment might have an impact on the diagnosis and treatment of illnesses (see fig. 17).

SOURCE: Translation by Robert Nau based on the Greek text from Jacques Jouanna, *Hippocrate, Airs, eaux, lieux* (Paris: Les Belles Lettres, 1996).

Chapter 1. 1. Medicine: anyone who wants to investigate it correctly must do the following. First, consider well what each season of the year can cause, for they are not at all similar to one another, but are different from each other and in their transitions. 2. Then, consider well the hot and cold winds [**pneumata**],[7] especially those common to all people and then those that are specific to each land. One must also consider well the properties of the waters. For, just as they differ in taste and in weight, so too does the property of each differ significantly. 3. Consequently, whenever someone arrives at a city and is unfamiliar with it, one must think through the city's position, namely how it is situated in relation to the winds and the risings of the sun. For whatever city faces the north wind does not have the same conditions as one that faces the south wind, nor one facing the rising sun as one facing the setting sun. 4. One must consider these things as thoroughly as possible, and also what their water is like, namely whether the inhabitants use marshy, soft waters, or hard waters from heights and rocky places, or salty and harsh waters. 5. And one must also consider whether the land is bare and waterless or thick with vegetation and well-watered, and whether it is low-lying and stifling hot or elevated and cold. One must also consider what sort of life the people enjoy, namely whether they like drinking, have more than one meal a day and are not given to hard work, or like exercise, labor, and prefer eating to drinking.

Chapter 2. 1. One must consider well each and every case arising from these circumstances. For if someone knows these things well—ideally all, but, if not, at least most of them—when arriving in an unfamiliar city, neither the local illnesses nor the nature of the body's **cavities** would elude him, so that he would not be at a loss in the treatment of their illnesses nor utterly fail. This is likely to happen if someone who does not know these things beforehand prejudges each of the illnesses. 2. As time and the year proceed, he would be able to tell what general illnesses are likely to afflict the city during the summer or winter, and the illnesses peculiar to each individual that are likely to be dangerous through a change in regimen. For by knowing in what manner the changes of the seasons and the risings and the settings of the stars happen, he would foresee what sort of year is coming. In this way, by searching out and learning beforehand the critical times, he would know a great deal about each case, and would for the most part succeed in securing health,[8] and would rightly win no small achievements in his art. 3. If someone believes that these are astronomical matters, if he should not change his mind, he would learn that astronomy contributes not

7. Throughout this text, the Greek word *pneuma* (plural: *pneumata*) is always translated as "wind(s)."

8. I.e., health for his patients.

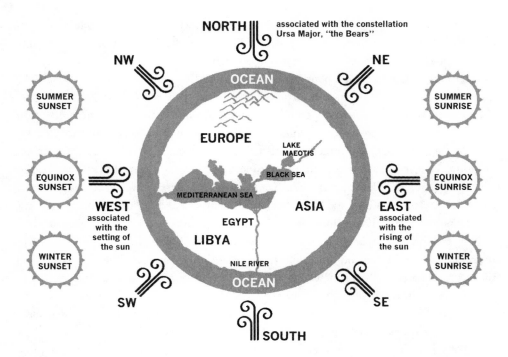

FIGURE 17 In antiquity, geographic orientation (north, south, east, west) was often pegged to the stars (for example, north was the location of the constellation Ursa Major, the "Bears"), even though thinkers like Aristotle recognized that stars' positions were not fixed, but were in different places in different seasons. For example, during the winter the sun rose in the southeast, arched across the sky further south, and set in the southwest; during the summer the sun rose in the northeast, arched across the sky further north, and set in the northwest. Because the stars were an imprecise landmark, other ancient thinkers pegged geographic orientation to winds: those that blew from different directions and that could also be differentiated by their characteristic qualities as warm or cold, and wet or dry. The Hippocratic author of *Airs, Waters, Places* assumes these views, stating, for instance, that southerly winds, which blow between the winter sunrise and the winter sunset, are typically colder than the warm northerly winds, which blow between the summer sunrise and summer sunset. The author also uses the varied conditions of different regions of the world to explain the varied temperaments of people who lived in these regions. (On this visualization, we have also included geographic landmarks mentioned in *Airs, Waters, Places*.) Created by Monica Hellström.

the least, but very much the greatest measure, to medicine. For as the seasons change, so do people's cavities.

Chapter 3. 1. I shall clearly explain how one must examine and test each of the things said earlier. A city that faces the warm winds—these are between the winter rising of the sun and its winter settings[9]—and for which these winds are normal and there is protection from the north winds, here there is a lot of brackish water that is necessarily at the surface.

9. Southeast to southwest.

During the summer the waters are warm, during the winter cool. 2. The people necessarily have heads that are moist and full of phlegm. Their body cavities are troubled constantly from the phlegm of the head flowing down upon them, and generally the people's physique is rather untoned and they are poor eaters and drinkers. Of course, those who have sickly heads would be poor drinkers, since drunken headaches oppress them more.

3. The following disorders are endemic. First, the women are sickly and suffer from unhealthy discharges. Next, many women are childless—not by nature but from sickness—and frequently miscarry. Children are afflicted by convulsions and shortness of breath and the things believed to cause the childhood illness and to be a sacred illness.[10] Men suffer from dysenteries and diarrheas and shivering fits and long-lasting winter fevers and many nighttime bouts of pustules and hemorrhoids. 4. **Pleurisies** and inflammation of the lungs and ardent fevers and all the illnesses considered severe do not arise very much. For where the body's cavities are moist, these illnesses cannot take hold. Inflammations of the eyes are runny, but are not serious and last a short time, unless some common illness strikes arising from a great change. When inhabitants are more than fifty years old, catarrhs originating from the head cause people to be paralyzed, whenever their head is suddenly warmed by the sun or chilled. 5. These are their endemic illnesses. Apart from these, they also are liable to some common illnesses arising from a change of the seasons.

Chapter 4. 1. The following conditions apply for cities that are situated opposite to these, facing the cold winds issuing between the summer settings and the summer rising of the sun,[11] for whom these winds are normal and which are protected from the south wind and from warm winds. 2. First, the waters are hard, cold, and for the most part sweet. The people are necessarily in good shape, lean. The majority of them have hard cavities that are liable to constipation below the diaphragm and cavities above the diaphragm that allow for an easier passage. They are necessarily more prone to bile than phlegm. They have healthy, hard heads but commonly suffer from internal ruptures. 3. These disorders are endemic: many pleurisies and the sicknesses considered severe. This is necessary whenever the cavities are hard. Because of the tenseness of the body and the hardness of the cavity, many abscesses arise from every cause. For the dryness and the water's coldness cause ruptures to happen. People with natures of this sort necessarily like to eat but are not fond of drinking, for it is impossible to have a great appetite for both food and drink. Inflammations of the eyes necessarily happen over time. The inflammations are hard and severe, and the eyes are ruptured immediately. Severe nosebleeds occur during the summer in men younger than thirty. The sicknesses called sacred are rare, but severe. More so than others these people are more likely to be long-lived. Their wounds do not become full of phlegm or malignant. The character of these people tends to be more aggressive than tame. 4. These are the endemic

10. Modern scholars commonly identify the "sacred illness" as epilepsy or other conditions involving seizures.

11. West northwest to east northeast.

illnesses for the men, apart from any common illnesses affecting them from a change of seasons. As for the women, firstly many become barren since the water is hard, difficult to digest, and cold, because their periods are insufficient but small and bad. Then they give birth with difficulty, but rarely miscarry. When they do give birth, they are unable to nurse the children, for their milk is dried up by the hardness and indigestibility of the waters. **Wasting ailments** happen often after deliveries, and its violence causes ruptures and strains. 5. As for the children, **dropsies** occur in their testicles while they are young, then disappear as they get older. In this type of city, they reach puberty late. So then, the effects of warm winds, cold winds, and these cities, are as described.

Chapter 5. 1. Concerning the cities situated facing the winds between the summer and the winter risings of the sun[12] and the cities opposite to these, it is as follows. 2. The cities facing the risings of the sun are likely to be healthier than those facing the Bears[13] and exposed to the warm winds, even if there is only a **stade** in between them. 3. First, the warmth and cold are more moderate. Next, all the waters that are open to the risings of the sun are necessarily clear, sweet-smelling and soft; and mist does not occur in this city, for the sun as it rises and shines down prevents this. The mist itself generally ceases each day in the early morning. 4. In appearance, the people have a healthy complexion and are rather vibrant unless some sickness prevents this. The people are clear-voiced and better in disposition and intelligence than those facing the north, just as the other things that grow there are better. 5. The city so situated is especially similar to spring for the moderation of its warmth and cold. Its sicknesses are fewer, weaker, and similar to the sicknesses in the cities facing the warm winds. The women there are quite fertile and give birth easily. Such are the features concerning cities thus situated.

Chapter 6. 1. Those cities facing the settings of the sun and that are protected from the winds blowing from the east, with the warm winds and the cold winds from the Bears blowing past them—these cities necessarily have the most unhealthy setting. 2. First, their waters are not clear. The reason is that early in the morning for a considerable time there is mist, which, when mixed into the water, destroys its clarity, for the sun does not shine directly upon these cities until it has raised itself high. In the early morning during the summer, cold winds blow and dews fall, and for the rest of the day the sun scorches the people through and through, as it descends. 3. Accordingly, the people are likely to be pale and sick and to have a share of all the aforementioned illnesses, since no one illness is peculiar to them. The people are likely to have deep voices and to suffer from hoarseness because of the mist, since generally it is impure and damp there, for it has not been separated out very much by the north winds which are not persistent. The winds that persist and cling to these

12. Northeast to southeast.

13. "The Bears" referred to the constellations Ursa Major and Ursa Minor, and was a way of indicating north (see fig. 17). The reference to constellations also hints at the impact that celestial bodies might have on human health.

cities are the wettest, since the winds of the west are of this sort. 4. Such a city's position is especially like autumn as far as the changes of the day go, for there is a great difference between the early morning and the afternoon. This is how it is with the favorable and unfavorable winds.

Chapter 7. 1. As for the rest of the waters, I wish to describe in full the ones that are harmful, the ones that are very healthy, and all the bad and good things that are likely to result from water, since it contributes a great amount to health. 2. The waters that are swampy, stagnant, and marshy are necessarily warm, thick, and stinking during the summer because they do not flow away. But, since they are always resupplied by fresh rain water and burnt up by the sun, they are necessarily colorless, unhealthy, and productive of bile. During the winter they are icy, cold, and cloudy from the snow and frost, so that they are most likely to cause phlegm and sore throats. 3. People who drink these waters necessarily always have big and hard spleens, hard, thin, and hot stomachs, and withered and wasted shoulders, collarbones, and faces because their **flesh** is dissolved to benefit the spleen, making them lean. People of this sort necessarily eat and drink to excess. Their cavities, above and below the diaphragm, are excessively dry, so that they require stronger drugs. This illness habitually afflicts them in the summer and winter. 4. In addition to these illnesses, very many and very deadly dropsies occur. For, during the summer, many dysenteries and diarrheas assail them and long-lasting **quartan fevers.** These illnesses, if prolonged, cause fatal dropsies in people with natures of this sort. These are the illnesses of the summer. 5. During the winter inflammations of the lungs and disorders accompanied by madness afflict the young, and ardent fever afflicts the old, because of the hardness of the cavity. 6. The women are swollen and have white, bloated skin; they are scarcely able to become pregnant and bear children with difficulty. Their babies are big and swollen, and then, over the course of being nursed, they are afflicted with the wasting ailment and are in a bad state. After childbirth, the women's discharge is not good. 7. Children especially suffer from hernias and men from the enlargement of veins and sores on the legs, so that people with natures of this sort must be short-lived and grow old before their proper time. 8. Further, the women seem to be pregnant, but when the birth is at hand, the fullness of the womb vanishes. This happens whenever wombs suffer from dropsy. 9. I judge that waters of this sort are worthless for every single use.

Second worst are those waters whose springs are from rocks (for their waters are necessarily hard) or from earth where the waters run warm or where there is iron, copper, silver, gold, sulfur, alum, bitumen or sodium carbonate (because these are all formed from the power of heat). Therefore, the waters from earth of this sort cannot be good, but are hard, cause fevers, are difficult to pass in urine, and obstruct excretion. 10. Best are the waters that flow from high places and from earthy hills, for they are sweet, clear and it is enough to add a little wine to them. They are warm during the winter and cold in the summer. They would be so, because they flow from very deep springs. I especially praise the waters with flows that burst forth towards the risings of the sun, and preferably towards the summer risings. They are necessarily brighter, good-smelling and light. 11. All waters that are salty, harsh, and hard are not good to drink, but there are some natures[14] and illnesses for which drinking waters of this sort is useful, about which I shall speak momentarily. Concerning the quality of these types of water it is so.

The very best waters are those whose sources face the risings of the sun. Second best are the waters between the summer risings and settings of the sun, preferably those facing the risings. Third best are the waters between the summer and winter settings of the sun. Worst are those facing south and the ones between the winter rising and setting. These are altogether bad under southern winds, but better under northern winds. 12. Spring waters should be used in the following way. A person who is healthy and strong does not have to deliberate but can drink whatever is at hand. But someone who because of a sickness wants to drink the most suitable waters could attain health by doing these things. People with cavities that are hard and easily heated benefit from waters that are sweetest, lightest and clearest. In contrast, people with stomachs that are soft, moist, and full of phlegm benefit from waters that are hardest, harshest, and brackish, for thus they would be dried out most effectively. 13. For the waters that are best for cooking and dissolving are also very likely to loosen the cavity and relax it. The waters that are harsh, hard, and worst for cooking are especially likely to contract and dry up the cavities. But people, through lack of experience, have deceived themselves about salty waters, in that it is believed that the brackish waters are laxative. But these are entirely the opposite to laxative: they are harsh and bad for cooking, so that the cavity is contracted by them rather than loosened. This is how it is with spring waters.

Chapter 8. 1. I shall speak about how it is with rain water and snow water. 2. Rain waters are lightest, sweetest, thinnest, and clearest. For, to begin with, the sun draws up and carries away the lightest and thinnest component of the water. 3. Salt makes this clear. For the brine is left behind due to its thickness and heaviness and becomes salt. The thinnest component, due to its lightness, is carried away by the sun. The sun draws up this part not only from the waters of marshes, but also from the sea and from everything in which there is any moisture, and there is moisture in everything. 4. And the sun even draws from people the thinnest and lightest component of their moisture. And there is a very great proof of this. Whenever a person walks or is sitting in the sun wearing a cloak, the skin that the sun shines on does not sweat, for the sun carries away any of the sweat that appears. What has been protected by the cloak, or by anything else, sweats, for the moisture is forced and drawn out by the sun, but is preserved by the covering, so that it does not disappear because of the sun. But, whenever one reaches shade, the entire body sweats equally, for the sun no longer shines upon it. 5. For these reasons, of all waters rain water also putrefies quickest and gets a bad smell, since it has been collected and mixed together from the most sources, so that it putrefies quickest. 6. What is more, whenever it is carried away and raised up, by being circulated and mixed in the air, its cloudy and murky components are separated out and are displaced and become mist and fog, and its clearest and lightest component is left and sweetened as it is burned and cooked by the sun. So too do all other things that are boiled

---

14. I.e., people with characteristics that would benefit from this type of water.

always become sweet. 7. As long as rain water has been scattered about and is in no way united, it is carried aloft. But whenever it has been gathered together somewhere and compressed suddenly in the same place by adverse winds, then it falls wherever it happens to have been compressed most. For this is very likely to happen when the clouds, stirred by the wind and on the move, suddenly strike against a contrary wind and other clouds. At that moment, the first clouds are compressed, and the ones behind come upon them and so are thickened, darkened, and compressed into the same place. There is a downpour because of the heaviness, and rainstorms. 8. In all likelihood, these waters are best, but they need to be boiled and to have their impurities removed. If not, they have a bad smell, and sore throats, coughs, and hoarseness afflict those who drink them.

9. Waters from snow and ice are all bad. For, whenever they freeze entirely, they no longer exist in their original condition, but their clear, light, and sweet components are congealed and disappear, and the thickest and the weightiest components are left behind. 10. One may observe this from the following. If you so wish, during the winter pour a measured amount of water into a vessel, and set it in the open where it is most likely to freeze. Then, on the next day, take it inside to a warm spot where the ice will easily melt. When it is liquefied, measure the water again. You will find it to be far less. 11. This is proof that the lightest and thinnest components disappear and are dried up by freezing, not the heaviest and thickest components, for that would not be possible. Thus I judge that waters from snow and ice, and waters similar to these, are the worst for all purposes. So then, these are the properties of rain, snow, and ice waters.

Chapter 9. 1. When people drink waters of all kinds, from great rivers into which other rivers flow, and from a lake into which many streams of all kinds arrive, and where people use foreign waters brought across a great, not a short, distance, they especially suffer from stones, kidney disorders, strangury, sciaticas, and hernias. 2. For one water cannot be like the other, but some waters are sweet, and some are brackish and contain alum, and some flow from warm sources. These, when mixed together in the same place, are at odds with one another, and the strongest always holds sway. The same water, however, does not always prevail. Sometimes one prevails, and sometimes another, depending on the winds. One has its strength from the north wind, another from the south wind, and the same principle applies for the rest. Such waters necessarily deposit dirt and sand in the bottom of their vessels. And from drinking these arise the illnesses mentioned previously. 3. But, I will show that this does not apply to all.

Those people with a healthy cavity that flows well, and a bladder that is not feverish with an unobstructed opening, easily pass urine and nothing solid forms in their bladder. 4. People with a feverish cavity necessarily have bladders that suffer from fever. For, when the bladder is warmed unnaturally, its opening is inflamed. When the bladder suffers these things, it does not expel its urine, but cooks and heats it together inside itself. The thinnest and purest components go through and are passed out in the urine, but the thickest and most turbid components are compressed and solidified. This is small at first, but then becomes bigger. For whatever is gathered thickly together is rolled about by the urine and combines with itself and so grows and hardens. When one urinates, the stone is propelled by the urine and falls against the opening of the bladder. This hinders urination and causes severe pain, so that boys who suffer from stones rub and tug their genitals, for it seems to them that the source of urination is from there. 5. There is proof that this is so. People suffering from stones pass the clearest urine, since its thickest and most turbid components are left behind and are compressed together. In most cases one suffers stones for these reasons. But a stone is also caused from milk if it is not healthy, but is too warm and productive of bile. For the milk thoroughly warms the cavity and the bladder, so that the urine suffers the same things by being heated up. And I say that it is better to give the most diluted wine possible to children, for it heats and dries the veins less. 6. Stones do not afflict women in the same way. For the bladder's urethra is short and wide, so that the urine is easily expelled. A woman does not rub her genitals with her hand as the male does, nor does she touch her urethra, for it is linked to the genitals by a channel. But men lack a connective channel that runs straight and on account of this their urinary channels are not wide. And women drink more than boys. So then, this, or something very close to it, is the explanation concerning these matters.

Chapter 10. 1. Concerning the seasons, a person can learn exactly what the year is likely to be, whether sickly or healthy, by considering well the following points. 2. For if the signs happen according to rule with the stars as they set and rise, if rains happen in autumn, if winter is moderate—neither excessively calm nor going beyond the proper time for cold—and if in the spring and in the summer rains happen seasonably, that year is likely to be healthiest. 3. But if the winter is dry with cold north winds and the spring very rainy with warm south winds, the summer necessarily produces fevers and causes eye inflammations and dysenteries. For whenever a stifling heat suddenly comes while the land is wet because of spring rains and the south wind, the heat is necessarily doubled, since the earth is thoroughly soaked and warm and is under a burning sun. Likewise, the cavities of people have not been contracted and their brains are not dry (for it is impossible during a spring of this sort for the body and its flesh not to bloat with fluid) so that very severe fevers fall upon all and especially those who have excess phlegm. Dysenteries are likely to strike women and people with the moistest natures. 4. And, if at the Dog Star's rising[15] a rainstorm[16] happens and the Etesian wind[17] blows, there is hope for respite and for there to be a healthy autumn. If not, there is danger that deaths will happen among children and women, but little chance of this among old men, and that the people surviving will end up with quartan fevers and, after quartan fevers, dropsies. 5. If the winter has warm south winds and is exceedingly wet and calm, and the spring has north cold winds and is dry and stormy, first the women who happen to be pregnant and expecting around spring are likely to miscarry. Those who give birth, give birth to sickly and weak children, so that they either die immediately, or live on thin, weak, and sickly. These things happen to women. 6. For the rest, there are dysenteries, dry inflammations of the eyes, and some have catarrhs from the head to the lungs.

15. The rising of the "Dog Star" (Sirius) was associated with the hottest summer days (whence comes the modern expression "dog days of summer").
16. Or a snowstorm.
17. The Etesian winds were strong, dry north winds that blew during the summer months.

Dysenteries are likely to occur in those who have excessive phlegm and also to women from phlegm that flows down from the brain because of the moistness of their nature. And dry eyes are likely to occur in those who have excessive bile, because of the heat and the dryness of their flesh, and catarrhs are likely to occur in the old, because of their veins' narrowness and deterioration, so that suddenly some perish and some become paralyzed on the right side. 7. For, whenever there is a hot winter with warm south winds, neither the body nor the veins are contracted, and when this is followed by a dry, cold spring with cold north winds, the brain hardens and is contracted at the time when it should have been relaxed with the spring and cleansed by a runny nose and sore throat. The result is that when summer suddenly follows accompanied by heat and great change, these illnesses strike.

8. The cities that are well situated in relation to the sun and the winds and use good waters are less sensitive to such changes. Cities that use marshy and swampy waters and are not situated well in relation to the winds and sun are more sensitive to such changes. 9. If the summer is dry, their sicknesses are shorter, but, if excessively rainy, they will be prolonged. If there is a wound, festering is likely to arise from every provocation. Also, as sicknesses come to an end, lienteries and dropsies follow because the cavities are not easily dried out. 10. If the summer and autumn are excessively rainy with warm winds from the south, the winter is necessarily sickly and ardent fevers are likely to strike those who have excessive phlegm and those older than forty. People with excessive bile are likely to suffer pleurisies and inflammations of the lungs. 11. If the summer becomes dry with warm south winds, and the autumn excessively rainy with cold north winds, in the winter headaches and suppurations of the brain are likely to happen, and, on top of this, coughs, sore throats, runny noses, and also wasting ailments in some. 12. But if there are cold north winds, it is rainless and showers come neither at the Dog Star nor at Arcturus;[18] this is especially beneficial to people with excess phlegm and moist natures and women, but most harmful to people with excessive bile, for they are dried up too much. Dry inflammations of the eyes and severe, long-lasting fevers afflict them. Some people are also afflicted by excess black bile, for the moistest and wateriest component of the bile is used up and the thickest and very acrid component of the bile is left—and so too with blood according to the same principle—from which these illnesses afflict them. But all these conditions are advantageous to people with excessive phlegm, for they are dried completely and do not enter winter bloated but dried up. [If the winter has cold north winds and is dry, and the spring has warm south winds and is excessively rainy, throughout summer there are severe inflammations of the eyes and fevers afflict children and women.][19]

Chapter 11. 1. By reflecting and reasoning with these principles, one would foresee most of the things that are likely to happen from the changes of the seasons. One must especially be on guard against the greatest changes of the seasons and neither willingly give a drug nor cau-

18. Arcturus is the brightest star in the constellation Boötes. When Arcturus became visible during sunrise (at which time it was called the "morning star"), it marked the end of summer. When Arcturus became visible in the evening twilight, it marked the beginning of spring.

19. The sentence in square brackets may not have been in the original Greek text.

terize or cut into the cavity before ten or more days pass. 2. The greatest and most dangerous transitions are as follows: both solstices and especially the summer; both of what are considered equinoxes, especially the autumnal. One must also be on guard against the risings of the stars, especially of the Dog Star, then of Arcturus, and also the settings of the Pleiades.[20] For on these days especially illnesses reach their **crisis.** Some illnesses cause death, others abate, and all the rest change into a different type and another state. So it is with these things.

Chapter 12. 1. Now I wish to speak about Asia and Europe and how they differ entirely from each other and how their peoples' physical appearance differ from one another.[21] An account of all these things would be too long, so instead I shall tell what I think are the greatest and most important differences. 2. I say that Asia differs most from Europe in the natures of their people and of everything that grows from their land. For everything is much more beautiful and bigger in Asia, and their region is milder than our region and the characteristics of its people are more gentle and more evenly tempered. 3. The cause for this is the blending of the seasons, since Asia lies towards the east between the risings of the sun[22] and further from the cold than Europe. What contributes most to growth and cultivation is when nothing dominates too much, but rather power over everything is shared. 4. Asia is not the same everywhere, but that part of the land situated in the middle of the hot and the cold is very fruitful, very rich in trees, and very mild, and has been endowed with the best waters from the sky and from the earth. For the land has not been too scorched by the heat, nor is it dried up by droughts and lack of water, nor overpowered by cold, nor is it damp and soaked through by many showers and snow. 5. Here the harvests are likely to be abundant, both those from seeds and whatever vegetation the land itself puts forth, whose fruits people use by cultivating them from the wild and transplanting them to suitable soil. The herds raised there are likely to grow well and especially to bear and produce very sturdy and very beautiful offspring. The people are also likely to be well nourished, very beautiful in appearance, very tall, and not very different in their looks and appearance from each other. 6. This land is likely to be closest to spring according to its nature and the temperateness of its seasons. Manliness, hardiness, industry, and good spirit could not arise in a condition of this sort [. . .][23] 7. neither of the same stock nor of a different stock, but necessarily pleasure rules. Accordingly, varied forms of animals exist. So then, with respect to the Egyptians and the Libyans, this is how I think it is.

Chapter 13. 1. Concerning those on the right of the sun's summer risings as far as Lake Maeotis,[24] for this is the boundary of Europe and Asia, it is as follows. 2. The peoples there differ more among themselves than those already described because of the changes of

---

20. The Pleiades are a group of stars in the constellation Taurus. The rising of the Pleiades marked the beginning of summer, while the setting of the Pleiades marked the beginning of winter.

21. For Greek authors, "Asia" referred primarily to Asia Minor, which is roughly equivalent to modern-day Türkiye.

22. I.e., between the rising of the sun in the winter and in the summer.

23. A section of the Greek text is missing here. When the text resumes, the author is discussing Egypt and Libya (which referred to any part of Africa other than Egypt).

24. Lake Maeotis is now called the Sea of Azov, located to the north of the Black Sea.

seasons and the nature of their lands. 3. It is with the earth just as it is with the people. For where the seasons cause the greatest and most frequent changes, there also the land is very wild and very irregular, and you will find that there are very many hills, bushy places, plains, and meadows. But where the seasons do not greatly change, the land is very flat. 4. That is how it is with people too, if one is willing to reflect upon it. For the natures of some people are similar to tree-covered, well-watered hills, others to sparse and waterless places, others to more meadowy and marshy places, and others to a plain and bare dry land. 5. For the seasons that change in the nature of one's physical form are different. And if the differences among the seasons are great, more pronounced differences also arise in people's appearances.

Chapter 14. 1. I shall omit the peoples that differ little. I shall instead speak about how the people that differ greatly either in nature or in custom fare. First, the Longheads. 2. For there is not another people that has heads at all like theirs. In the beginning, the length of the head was caused mostly by custom, for they consider people with the longest heads to be noblest, but now their nature also contributes to the custom. 3. Concerning their custom, it is so: as soon as possible when the child is born, they reshape its head by hand while tender and force it to be increased in length by applying bindings and suitable devices, by which the head's spherical shape is destroyed, and the length is augmented. And so in the beginning custom was at work, so that a nature of this sort existed by force. 4. Over time, it began to arise naturally, so that custom was no longer the driving force. For the seed comes from everywhere in the body, the healthy seed from healthy parts and sick seeds from sick parts. So if bald-headed people come from bald-headed parents, and grey-eyed children from grey-eyed parents, and squinting children from squinting parents, and for the most part the same principle holds for other differences in form, what stops a long-headed child from being born from a long-headed parent? 5. But now this no longer happens to the same degree as earlier, for the custom is no longer influential on account of their intermingling with other people. So then, with respect to these people, this is how I think it is.

Chapter 15. 1. As to those on the river Phasis,[25] that land is marshy, warm, watery, and wooded. Many violent rains fall there every season and the people dwell in the marshes and in wooden and reed dwellings built amid the waters. They hardly travel by foot through their city and harbor but sail up and down throughout it in dug-outs, for there are many canals. They drink warm and standing waters that have been corrupted by the sun and swollen by rains. The Phasis itself is the most stagnant with the gentlest flow of all rivers. The fruits produced there are all small, too soft, and incomplete because of the overabundance of water and for this reason they do not ripen. Much mist from the waters clings to the place. 2. For these reasons, the people of Phasis differ in appearance from other people. For they are tall in stature, and are overly fat. As far as being fat goes, neither their joints nor veins are visible and they have yellowish skin just as if they were afflicted with dropsy. Compared to other people they have the deepest voices, since they are subject to air that is not clear, but southerly and wet. In terms of

25. The Phasis is the modern-day Rioni River. It flows into the Black Sea on its eastern coast, and in antiquity was sometimes considered the border between Europe and Asia (see fig. 17).

physically enduring hard labor, they are rather inactive by nature. 3. Their seasons do not change much in terms of stifling heat or cold. Their winds are mainly damp, except for one native wind. This blows from time to time strong, violent, and warm. They name this wind the *kenchron*. The north wind does not come very much, but whenever it blows it is weak and slight. Concerning the difference in nature and shape of the people in Asia, it is so.

Chapter 16. 1. As to the people's lack of spirit and unmanliness, their seasons are very much to blame for the Asians are as unwarlike as can be compared to the people of Europe and rather tame by disposition, for instead of causing great changes towards heat or cold they are nearly identical. 2. Asians do not experience shocks to their mind nor severe changes to the body, which are likely to make one's temperament fierce and to make them be more reckless and high-spirited than if they were always in the same state. For there are changes in all things and these always stir up people's temperament, not allowing it to remain at rest. 3. For these reasons it seems to me that Asian peoples are unwarlike, as are their customs, for the majority of Asia is ruled by kings. Where people are not masters of themselves nor autonomous, but are ruled by despots, they are uninterested in practicing warfare, but rather in seeming to be unwarlike. 4. For the dangers they experience are not the same. The subjects are likely, out of necessity, to go to war and endure hard labor and die on behalf of despots while away from children, wives, friends, and family. The despots make themselves rich and prosper from the many worthy and manly deeds they do, but the subjects themselves harvest dangers and deaths. In addition, the land of such people is necessarily made barren because of hostilities and their idleness, with the result that even if someone is naturally manly and stout of heart, his inclination is diverted by their customs. 5. There is a great proof of this. All the people in Asia, whether Greeks or barbarians, who are not under despotic rule but are autonomous and endure hard labor for their own benefit, are, of all people, most warlike. For they risk dangers for themselves and they take away the prizes of manliness and likewise the penalty of cowardice. You will also find that Asians differ from each other, some being better and some being worse. The changes of the seasons are the cause of this, just as I said in the earlier accounts. Thus it is concerning people in Asia.

Chapter 17. 1. In Europe there is a Scythian people that lives around Lake Maeotis and differs from other peoples. They are called Sauromatae. 2. For as long as they are virgins, their women ride horses, are archers, throw javelins from horseback, and fight in battles. They do not abandon their virginity until they kill three people in battle, and they do not live with men before they make their customary sacrifices. A woman who takes a husband for herself stops riding, unless compelled by a campaign requiring everyone's efforts. 3. They lack their right breast. For their mothers, while the children are still infants, thoroughly heat a bronze instrument that has been devised for this very thing, and apply it to the right breast. It is burnt away so that its potential to grow is destroyed and it gives all its power and mass to the right shoulder and arm.

Chapter 18. 1. Concerning the physique of the rest of the Scythians, in that they are alike to one another and not at all alike to others, the same principle applies to them as to the Egyptians, except that the Egyptians have been oppressed by the heat and the Scythians by the cold. 2. What is called the Scythians' desert is level, grassy, elevated, and moderately watered, for there are great rivers that draw off the waters from the plains. There the Scythians live, and they are called nomads since they do not have houses but live in wagons. 3. Some wagons are very small with four wheels, and others, the largest, have six wheels. These are enclosed by felt and are built just like houses with some having a single chamber and others three. These are shelters against rain, snow, and the winds. Two pairs of yoked hornless oxen draw some wagons and three pairs of yoked hornless oxen others. They have no horns because of the cold weather. The women conduct their lives in these wagons, but the men ride horses, with the sheep that they have following them, along with their cattle and horses. The Scythians remain in the same place for as long as the feeding ground provides for their herds. When it no longer meets their needs, they move on to another place. They consume boiled meats, drink mares' milk, and eat *hippakē,* a cheese from mares' milk. Thus it is with their manner of life and customs.

Chapter 19. 1. Concerning their seasons and their physique, the Scythian people differ much from the rest of humankind but, like the Egyptian people, are homogenous among themselves. They are least fertile and their land supports the smallest and fewest wild animals. 2. For their land is positioned below the Bears and the Rhipaean mountains,[26] from which the north wind blows. The sun as it ends its journey is nearest to the mountains when it comes to its summer circuits, and then warms them for a short time, but not very much. The winds blowing from warm regions only come occasionally and are weak, but winds blow from the north that are always cold from snow, frost, and many waters. These winds are never absent from the mountains, which are uninhabited because of them. For much of the day, fog clings to the plains, on which the Scythians spend their lives, so that it is always winter and summer (though not very summery) only for a few days. For the plains are high, bare, and are not circled by mountains, apart from the northern side. 3. There the wild animals are not large in size, but the kinds that are able to shelter themselves underground, for winter and the barrenness of the land stunt their growth, since there is neither warmth nor protection. 4. The changes of seasons are neither great nor severe, but the seasons are similar and change little. For this reason the people are similar to each other, since they also always use the same kind of food and clothing in summer and winter, and they breathe the watery thick fog and drink the waters from snow and ice, while not engaging in hard work. For, where the changes are not severe, neither the body nor the spirit can endure hard labor. 5. Because of these constraints, in appearance they are stout, fleshy, without visible joints, soft and slack, and their cavities below the diaphragm are as wet as they can be. For the belly cannot be dried up in a land of this sort, with such a condition and type of season, but their flesh is forever fat and hairless. Their appearances are similar to one another, men are similar to men and women to women. Since the seasons are so alike the coagulation of the seed

26. The Rhipaean mountains were a range of mountains believed by Greek and Roman writers to rise at the world's northern edge (see fig. 17). Which mountain range they had in mind is uncertain, if the Rhipaean mountains existed at all.

does not have corruptions and ill effects,[27] unless through the misfortune of some violent force or sickness.

Chapter 20. 1. And I shall provide a great proof of their moistness. For you will find that most Scythians, all who are nomads, have had their shoulders, arms, wrists of their hands, chest, and loins **cauterized** for no reason other than their nature's moistness and softness. For they cannot draw taut their bows nor throw a javelin from the shoulder with a soft and untoned nature. But when they are cauterized the excess moisture is dried up from the joints and the bodies become more toned, and visibly jointed. 2. Their bodies become flabby and broad, firstly because they, unlike the Egyptians, do not have the custom of swaddling so that they may ride a horse well, and secondly, from their sedentary lifestyle. For, because of their migrations and travel, because the men (until they are able to ride a horse) sit in the wagon for most of the time and because they rarely walk. In appearance, the women are wondrously flabby and slow moving. 3. The Scythian people have red skin from the cold, not because of the force of the sun, but because their skin's whiteness is burned up by the cold and becomes red.

Chapter 21. 1. A nature of this sort cannot produce many offspring. A man has little desire for intercourse because of the moistness of his nature and his belly's softness and coldness. A man with these conditions is quite unlikely to lust. In addition, since they are always being jolted by their horses, they become too weak for intercourse. These are the reasons why men are infertile. 2. For women, it is their body's obesity and moistness. Their wombs are no longer able to receive the seed. Neither is their monthly menses as it should be, but is slight and intermittent. The opening of their wombs is closed together by fat and does not accept the seed. The women themselves are not hard-working and fat, and their cavities are cold and soft. 3. The Scythian people are not fertile because of these constraints. Their slave-girls provide great proof, for when they come to a man, as soon as they arrive, they become pregnant owing to their life of hard labor and their flesh's leanness.

Chapter 22. 1. What is more, many men among the Scythians are like eunuchs. They labor at women's work and speak to one another as women do. They are called *Anariees*. 2. The natives attribute the cause to a god and they worship these people, each fearing for himself. 3. I also think that these conditions are divine, as are all others, and that not one is more divine than another nor more human, but all are alike and all are divine. Each of these conditions has a nature and no condition happens without a natural cause. 4. I shall state how I think this condition happens. There are swellings at the joints from horse-riding, since their feet are always hanging from their horses. Then those who suffer severely become quite lame and suffer sores at their hip joints. 5. They heal themselves in the following way: when the sickness starts, they cut the vein behind each ear, and when the blood flow ceases, in their weakness, sleep suddenly takes hold and they sleep. Then they wake up, some healthy, some not. 6. I think that, through this cure, their seed is destroyed. For alongside the ears are veins and those whose veins have been cut become sterile. I think that the Scythians are cutting these veins. 7. After this, when they come to their wives and cannot have sex with them, at

27. This description refers to the formation of an embryo in the womb.

first they are unconcerned and undisturbed. But when nothing different happens after trying two, three, and many times more, they believe that they have in some way wronged the god, whom they hold responsible, and they put on women's clothes. In sentencing themselves to unmanliness they act as women and labor with the women at their work.

8. Because of riding horses, those who suffer this most are wealthy Scythians and men who are best born and endowed with the most strength, not men who are worst off. But the poor suffer this less, for they do not ride horses. 9. If indeed this sickness is more divine than the rest, it would not attack the best born and wealthiest Scythians only, but all equally and more so if the gods delight in being worshipped by humankind and bestow favors in return, attacking those owning little, not those already honored. 10. For the wealthy are likely to sacrifice much to the gods and to dedicate their goods and honors as offerings, but the poor do this less often since they lack these. Consequently the poor blame the gods for not giving them wealth, so that naturally those who have little suffer the punishments for these wrongs more so than the wealthy. 11. But indeed, just as I said earlier, these conditions are as divine as others, with each arising according to its nature. This kind of sickness afflicts the Scythians from a cause of this sort, as I have said. 12. Throughout the rest of humankind it is the same. Wherever people ride horses with great regularity and frequency, they are attacked by swellings of the joints, sciatica, gout, and they are the least capable of having sexual intercourse. 13. These issues are present among the Scythians and they are the most eunuch-like of men for the reasons already stated. Also, because they always wear trousers and spend most of their time on horses, they do not handle their genitals; and because of the cold and being jolted about, they forget about desire and intercourse. Before they reach manhood they are no longer passionate. So it is then with the Scythian people.

Chapter 23. 1. The remaining peoples in Europe vary in size and shape because of the great and frequent changes of the seasons, with severe warm spells, strong winters, frequent rain and then long-lasting droughts, and winds that cause many changes of many kinds. From these conditions one is likely also to perceive that generation is different with respect to the coagulation of the seed and that the same process does not happen to the same seed in the summer and in the winter, nor in a rainstorm and in a drought. 2. And for that reason I think that Europeans differ more in appearance than the Asians, and, amongst themselves from city to city, they differ most in height. For, with frequent changes of the seasons, more corruption in the coagulation of the seed happens than in seasons that are similar and uniform. 3. The same principle holds for character. In such a climate arises wildness, unsociability, and high spirits. For the frequent shocks to their temperament produce wildness and destroy gentleness and mildness. For this reason, I believe that people living in Europe are more courageous than people in Asia. For where there is always consistency, complacency is abundant, but where there is change, there is endurance for the body and the soul. Cowardice will be developed from peacefulness and ease, but virtues will be increased from hard work and toils. 4. Inhabitants of Europe are more warlike for this reason, and also because of their customs, since they are not ruled by kings as the Asians are. For where people are ruled by kings, the people there are necessarily most cowardly. I said this earlier too. For their spirits are enslaved and they will not willingly take on risks for someone else's power. Those who are autonomous, undertaking risks not for others but for themselves, willingly exert themselves and come into danger, for they themselves carry off the noblest prizes of victory. Thus customs to no small degree fashion courage. This is how it is generally and overall with Europe and Asia.

Chapter 24. 1. The abundant peoples in Europe differ in height, form, and manliness. The differences are the same as those that I have mentioned earlier. I shall describe them yet more exactly. 2. People who inhabit mountainous, rugged, elevated, and well-watered land where the seasons' changes differ greatly are likely to be large in size and have a nature suitable for hard labor and manliness. Natures of this sort have much wildness and ferocity. 3. People who inhabit lands lying in meadowy, stifling-hot hollows and lands with more warm than cold winds, and who use warm waters, would not be large or well-made, but are by nature broad, fleshy, dark-haired, dusky rather than fair, and with less phlegm than bile. Manliness and endurance are not present naturally in equal measure, but could be produced with the force of custom applied, as if that were one's type, even though it is not. 4. If there are rivers in the region to draw off standing water and rain water, the people will be healthiest and without blemish. If, however, the rivers are not abundant, and the people drink spring water, standing water, and marshy water, they will necessarily have protruding bellies and spleen ailments. 5. People who live in elevated, level, windy well-watered land, would be large in size, similar to one another, and inclined to be rather unmanly and somewhat submissive. People in a temperate land who enjoy the best and abundant waters have a noble character and form, being stout, tall, and similar to one another. 6. People who live on thin, waterless, and bare soil that have sharp changes of seasons are likely to be well toned and more fair-haired than dark in appearance, and willful and single-minded in their character and passions. For where the seasons' changes are most frequent and differ most from each other, there you will find the greatest differences in appearances and natures. 7. These are the greatest influences on differences in the nature of humans, followed by the land in which one is raised and the waters. For you will find that, for the most part, the appearances of peoples and their ways follow the nature of the land. 8. For where the land is rich, soft, and well-watered and the waters are very close to the surface, so that they are warm during the summer and cold during the winter, and the land is favorably positioned in its seasons, then also the people are fleshy, without visible joints, moist, intolerant of hard work and generally cowards. Light-heartedness and sleepiness are common among them and in arts and skills they are thick-headed and neither refined nor clever. 9. Where the land is bare, waterless, rugged, distressed by winter and burnt by the sun, there you will find people who are hard, lean, well jointed, well toned, and hairy. In nature of this sort, quick-witted industriousness is abundant and their characters and passions are marked by stubbornness and single-mindedness, and they are more wild than tame, and in arts and skills they are sharper, more intelligent and better at matters of war. The other things produced on the land all follow the natures of the land. 10. Such are the most opposed natures and appearances. Using these observations as your guide, you will not go wrong when you make conclusions about the rest and you will not make mistakes.

FIVE

The Art and Science of Medicine

Although in many parts of the world today, medicine is a prestigious field and physicians are esteemed, this was not always the case. When the professional field of medicine emerged in the fifth century BCE, physicians had to convince sick and suffering people to hire them instead of turning to others in the healing marketplace. And early on, medicine appears to have been a tough sell.

Channeling the perspectives of ancient people, we see why medicine could have been perceived as an unreasonable risk. People were accustomed to seeking help from religion, whether they petitioned **Asclepius** and **Hygieia** to address their health concerns (see chapter 2), or other gods who were thought to hold power over specific ailments (such as Hera for issues related to childbirth). Because they understood suffering and illness as a sign of the gods' displeasure or punishment, they likewise believed that health could only be restored once the gods were appeased. To understand illness in terms of material causes and to seek out help from a physician, therefore, must have seemed like a risky circumvention of the gods, a move that might further anger the gods and cause even greater peril. Sick and suffering people also sought help from drug sellers (*pharmakopōlēs;* see chapter 10, on pharmacology), **obstetricians**, and ritual experts (so-called magicians), all of whom were trusted for their wealth of hands-on experience. Why, some must have asked, would they risk trying the new, unproven science of physicians over these experienced professionals with a record of past success?

In early medical texts like the Hippocratic *On the Art of Medicine* (Text 3), we see the skepticism and criticism leveled against the fledgling field of medicine. Some skeptics questioned whether medicine was in fact a real science, a totalizing system of knowledge that could explain a wide variety of illnesses. Other critics disputed the science's efficacy, observing that some people who were treated by physicians failed to recover and some people who did not consult physicians got well without them. Still other critics pointed to physicians' refusal to treat some illnesses, a decision that, at best, demonstrated the limits of the science's power and, at worst, alluded to the possibility that medicine was merely taking credit for recoveries of simple illnesses that would have occurred on their own.

In response, the Hippocratic author argued vigorously for the truth and effectiveness of the science, contending that medical logic was at play even in the treatments not prescribed by physicians and even if treatments were called something other than "medicine." And when medicine failed, the Hippocratic author explained, it was due to human error or lack of resources, not because of any deficiency in the science itself. The Hippocratic author punctuated his defense of medicine by urging critics and skeptics to marvel at the success of medicine despite the myriad challenges faced by physicians. For example, unlike other arts, such as woodworking or metalwork, physicians conducted their work without being able to see what was hidden inside the body. They were forced to read signs on the surface of the body and apply their reason to infer the nature of the ailment within. Such an art, the Hippocratic writer concluded, was worthy of respect not criticism.

By the first century BCE, when **Celsus** wrote his history of the origins of medicine (Text 4), the field had earned some hard-won prestige. Celsus's narrative erases the tensions and criticisms we find in early medical sources. He prefers a more positive spin: a story in which medicine was the inevitable heir apparent of philosophers and metaphysics.

As early proponents labored to build a reputation for medicine, they also worked to define medicine as both a science and an art. In terms of the former, Hippocratic authors asserted that the science of medicine was nothing more than the study of nature and an understanding of the natural laws of the body and the world. There was, they explained, a coherent logic to the natural operations of the body; and if one understood the body's logic, one could likewise understand why bodies fell ill and how to restore their health. In short, the science of medicine was an attempt to grasp this inherent body logic, the natural order of bodies. Medical thinkers sought to reconstruct this logical system by studying, recording, and organizing their observations about how bodies worked, paying particular attention to patterns. At the same time, medical thinkers also studied the remedies found in nature, observing the healing properties of plant and animal products and attempting to systematize the logic of their efficacy relative to the logic of the body.

If the *science* of medicine focused on systematizing knowledge, the *art* of medicine focused on applying such scientific knowledge in practice.[1] As physicians were faced with a wide variety of patients and illnesses, in a variety of contexts, they were forced to adapt what they had learned in theory to the specific patients in front of them. Physicians were required to distill all of the symptoms they observed in their patients and match them with their previous studies and past experience in order to make their best guess of a diagnosis and

---

1. These two sides of the coin were sometimes referred to as the theoretical and practical aspects of medicine.

treatment plan. And, as an illness progressed, physicians were required to stay open to other possibilities they had not considered and to revise their course of action as needed. The intellectual flexibility and creative reasoning required in clinical practice was regarded as an "art." Calling medicine an "art" aligned it with the other "liberal arts"—the areas of study thought to be essential for any educated free person: astronomy, arithmetic, geometry, and music—thus putting medicine on equal footing with other prestigious fields.

The Greek term *technē* used in the title of Text 3 (the Hippocratic *On the Technē of Medicine*) captures the sense of both science and art. In the fifth century BCE, this term was at times juxtaposed against the similarly sounding Greek term *tuchē*, which referred to the goddess of chance or, more generally, to random acts that defy logical explanation. The *technē* of medicine, the author appears to assert, requires a skilled practitioner who has mastered theory and practice (both the science *and* art of medicine), and whose work is grounded in a system of logic that cannot be reduced to chance.

TEXT 3. HIPPOCRATIC CORPUS, *ON THE ART OF MEDICINE*

On the Art (Technē) of Medicine was attributed to **Hippocrates***, but as with all the texts in the Hippocratic corpus, the authorship is uncertain. The text was likely written in Greece during the later part of the fifth century BCE. The author displays knowledge of medical practice and human anatomy, plus familiarity with the types of debates engaging philosophers and sophists in Greece during the fifth century. The author's primary task was to defend medicine against those who doubted its status as an art and who questioned its effectiveness. Though medicine cannot save everyone, the author argues that it is a legitimate field of study, and not merely based on luck or inevitability.*

SOURCE: Translation by Joel E. Mann based on the Greek text from Jacques Jouanna, *Hippocrate, Des vents, De l'art* (Paris: Les Belles Lettres, 1988). First published in *Hippocrates, On the Art of Medicine,* Studies in Ancient Medicine 39 (Leiden: Brill, 2012). Reprinted with permission of Brill.

Chapter 1. 1. There are some who make an art of demeaning the arts, so they think, not achieving the result I just mentioned, but rather making a display of their special 'skill.' 2. But it seems to me that to discover fully something that has not yet been discovered and which, once it has been discovered, is better than if it had not been fully discovered, is an object and occupation of the intellect, as is likewise to accomplish fully what has been accomplished only in part. In contrast, the eagerness to debase the discoveries of others by an art of mean discourse, not suggesting any improvements but instead slandering the discoveries of those who have knowledge in front of those who do not—this no longer seems to be an object or occupation of the intellect, but rather an indication of a mediocre nature or a lack of art. For indeed, such business is fit for the artless alone, namely, serving the mediocrity of those with ambition but utterly without power in slandering their fellows' achievements when they are right or criticizing them when they are not. 3. As for those who attack the other arts in this way, let those who are able deter such attacks when and where they care to. The present discourse will oppose those who thus march against medicine, emboldened on account of these invaders, whom it blames; well equipped through the art to whose rescue it comes; and powerful through wisdom, in which it has been trained.

Chapter 2. 1. It seems quite clear to me that, on the whole, there is no art that is not, since it's just absurd to believe that one of the things-that-are is not. For what being could anyone observe of the things-that-are-not and report that they are? For if indeed it is possible to see the things-that-are-not, just as it is to see the things-that-are, I do not know how anyone could believe of those things that it were possible both to see with his eyes and to know with his mind that they are, that they are not. 2. Is it not rather more like the following? Whereas the things-that-are always are in every case seen and known, the things-that-are-not are neither seen nor known. Accordingly, the arts are known only once they have been taught, and there is no art that is not seen as an outgrowth of some form. 3. In my opinion, they acquire their names, too, because of their forms. For it's absurd—not to mention impossible—to think that forms grow out of names: names for nature are conventions imposed by and upon nature, whereas forms are not conventions but outgrowths.

Chapter 3. 1. Concerning these matters, then, should anyone not have reached a sufficient understanding from what has been said, clearer instruction may be given in other discourses. Concerning medicine—as this is the subject of the discourse—about this, then, I will now give a demonstration. 2. First, I will define what I think medicine is, namely, totally removing the sufferings of the sick or alleviating the violent effects of their diseases, as well as not handling the sick who have been overwhelmed by their diseases, knowing that all these things are in medicine's power. 3. That it does these things and always is able to do so will be the focus of my discourse from this point forward. In giving this demonstration of the art, I will at the same time refute the arguments of those who think they are demeaning it, and on the very points where any one of them happens to think they are accomplishing something substantial.

Chapter 4. 1. Now my discourse starts from the following premise, which will be accepted by all. That some of those who have been treated by medicine fully recover is generally accepted. But, in light of the fact that not all recover, the art is now criticized, and those who speak more meanly of it on account of those defeated by their diseases claim that those who escape them do so by chance and not because of art. 2. I myself do not deprive chance of its accomplishment; however, I do believe that for the most part misfortune follows upon the poor treatment of a disease, while good fortune follows upon good treatment. 3. How, then, could those who fully recovered hold something other than the art responsible for this, if indeed they did so while using and submitting to it? For in turning themselves over to the art, they did not wish to observe the form of pure chance, 4. and as a result they are freed from their reliance on chance, though their debt to the art is not discharged. For they turned themselves over to the art and put their faith in it; in this, they observed its form and, once the work was accomplished, they came to know its power.

Chapter 5. 1. Now he who makes the opposite argument will say that many who were sick have recovered even without consulting a physician, and I do not doubt the claim. 2. It seems to me, however, that it is possible even for those who do not consult a doctor to chance upon medicine. This does not, of course, actually result in their knowing what is correct in it and what is not, but rather in their hitting upon by chance the very treatments that would have been applied had they consulted a doctor. 3. And this is powerful evidence of medicine's being—evidence that it both is and is powerful—that even those who do not believe that it is are evidently saved by it. 4. Even those who did not consult a doctor but recovered after falling sick surely must know that they recovered by doing or not doing something. For it was by fasting or by overeating, by drinking much fluid or by abstaining from it, by bathing or by not bathing, by vigorous exercise or by rest, by sleep or by wakefulness, or by using some combination of these that they recovered. 5. In virtue of having been benefited, they surely must have known what it was that benefited them; and likewise, if they were harmed somehow, then, in virtue of being harmed, what it was that harmed them. For is not everyone capable of knowing the things determined through his benefit or harm? So if the sick person knows how to praise or blame any of the components of regimen by which he recovered, then all these belong to medicine. The mistakes of medicine, too, no less than the benefits, are testimonies to its being. For what is beneficial brings benefit through correct application, while what is harmful causes harm through incorrect application. 6. And where the correct and incorrect each has its own determination, how could this not be art? There is artlessness, I claim, where there is neither correctness nor incorrectness; but where each of these is present, the work of artlessness would be absent.

Chapter 6. 1. Still, if doctors and their art brought about cures only by means of purgative and binding **drugs**, my argument would be weak. 2. But in fact it is evident that the most highly praised doctors heal by regimen and other forms of treatment that nobody, neither doctor nor unknowledgeable layperson (provided the latter had even heard of them), would claim did not belong to the art. 3. So nothing is useless for good doctors or for medicine itself; rather, forms of treatments and drugs are present in most things, both natural and synthetic. Hence, by a correct account, not a single person who has recovered without a doctor can still give the credit to spontaneity. 4. For, upon examination, it is evident that spontaneity is nothing at all since everything that comes to be would be discovered to do so because of something, and it is in virtue of this 'because of something' that spontaneity evidently has no being other than a name. But medicine evidently has and always will have being, both in virtue of things that come to be 'because of something' and in virtue of things known in advance.

Chapter 7. 1. Someone could make such arguments against those who attribute health to chance and discredit the art. I am further surprised at those who base their denial of the art on the misfortunes of those who died. By what sufficient argument are they moved to exculpate the weakness of those who died while holding responsible the intellect of medical practitioners, as though it were possible for doctors to give the wrong orders but impossible for the sick to deviate from the orders they are given? 2. In actual fact, it is far more probable that the sick are powerless to follow the orders they are given than it is that doctors give the wrong orders. 3. For the latter handle the situation with healthy mind and body, reasoning about the present condition as well as conditions in the past similar to those in the present, so that they can tell how they were cured once they were treated. The former, however, while knowing neither what they suffer nor because of what they suffer, nor what will come of their present condition, nor what comes of similar conditions, are given orders. Pained in the present and fearing for the future, they are full of disease but empty of food, consenting at last to admit those things that promote disease rather than those that promote health, not because they desire death, but because they are powerless to endure. 4. Which is more likely—that people in such a state do what their doctors ordered, or that they do things that were not ordered? Or is it likely that doctors, in the state mentioned earlier, give the wrong orders? 5. Is it not much more likely that doctors give the right orders, but that in all probability the sick are powerless to obey them, and by not obeying them meet their deaths? And also that those who reason incorrectly attribute responsibility for these deaths to those who are not responsible, thereby setting the guilty free?

Chapter 8. 1. There are some, too, who criticize medicine on account of those who do not consent to handle people who have been overcome by their diseases: they say that doctors make an attempt to heal diseases that would resolve themselves on their own but do not touch those in great need of help. But if indeed medicine is, it ought to try to heal all alike. 2. Now if such people criticized doctors for ignoring them because they were out of their heads, then their criticism would be more plausible than it is. For if a person expects art to have power in matters where art is not, or expects nature to have power in matters where it is not present, then he is ignorant of an ignorance more in tune with madness than with lack of learning. 3. For of those things that we can master using the instruments of art and nature, we can be craftsmen. Of other things, we cannot. Thus, whenever a person suffers some evil that is stronger than the instruments of medicine, he should not expect medicine to be able somehow to overcome this. 4. For example, fire burns the most intensely of all the caustics used in medicine, but there are many others that burn less so. Clearly, then, things that are stronger than the lesser caustics are by no means untreatable. But is it not clear, too, that things stronger than the most powerful caustics are untreatable? As for the things that fire does not work on, is it not clear that if undefeated by it they require an art other than the one of which fire is an instrument? 5. My argument is the same on behalf of all other instruments allied with medicine. I claim that if the doctor is unsuccessful with each of all these, he ought to hold responsible the power of the affliction, not the art. 6. So people who criticize doctors for not handling those who have been overcome are demanding that they touch what is improper no less than what is proper. And while in making these demands they gain the admiration of those who are doctors in name, they are ridiculed by those who are doctors also in virtue of their art. 7. Those experienced in this craft have no need for criticism or praise that is so senseless. Instead, they need people who have rationally considered in relation to what the products of craftsmen are fully finished; in what respect imperfect products are deficient; and further, concerning these deficiencies, which are to be attributed to the craftsmen and which to the things being crafted.

Chapter 9. 1. Demonstrations concerning the other arts will take place at another time and with another discourse. But concerning medicine—that is, what sorts of things it involves and how they are to be judged—the first half of this discourse has elucidated in part, and from here forward it will address the remaining issues. 2. According to those with sufficient knowledge of this art, some diseases are located where they are not hard to see—though these are few—while others are located where they are not easy to see, and these are many. 3. Things that erupt on the skin are evident by their color or swelling. They offer us the opportunity to perceive their solidity and liquidity by our senses of sight and touch, as well as which of them are hot and cold, these diseases being the sorts of things they are through the presence or absence of each of these. 4. In all cases, then, the treatments for diseases of this sort ought to be free from error, not because they are easy, but rather because they are fully discovered, such discoveries being made not by those who have merely the desire, but by those who have also the power. And power is available to those whose training is not lacking and whose natures are not indolent.

Chapter 10. 1. With respect to evident diseases, then, the art ought to be thus well equipped. But neither ought it be unequipped with respect to less evident diseases, namely, those affecting the bones and the bodily **cavity**. 2. Actually, the body does not have just one cavity, but many. There are two that take in and expel food, for example, and there are many others that are known to those who care about these matters. 3. For all of the limbs surrounded by **flesh** (so-called "muscle") have a cavity. For everything that is not grown together, whether covered by skin or flesh, is hollow, and when healthy is full of breath [*pneuma*];[2] when weak, of fluid. Accordingly, the arms have this kind of flesh, as do the upper and lower parts of the legs. 4. Moreover, the sort of cavity shown to exist in the flesh-covered parts is found also where there is no flesh. For the so-called trunk encases the liver and the round part of the head contains the brain; next to the back are the lungs. None of these is not itself empty, each being full of natural fissures, and in these cases nothing prevents the presence of receptacles for many things, some of which are harmful to their possessor, and some of which are beneficial. 5. In addition, there are numerous vessels, as well as sinews that are not on the surface of the flesh but rather are stretched out along the bones and form a bond for the joints, and also the joints themselves, in which the balls of the moving bones circle round. None of these does not have a viscous quality, each being surrounded by chambers that are indicated by fluid, which issues forth copiously when the cells are completely ruptured, causing a great deal of pain.

Chapter 11. 1. Of course, it is impossible for a person who sees only with his eyes to know any of the things just mentioned. For this reason, I have given them the name 'non-evident,' and so they have been judged by the art. However, they have not prevailed just because they are non-evident; rather, they have been prevailed over where possible. And it is possible insofar as the natures of the sick submit to examination and the natures of those searching for the non-evident are well suited to the role. 2. For they are known with no less time and with even greater effort than they would have been if seen with the eyes. For what eludes the sight

---

2. Throughout this text, the Greek word *pneuma* (plural: *pneumata*) is always translated as "breath."

of the eyes is captured by the sight of the mind. 3. And if the sick suffer from a lack of speed in being seen, it is not those providing treatment who are responsible, but rather nature, specifically, the nature of the sick person as well as the nature of the disease. For the former, since it was possible neither to see the problem with his sight nor to learn about it by hearing, tried to pursue it using reason. 4. After all, even the reports that those who are sick with non-evident diseases attempt to give to their doctors are based on opinion rather than on knowledge. For if they had knowledge, they would not have run afoul of these diseases, since knowing the causes of diseases and knowing how to treat them by all the means that hinder their progress belong to the same intellect. Now as it is impossible to achieve perfect clarity by listening to these reports, the doctor must look to something else. 5. Thus, it is not the art that is responsible for slowness, but rather the nature of human bodies. For the art sees fit to provide treatment only after it has perceived the problem, taking care that its treatments are applied not rashly, but, rather, thoughtfully, and gently rather than violently, while the nature of the human body, if it can hold out until it is seen, will hold out long enough to be healed, as well. But if, in the time it takes for this to be seen, the sick person is overcome, whether on account of his slowness in going to the doctor or the speed of the disease, he will be lost. 6. For if it starts the race from the same mark as treatment, disease is not the swifter, though it will be swifter if given a head start. And it gets a head start both from the impenetrability of human bodies, which diseases occupy without being seen, and from the negligence of the sick, which they impose upon themselves. For they consent to treatment only once their diseases have taken hold, and not before. 7. So then the power of the art is worthier of admiration when it restores those sick with non-evident diseases than when it does not handle impossible cases? Surely such is not the case in any of the other crafts that have been discovered up to now. Instead, those that work with fire cannot function when it is not present, and those that work with materials that are visible and malleable—for example, those that work with wood, or with leather, or the numerous others that work with bronze or iron or similar metals—as I was saying, though the things crafted from and with these materials are easy to work with, all the same they are crafted not with mere speed in mind, but with regard for what is required and without skipping any steps, and if ever one of the tools is missing, all work ceases. And though even in these crafts slowness is an obstacle to turning a profit, nonetheless it is paid greater respect.

Chapter 12. 1. But medicine, though deprived of seeing any of the abscesses, whether of the liver or the kidneys, or indeed any of all those diseases located in the bodily cavity, with the eyesight—by which all people see all things most adequately—nonetheless discovered other resources to work with. 2. From the clarity or scratchiness of voice, from the speed or slowness of breath, and from each of the fluids regularly discharged through the orifices (gauging some on the basis of their smell, others by their color and still others by their thinness and thickness), it makes an inference to the conditions of which these things are signs, including what has already been suffered and what it is possible yet to suffer. 3. And whenever nature herself does not willingly relinquish these informants, medicine has discovered devices of compulsion by which nature is forced—without injury—to surrender them. She is released once she has made it evident to those knowledgeable in the art what should be done. 4. For example, using acrid food and drink the art forces fever to melt the congealed phlegm in order to draw an inference about what it was unable to see based on what has been seen. In turn, by running up steep roads the art forces breath to bring a charge against those things of which it is the accuser. Inducing sweats by the aforementioned means and by the vapors of hot water, the art makes an inference. 5. There are things that, in passing also through the bladder, are better suited for making the disease evident than when they pass out through the flesh. Accordingly, medicine has discovered food and drink that become hotter than the sources of heat, melting them and causing them to pass from the body along a route by which they never would have passed had they not been subjected to this. 6. Thus, the things that escape the body and betray its secrets differ with respect to the different routes they take and the different information they carry, so that it is no surprise that the time spent coming to some conviction about them exceeds that left for action, especially since their interpretation must pass through foreign translators on its way to the intellect that provides treatment.

Chapter 13. 1. The discourse given here makes it evident that medicine has well equipped arguments of its own to help in its fight. It rightly does not handle diseases that cannot be remedied, and, when it does handle a disease, it does so without making mistakes. This is made evident also by the displays of those knowledgeable in the art, for whom it is easier to give a display in action rather than in word, since they have not made a study of speaking. Instead, they hold that the majority of people are more apt to be convinced by what they see rather than by what they hear.

TEXT 4. CELSUS, *ON MEDICINE* SELECTION (PREFACE 1–57)

*On Medicine, written by Aulus Cornelius **Celsus** (first centuries BCE and CE), was originally part of an encyclopedia that covered a range of topics, including agriculture, medicine, rhetoric, philosophy, and military science. The section on medicine, the only one to survive, is organized around the three major divisions of ancient medicine: regimen, pharmacology, and surgery. Scholars debate whether Celsus was himself a practicing physician, but his text offers hints of real experience, especially in the sections on surgery. In the selection below Celsus sketches an overview of the early history of medicine up to the first century BCE, and summarizes a debate between physicians of his time about whether hands-on experience or rational theorizing was more important for medicine. The selection concludes with Celsus's account of the controversial "Methodist" school of medicine that was becoming prominent in his time.*

SOURCE: Translation by Jared Secord based on the Latin text from Philippe Mudry, *La préface du "De medicina" de Celse* (Rome: Institut Suisse de Rome, 1982).

Preface. 1. Just as agriculture provides food for healthy bodies, so too does medicine provide health for the sick. Nowhere is medicine absent, since even the most uncivilized peoples are familiar with herbs and other things at hand for helping wounds and illnesses. 2. Yet medicine has certainly been developed much more among the Greeks than among other peoples, though not even among the Greeks from their earliest origin, but only a few generations before us. Thus **Asclepius** is honored as medicine's most ancient founder. He was received among the gods because he developed what was as yet primitive and common knowledge with a little more exactness. 3. Afterwards his two sons, Podalirius and Machaon, who accompanied their commander Agamemnon during the Trojan War, brought considerable help to their comrades.[3] Homer related, however, that Podalirius and Machaon offered no help for the pestilence[4] or for various types of illnesses, but that they tended only to heal wounds with a knife and **drugs**. 4. From this it is apparent that only these parts of medicine were practiced by these men, and that these parts are the most ancient.

From the same author, to be sure, it can be learned that illnesses were at that time attributed to the anger of the immortal gods, and from them help used to be sought. It is likely to be true that, despite no remedies for poor health, health was nevertheless generally good on account of good habits, spoiled by neither laziness nor extravagance. 5. These two things have damaged bodies, first in Greece, and later among us. Therefore, this complex type of medicine which was neither necessary in the past, nor among other peoples, leads hardly any of us now to the beginnings of old age.

Now, after those I mentioned, no famous people practiced medicine until the study of literature began to be pursued with greater zeal. 6. This study is as necessary for the mind as it is harmful to the body. At first the knowledge of healing was considered to be part of philosophy, so that both the treatment of illnesses and the contemplation of the natural world originated from the same founders. 7. Of course, those who had weakened the strength of their bodies with sedentary[5] thinking and nocturnal wakefulness especially needed this knowledge. Therefore we learn that many of those who professed philosophy were experienced with medicine, the most famous of these being **Pythagoras, Empedocles**, and **Democritus**. 8. But it was, as some people believe, a student of Democritus, **Hippocrates** of Cos, who was the first of all to be worth remembering, and a man distinguished in both knowledge and eloquence, who separated this discipline from the pursuit of philosophy. After him, **Diocles of Carystus**, then **Praxagoras** and **Chrysippus**, and next **Herophilus** and **Erasistratus**, practiced this art in such a way that they made advances in various ways of treatment.

9. In the same times medicine was divided into three parts. One healed through diet, another through drugs, and the third by hand. The Greeks called the first "dietetic,"[6]

---

3. Homer, *Iliad* 11.833.

4. Homer, *Iliad* 1.61. The "pestilence" Celsus mentions here is the epidemic inflicted by the god **Apollo** on the Greek army besieging the city of Troy.

5. The Latin manuscripts of Celsus differ on this word. Most manuscripts have *quieta* ("sedentary"), but one has *inquieta* ("restless").

6. In Greek, *diaitētikēn*.

the second "pharmaceutical,"[7] and the third "surgery."[8] But by far the most famous authorities of dietetics, trying to pursue certain topics more deeply, also claimed for themselves an understanding of nature, as if medicine would be lacking and weak without this. 10. After them, **Serapion** was the first of all to declare that this type of theoretical learning had no relevance for medicine. He held that medicine was based only on practice and experience. **Apollonius, Glaucias** and, much later, **Heraclides of Tarentum**, and some other men of significance followed Serapion, and, in accordance with their views, called themselves Empiricists. 11. Thus the type of medicine that treats by diet was divided into two parts, with some claiming it was a theoretical type of knowledge, and others that it was based only on practice. But, after the people discussed above, no one caused a disturbance in what was passed down, until **Asclepiades** significantly transformed the method of healing. **Themison**, one of his successors, recently changed this method in some respects during his old age. And it is through these men especially that this healthful profession of ours has developed.

12. Since, however, the most difficult and also the most distinguished of the three parts of medicine is that which heals illnesses, it must be spoken about before all others, because in this first part of medicine there is a disagreement. Some assert that the only thing necessary is derived from experience, but others propose that practice is insufficiently capable without a verified theory of bodies and nature. So that our own opinion can be interposed more easily, I must indicate the most significant things said by both sides.

13. Consequently, those who declare that medicine is theoretical propose that these features are necessary: familiarity with the hidden causes that form the basis for illnesses, then the evident causes, and after these natural actions, and finally the internal organs.

14. They call "hidden causes" those in which there is investigation into the elements that make up our bodies, and what is favorable for and what is against good health. For they believe that someone who is ignorant of where illnesses come from cannot know how to treat them appropriately. There is no doubt, they say, that there is a need for one type of treatment if some abundance or deficiency of the four elements causes poor health, just as some who teach philosophy have said. 15. They say there is a need for another type of treatment if all the fault is in the **humors,** as it seems to Herophilus; and another type, if the fault is in the breath, according to Hippocrates; and another type, if blood is transfused into the blood vessels that are adapted for the breath, and causes inflammation (which the Greeks call *phlegmonēn*), and that inflammation brings about the type of disturbance that there is in a fever, as seemed right to Erasistratus. 16. They say that, if tiny particles flowing through invisible pores block passage by being stopped, there is a need for another type of treatment, as Asclepiades argues. They say that the person who has not been mistaken in identifying the primary source of the cause will perform treatment correctly.

They do not deny that experience is also necessary, but they assert that it is impossible to arrive at an opportunity for this without some theorizing. 17. For the more ancient physi-

---

7. In Greek, *pharmakeutikēn.*
8. In Greek, *cheirourgian.*

cians, they say, did not force anything on sick people, but reflected on what would be most appropriate, and put what the previous conjecture had suggested to the test by experience. It made no difference, they said, whether now most remedies had already been investigated if they nevertheless began with reasoning. And, they say, this has in fact happened in many cases. Indeed, they say that new types of illnesses often occur, and experience reveals nothing about these yet, making it necessary to examine where these illnesses originated. Without this, no mortal would be able to learn why one remedy rather than another should be used. And for these reasons the hidden causes are investigated.

18. They call "evident causes" those concerning which they seek to find out whether heat or cold, hunger or fullness, and other similar things, cause the beginning of an illness. For they say that the person who knows the origin of the problem will counteract it.

19. They call "natural actions" of the body those through which we inhale and exhale breath, take in and digest food and drink, and also those through which food and drink are distributed into all of the body. Moreover, they also investigate how our blood vessels sometimes subside and sometimes expand, and what is the explanation for sleep and wakefulness. Without familiarity with these things they judge that no one can counteract or heal illnesses that arise from these functions. 20. Because digestion seems out of all these to be especially important, they deem it most significant. Some of them, following Erasistratus, assert that food is ground up in the stomach. Others, following **Pleistonicus**, the student of Praxagoras, assert that food rots. Others trust Hippocrates that food is digested by heat. There are also the followers of Asclepiades who propose that all these ideas are false and unnecessary, and that no food is digested but instead is pulled through the whole body in the raw state it had when it was swallowed. 21. There is little agreement among them about these points. But there is at least consensus that one type of food should be given to those in distress if one idea is true, and another type of food if the other is true. For if food is ground up internally, the food that can most easily be ground up must be sought. If food rots, the food that does this most expeditiously must be sought. If heat digests food, the food that especially provokes heat must be sought. 22. But, if nothing is digested, none of these types of food must be sought, and those that remain as they were when they were swallowed must be sought. By the same reasoning, when breathing is heavy, when sleep or wakefulness are imminent, they judge that someone who has previously learned how these states happen is able to heal.

23. Besides this, since both pains and various kinds of illnesses arise in the inner parts, they judge that no one who does not know these inner parts can apply remedies to these. Therefore they judge it necessary to cut open the bodies of the dead and to examine their viscera and intestines. And they say that Herophilus and Erasistratus did this in by far the best way, cutting into still-living criminals they received from the kings out of prison,[9] 24. and, while they were still breathing, inspecting the parts that nature had previously concealed:

9. The kings mentioned here must be the early Ptolemies, Greek rulers of Egypt from the fourth to the first century BCE.

their position, color, shape, size, arrangement, hardness, softness, smoothness, points of contact, the processes and recesses of each, and whether any part is inserted or accepted into another. 25. For, when pain occurs internally, they say that the person who does not know the position of each organ and intestine cannot know what is causing the pain, and neither can the diseased part be treated by someone who does not know what it is. And when a person's viscera are exposed through a wound, they say that a person who does know the color of the part when it is healthy may not know which part is uninjured and which is damaged. 26. Thus, they say, he cannot help the damaged part. They say that external remedies can be applied more effectively when the positions, shapes, and sizes of inner parts are known. And they say that similar rules hold for all the cases mentioned above. They say that it is not cruel, as most people suggest, that remedies be sought from the sufferings of criminals, and a small number of them at that, for the benefit of innocent people of all future generations.

27. In opposition, those who call themselves Empiricists from their experience regard evident causes as necessary, but they assert that inquiry regarding hidden causes and natural actions is unnecessary because nature is not comprehensible. 28. They say it is obvious that nature cannot be comprehended from the disagreement of the people who have debated these topics, since on this subject there is no agreement among teachers of philosophy or physicians. For why should someone trust Hippocrates rather than Herophilus? Why trust Herophilus rather than Asclepiades? 29. If a person wants to adhere to theories, the theories of all of them can seem probable. If a person wants to adhere to treatments, sick people have been led to health by all of them. They consequently say it is unfitting for anyone to be disparaged, in argument or in authority. If theorizing made a physician, they even say, students of philosophy would be the greatest physicians. As it is, they say that these students of philosophy have an excess of words, but they lack knowledge of healing. 30. They also say that the types of medicine differ according to the nature of places, and that there is a need for different methods in Rome, Egypt, and Gaul.[10] But, they say, if the causes that produce illnesses were the same everywhere, the remedy also should be the same. Often, they say, the causes are apparent, as for instance in an inflammation of the eyes or a wound, but a remedy is not apparent from these causes. 31. If an evident cause does not reveal this knowledge, how much less can it reveal a cause that is in doubt.

Since, therefore, the cause is as uncertain as it is incomprehensible, protection must be sought rather from things that are certain and explored, that is, what experience has taught in the treatments themselves, just as in all the other arts, for even a farmer or a helmsman is made not by debate but by experience. 32. That such reasonings have no relevance for medicine is also learned, they say, from the fact that people think different things on these topics, but nevertheless guide people to the same state of health. This has happened, they say, not because they derived ways of healing from hidden causes or natural actions, about which they disagreed, but from experiences that had succeeded.

10. Gaul was the Roman name for modern-day France.

33. They say that even during its earliest phases medicine wasn't developed from such inquiries, but from experience. For, they say, the sick people who were without physicians took food immediately in the first days, on account of their appetite. But, they say, others abstained from food on account of distaste. They say that the illness was alleviated more in the people who abstained from food. 34. Likewise, they say that some people ate something while still feverish, while others ate a little before the fever, and yet others after its remission. They say that those who did this after the end of the fever had the best results. Similarly, they say that some people enjoy a rather full diet immediately during the beginnings of the fever, while others had a meager diet. They say that those people who filled themselves up had more pain. 35. When these and similar things happened day after day, they say that careful people noted what generally had a better result, and they began to prescribe this to sick people. Thus was the origin of medicine, which, from the pattern of health for some people and death for others, distinguished dangerous from healthful actions. 36. After remedies had been discovered, they say that careful people began to discuss theories. They say that medicine was invented not from theory, but that theory was sought out after medicine was invented.

They also ask if theory teaches the same thing as experience, or something else. If it teaches the same thing, it is unnecessary. If it teaches something else, it is incompatible with experience. Nevertheless, they say that remedies initially had to be tested with the greatest care. Now, however, they say that they have already been tested. They say that new types of illnesses are not being discovered, and that a new kind of remedy is not needed. 37. Now, even if some unknown type of problem arose, physicians would not have to ponder obscure topics but would immediately see what illness it was most similar to and then test remedies similar to those that often help the illness that was close to it, and through the similarities obtain help. 38. They say that a physician would still need to deliberate, and that an irrational animal could be capable of excelling in this knowledge, but that these conjectures about concealed matters are not relevant to the matter at hand, because it does not matter what causes the illness, but what removes it, nor is it relevant to the matter at hand how digestion happens—whether digestion happens from this cause or that, and whether the process is digestion or only the distribution of assimilated food in the body—but what is digested most easily. 39. They say that there should be no inquiry about how we breathe, but about what relieves heavy and slow breathing; nor what moves blood vessels, but what the types of motion mean. They say, moreover, that in all thinking of this type it is possible to argue both sides, and that these things are to be learned by experience. Thus they say that cleverness and eloquence triumph, but that illnesses are treated not by eloquence, but by remedies. A person lacking eloquence who has learned well with wise practice would be a considerably better physician than someone who, lacking practice, has polished his speech.

40. And they say that these matters just discussed are unnecessary. But it remains to be said that it is cruel for the belly and chest of living people to be cut into and to inflict on the art—that is the protector of human health—not only someone's death, but also death in a most savage way. This is especially true when, of the things being sought with so much

violence, some cannot be discovered at all, and others can be discovered without wickedness. 41. For color, smoothness, softness, hardness and all the other similar things would not be the same with the body cut open as when it was untouched. Because features of uninjured bodies are often changed from fear, pain, hunger, indigestion, exhaustion, and a thousand other common conditions. It is much likelier to be true that the internal parts, which are much softer, and for which the light itself is a new thing, are changed by the most serious wounds and the savagery of the killing. 42. Nor is anything more foolish, they say, than to suppose that a living person is the same as a dying person, much less someone who is already dead. For, they say, the abdomen, which is less important, can be spread open with a person still breathing. But as soon as the blade approaches the chest, and there is a severing of the transverse septum, which is a type of membrane that separates the higher parts from the lower (the Greeks call it a "diaphragm"[11]), they say that a person dies immediately. Thus the chest and all the organs of only a dead person come into the view of the criminal physician, and these are necessarily those of a dead, not a living, person. 43. Therefore, they say, it follows that the physician does not learn about the type of viscera we have when we are alive, but rather cruelly butchers a person. If, however, there is something to learn from a still-breathing person being exposed to view, they say that chance often presents this to people providing treatment. For, they say, sometimes a gladiator in the arena, or a soldier on the battlefield, or a traveler ambushed by criminals is wounded in such a way that some interior part of his may be revealed, and another interior part of another person. Thus they say that a sensible physician learns the location, position, arrangement, shape, and other similar things by laboring for health, not murder, learning through compassion what others would come to know from terrible cruelty. 44. For this reason, since most parts in dead people are of a different character, some say that even the dissection of the dead is not necessary, which, although it is not cruel, is nevertheless loathsome. Treatment itself reveals how much can truly be learned from living people.

45. Since these issues have often been discussed and are still being discussed by physicians in many books and debates of great controversy, the view that may seem closest to the truth must be supplied. This is not awarded to one side or the other or much different from them, but is in a certain sense a middle ground between the different ways of thinking. One may recognize this in most controversies when people are searching for the truth without bias, as in the present matter.

46. For, in the end, not even teachers of philosophy understand exactly, but pursue by conjecture, the causes that make for good health or stir up illnesses, and how breath is drawn in or food is digested. When there is no certain familiarity with something, opinion cannot find a certain solution. 47. And it is true that nothing conveys more to the theory underlying treatment than experience. Although, therefore, there are many things not directly relevant to the arts as such, these nevertheless help by stimulating the capacity of those who practice them. Accordingly, this contemplation of the nature of things, although

11. In Greek, *diaphragma*.

it does not make someone a physician, nevertheless makes someone more suitable for the practice of medicine. And it is likely to be true that Hippocrates, Erasistratus, and certain others—not content only to meditate on fevers and sores, but also to a certain extent investigated the nature of things—did not, on account of this, become physicians but, on account of this, truly became better physicians. 48. Theory, however, is nevertheless often needed for medicine itself, although not among hidden causes and natural actions. For this art is conjectural, and not only conjecture but also experience often fails to provide an answer, and sometimes neither fever, nor food, nor sleep behave as they normally do.

49. Less often, but occasionally, an illness is actually new. That this does not happen is clearly untrue, since in our time a certain woman died within a few hours when **flesh** from her genital parts prolapsed and was stuck together,[12] such that the most famous physicians discovered neither the type of the injury nor a remedy. 50. I judge that they attempted nothing because no one, on account of their illustrious reputations, wanted to endanger himself with a conjecture and seem to kill her if he did not save her. It is nevertheless likely to be true that someone could have devised something, and perhaps solved the problem, if such embarrassment did not prevent them from trying. 51. For this type of medicine, a similarity is not always useful, and even when it is, some reasoning has nevertheless taken place to consider which drug may be most effective to use among similar types of illnesses and remedies. When, therefore, such a situation happens, it is appropriate for a physician to contrive something that perhaps may not provide a solution, but more often nevertheless will. 52. The physician, however, will seek any new plan from things that can be tested, that is, evident causes, not from hidden matters—for these are dubious and uncertain. For there is a difference if an illness is caused by tiredness or thirst, cold or heat, wakefulness or hunger, an abundance of food and wine or intemperance in lust. 53. Nor is it appropriate for the physician to ignore this: what is the nature of the sick person, whether the sick person's body is rather moist or rather dry, if the sick person's nerves are strong or feeble, whether the sick person's adverse health is frequent or rare, and, when the sick person is in adverse health, whether this tends to be severe or light, short or long, what type of life the sick person has pursued, laborsome or quiet, with luxury or with frugality. For from these and similar things, one may often derive a new method of treatment.

54. Nonetheless, these statements should not be neglected as if they are not debatable. For even Erasistratus has said that illnesses are not produced from those circumstances because other people, and even the same person at different times after this, did not become feverish from them. And certain physicians of our time, influenced by Themison, as they wish it to seem, assert that there is no cause with which someone may become familiar that has anything to do with treatment, and that it is enough to consider that there are some common features of illnesses. 55. Accordingly they say that there are three types of illnesses: one kind is constricting, another is a flux, and a third is a mixture of the first two. For they say

12. An alternative reading in the Latin here would mean that the woman's genitals were dried out, rather than stuck together.

that sick people sometimes excrete too little, sometimes too much, and sometimes too little from one part and too much from another. They also say that these kinds of illnesses are sometimes acute, sometimes long-lasting, and that they sometimes are increasing, sometimes remaining the same, and sometimes diminishing. 56. Once, therefore, it has been recognized which of these illnesses it is, they say that the body must be relaxed if it is constricted. If the body is in distress from a flux, they say that it must be contained. If the body has a mixed condition, they say that the more serious harm must be opposed immediately. They also say that there must be one type of healing for acute illnesses, another for chronic; one for increasing illnesses, another for diminishing illnesses; and another for illnesses already turning towards health. 57. They assert that medicine is the observation of these features. They define medicine as a sort of way that they call a "method,"[13] and assert that medicine is something that contemplates the features that are common in illnesses. They do not want to be classified with theorists or those who consider only experience. They differ in name from the former because they do not want medicine to be the inference of hidden things, and from the latter because they believe that the art of medicine is hardly concerned with the observation of experience.

---

13. In Greek, *methodon*. The term refers to the school of physicians called "Methodists."

SIX

Theories of Health and Illness

Although seemingly straightforward, it is actually quite difficult to define "health" and "illness." Our initial impulse might be to think of health and illness as opposites, with health being defined as the absence of illness, and vice versa. But the simple opposition of health and illness is quickly complicated by a number of considerations. First and foremost, what it means to be healthy or sick is often neither clear-cut nor an absolute state. For instance, someone may possess an unhealthy bodily condition such as high blood pressure or a tumor, but these conditions may not yet have impaired their normal daily functioning. Meanwhile someone else may experience chronic pain that affects their daily routines, but at the same time be perfectly healthy in terms of the proper functioning of their body. People can have an illness but not feel unwell (i.e., the illness may not manifest in symptoms, such as pain), and, vice versa, people may feel unwell but not be sick. Second, the understanding of health and illness is also determined, in large part, by sociocultural context. For instance, in certain times and places lovesickness and homosexuality have both been labeled illnesses (associated with states of body or mind that people deem abnormal or a malady), while in other contexts they are normalized or even celebrated, thus revealing the sociocultural subjectivity involved in categorizing "sickness."

Some argue that health should be defined in terms of "normal" bodily functioning, where illness or injury is defined by, for instance, a limb or bodily system whose functioning falls outside the statistical "norm." But this definition has been critiqued by disability studies scholars and advocates of people with impairments, who argue that one's ability to function has as much to do with one's environment as it does with one's body. For instance, a person who has less than 20/20 vision or a person with impaired mobility can nonetheless function as ably as another person when they are given eyeglasses or mobility aids (such as a wheelchair, cane, or prosthesis, and spaces outfitted with ramps and handrails). As disability studies explain, impairments only become "disabling"—that is, hindering the ability of people to function in society—when societies do not normalize accommodations. Moreover, with or without such accommodations, many people with bodily impairments would still be regarded as "healthy."

These points are helpful to our study of ancient pathology (theories of illness) because, for the most part, people in antiquity also assumed that there was nothing inherently "unhealthy" about people with impairments. In fact, in antiquity there did not exist an identity category, nor Greek and Latin terms, analogous to our notion of "people with disabilities," in part because bodily impairments and disfigurements were far more common and normalized. As we discussed in chapter 3, archaeologists find that the majority of human remains from antiquity have evidence of some injury or illness, indicating the prevalence of bodily impairments. And a wide range of these impairments or deformities—such as broken bones that had healed poorly, baldness, and the female body in general (see chapter 9, on women's illnesses)—were not medicalized in antiquity; physicians did not see them as something that needed medical treatment.

So how did ancient Greeks and Romans conceptualize health and illness? There were several different, often competing, understandings of health and illness, as well as different ideas about what caused each. At the most basic level, though, most people agreed that health was a primary good and a blessing without which other goods—such as wealth, family, friendship, education, and other pleasures—could not be fully enjoyed. We find this sentiment repeatedly expressed in ancient poems and hymns. For example, the *Orphic Hymn to* **Hygieia** talks about how, without health, all human efforts are to no avail, and wealth and abundance are meaningless. The poet Ariphron of Sicyon (fourth century BCE?) is also reported to have said that without health, no one can be happy. And **Herophilus** said that "in the absence of health, wisdom cannot be displayed, science is non-evident, strength not exerted in contest, wealth useless, and rational speech powerless" (T230 von Staden).

Just as many people in the ancient world believed that health was a gift of the gods, so did many believe in the supernatural origins of illness. Ancient Greek poets recorded various myths of how suffering and illness were first introduced into the world. For example, **Hesiod** tells the myth of Pandora. In the story, Prometheus incurred the rage of the gods when he stole fire from them. In response, Zeus sent Pandora, the ancestor of all women, to the realm of human men. She brought with her suffering, illness, and death. In another account, Hesiod described a happy Golden Age of humanity, a time when humans were preternaturally healthy and happy, but, after generations, matters devolved and declined, with humans becoming not only less moral, but also far weaker and more prone to illness, shorter lives, and death. Finally, Jews and Christians told a story of Adam and Eve's disobedience to their creator God, for which they were exiled from the perfect conditions of the Garden of Eden and, as a result, began to experience suffering, illness, and death.

Following these myths about the introduction of suffering and sickness into the world, many people in antiquity thought that the gods, goddesses, and other immortal beings afflicted humans with suffering—often taking the form of sickness—as punishment for wrongdoing. For example, from as early as the Homeric epic the *Iliad*, the god **Apollo** is depicted sending arrows laden with illness against the Greeks who angered him, resulting in an epidemic and mass death. We also hear that the gods, enraged by the insurrectionist Cylon of Athens, who set out to seize control of the Acropolis, dispatched a plague upon the city in retribution. And the historian Herodotus suggests that the gods were punishing multiple generations of Scythian people with reproductive ailments for an offense committed by their ancestors: robbing the temple of Venus at Ascalon. These stories illustrate the widely held belief that the gods sent sickness when individuals or a collective slighted them or offended the proper order of things.

In addition to the gods, many also thought that sickness was the result of oppression or possession by capricious, dangerous, or evil spirits. Daemons (*daimones*), immortal spirits akin to angels, were positioned above humans but below the gods. They could be beneficent or malevolent, helpful or harmful spirits (*kakodaemones*). In the second century CE, the Greek philosopher Plutarch identified "powerful daemons" as the cause of sickness and plagues, as did the philosopher Porphyry in the third century. Similarly, some Christians also believed that evil daemons caused illness, spiritual and physical. According to the African Christian writer Minucius Felix (third century CE), evil daemons were behind deceptive religious beliefs, drawing people away from the true Christian god, and they also deceived people by producing and then curing illnesses. Evil spirits, Minucius explains, were able to enter humans' bodies because the bodies of these spirits were made of fine matter more like air than the earthy **flesh** of human bodies. Once they inhabited humans' bodies, they engendered both physical and psychological symptoms in their victims, causing illness and distress. The goal of evil daemons was to induce humans to offer burnt sacrifices to the gods in hopes of being cured, so that the evil daemons could feast on the smoke and vapors, sating their appetites. Once satisfied, Minucius concludes, the daemons would leave their host, and the symptoms would abate.

Finally, still others believed that the envy and negative feelings of other people, expressed, for example, through the evil eye or curse tablets, could cause withering and the drying up of good things, including health. For instance, many ancient parents would adorn their children with amulets bearing symbols meant to ward off the evil eye. And many people would use similar images to protect homes and other property. One mosaic from Antioch depicts an eye being attacked by all of the following: a man with horns and a very large erect penis, a rabid dog, a bird, a trident, a sword, a centipede, a cat, and a snake (see fig. 1).

Philosophers and physicians had their own views about the causes of illness. An author now called **Anonymus Londiniensis** (late first or early second century CE) provided a synopsis of the pathological theories of twenty thinkers, dividing them into two categories: those who thought that illnesses resulted from residues left over from digestion, and those who thought illnesses were caused by the elements and qualities that made up the body (air, water, fire, earth; hot/cold, wet/dry). With regard to residue theories, the fifth-century BCE physician **Euryphon of Cnidus** envisioned illness arising from improper digestion, and what even seems like constipation: "When the **cavity** does not discharge the nourishment that has been taken, residues are generated, which then rise up to the areas around the head and produce illnesses. But when the cavity is clear and not bloated, **concoction** happens as it should" (Anonymous Londiniensis 4.33–40).

Among those who thought that illness was caused by the elements and qualities that made up the body, we can point to the medical writer and philosopher **Alcmaeon of Croton** (fifth century BCE), who identified pairs of powers in the human body (and in the cosmos)—namely, hot and cold, dry and wet, and sweet and bitter. He defined health as the equality or balance of these qualities of the body. Using a political metaphor, he thought of illness as the monarchy of any one of these over the others (for example, an overly hot body was governed by heat, and an overly dry body was governed by dryness). Later thinkers would adopt Alcmaeon's definition of health as "balance" and illness as "imbalance"; yet in the years to follow they would continue to debate whether balance and imbalance were related to causal powers (hot, cold, wet, dry), or to the **humors** of the body (blood, phlegm, yellow bile, and black bile), or to the tension and slackness of the body.

Plato drew and expanded on preceding theories in his discussions of the causes of health and illness in the human body. First, he advanced the view that health was a state of balance among the substances that make up the body—namely, the elements (earth, water, air, and fire). Illness was a result of these elements being in some state of imbalance: an excess or deficiency of a particular element, an unsuitable mixture of elements, or a displacement of element(s) (i.e., they were not located where they were supposed to be in the body).

Plato went further in his account of illness to explain that in the process by which various parts of the body were generated (blood, flesh, sinews, bone, marrow, veins, and so forth), their development was sometimes interrupted and might even reverse itself. When this happened, noxious substances like rot (gangrene), certain kinds of bile, pus, and other waste materials were by-products of this degeneration. These substances could then corrupt the body parts with which they came into contact. For example, the heat and bitterness of gangrene burned, blackened, and ate away the flesh that it touched.

Finally, Plato articulated the view that health was a state in which all parts of the body were able to fulfill their potential and function as intended (in other words, according to their true end or *telos*). For example, a healthy body engaged in breathing as intended (in terms of the movement of respiration and of *pneuma*, the enlivening spirit of the body). Yet the body would be considered unhealthy if the proper functioning of respiration—if the actualization of a healthy body's potential functioning—was impaired or obstructed.

In a number of Hippocratic texts, writers adopted Plato's understanding of illness as the result of displacement or blockage of fluids, elements, and humors in the body. Other Hippocratic texts followed Alcmaeon, understanding illness as an imbalance of the causal powers (hot/cold, dry/moist). Yet, in the text *Ancient Medicine,* for instance, the Hippocratic author revises the pairs of causal powers beyond those of Alcmaeon, to include not only hot and cold, dry and moist, but also "salt and bitter, sweet and acid, **astringent** and insipid, and a vast number of other things" (Hippocratic Corpus, *Ancient Medicine* 14). Still other

Hippocratic texts, such as *On the Nature of Humans* (Text 5), defined health as the balance of the four humors: blood, yellow bile, black bile, and phlegm.

Whether focusing on the elements of the body (earth, water, air, and fire) or causal powers (hot/cold, dry/moist) or humors (blood, yellow bile, black bile, and phlegm) or other substances or qualities of the body, most Hippocratic thinkers regarded balance as the defining characteristic of a healthy state. Yet they also acknowledged that what it took to achieve balance was idiosyncratic. In other words, no one person's constitution—their unique makeup of elements, causal powers, and humors, as well as the unique ways in which their body typically functioned—was the same as any other person's constitution. Certainly there were types of people who shared common bodily constitutions as, for example, a function of environment (as we see in Text 2, the Hippocratic *Airs, Waters, Places*) or in terms of people in the same age bracket (see Texts 47 and 48). But every individual's constitution was a function of a complex mixture of heredity, development in utero, and early childhood experiences. Thus, physicians aimed to determine information about their patients' typical constitution in order to anticipate the kinds of ailments a patient was prone to experience and as a baseline against which to diagnose abnormal states (i.e., illness).

The Methodists also defined health using the principle of balance, but they did so not with reference to bodily substances like the elements or humors, but with reference to looseness and constriction. The lax and tense states of the body, they argued, were the result of atoms in the body being either too close together or too far apart, which in turn affected the atoms' movement through the body. Problems arose when the atoms became obstructed in the channels of the body or moved too freely through them. Methodist pathologists, therefore, classified illnesses according to three categories: those that were the result of too much constriction (for example, constipation or epileptic seizure), too much looseness (for example, diarrhea or excessive sweating), or a combination of both (for example, catarrh, which featured the looseness of a runny nose and the tightness of sinus pain and a sore throat).

Another loosely affiliated group of physicians traditionally called "Pneumatists" (first and second centuries CE), defined health as balance, but focused on imbalances of the body's **pneuma** (literally meaning "air," "breath," or "enlivening spirit"), which they regarded as something that held together and regulated the body. External and internal factors (such as weather conditions and drugs) could cause the body's *pneuma* to be poorly mixed. The *pneuma* would then be unbalanced, making it too cold, hot, wet, or dry, and leading to illness. Whereas other physicians focused on blockages that prevented *pneuma* from moving around the body, Pneumatists thought that illness was caused by changes to the *pneuma* itself. On these grounds, they believed that the *pneuma* needed to be "renewed and rekindled" by adding or removing heat to restore its equilibrium and balance.

Galen's writings further complicate definitions of health and illness. In some instances, Galen thinks about health and illness in terms of the balance of the four qualities of the four humors (hot/cold, wet/dry). But Galen also learned from the anatomical experiments in Alexandria, so in other instances he defines illness in terms of problems with the functioning of bodily structures. For Galen, an impairment of function could happen on several

A **crisis** was a critical turning point in an illness, for instance days in which an illness took a sharp turn for the worse or the better. A crisis sometimes occurred in conjunction with pronounced symptoms (called a **paroxysm**), such as a spike of fever, heightened delusion, increased inflammation, or sudden, violent, or heavy bodily emissions (e.g., bleeding, bowel movements, etc.); and sometimes a crisis occurred when symptoms ceased or lessened, such as when a fever broke. A crisis was followed by a period of respite in the course of the illness, or recovery, or death.

Critical days segmented an illness into uniform units of time, though the number and duration of those segments varied across illnesses. Ancient physicians observed that in some cases people experienced only one crisis, whereas in other cases people experienced multiple crises before their illness resolved. When multiple crises occurred, they could be paced at intervals of one, two, three, or more days apart depending on the illness.

Physicians were tasked with monitoring illnesses carefully to detect such patterns and use these patterns to inform their diagnoses and treatments (see Text 6).

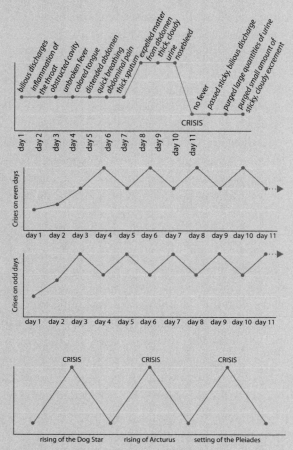

FIGURE 18A Example of an illness with a single crisis (*On Epidemics*, Book 2, Case 3.11).

FIGURE 18B The Hippocratic author of *On Epidemics* 1.26 explained that some illnesses had a pattern of crises on even days or odd days. In these cases, each crisis either could be regarded as a regular pattern of the illness or could signal that the illness was coming to a resolution. A crisis that occurred outside of the pattern, however, was often a bad sign, signaling that the person would die.

FIGURE 18C The Hippocratic author of *Airs, Waters, Places* 11 warns that crises can be triggered by the position of the stars (Text 2). Examples can be seen in Text 8, *On Epidemics*, Book 4, Case 20e and Book 5, Case 73.

levels, on the level of what he calls the "uniform parts" (for example, nerves, arteries, veins, bones, cartilage, membranes, flesh), on the level of the organs (for example, the heart, liver, spleen, eyes, kidneys), or on the level of the whole body (that is, the intersection of tissues, organs, systems of digestion, respiration, perception, etc.). In short, Galen offers the following definitions in *On the Differences of Illnesses*: people understand themselves to be healthy "whenever the parts of their body are functioning perfectly to serve the actions of life," and "they consider themselves to be sick in a part of the body whenever they are damaged in any one of these functions" (2.1 [6.836–37K]).

When discussing theories of illness, we must keep in mind that ancient thinkers believed that an illness originating or concentrated in one part of the body might affect other parts of the body. For example, Galen discusses the "sympathy" between the eyes and the brain, explaining how illnesses related to the former manifest as symptoms in the latter. He cites the example of hallucinations that arise from imbalance in the stomach, and explains how to distinguish these from hallucinations that arise from cataracts (see Text 14, *On the Affected Parts* 4.2).

We also have to keep in mind the close connections ancient theorists believed to exist between the body and the soul or mind. On many occasions, physicians entertained the possibility that certain physical symptoms were the result of psychic or mental distress. Galen, for instance, diagnosed excessive passion (what today we would call "strong emotion"), such as the lovesickness of an elite woman for a theater performer or a slave's anxiety over his misappropriation of funds, as the cause of such illnesses.

A final aspect of ancient theories of illness relates to the course or periodization of illnesses. Medical writers tended to chart illnesses in terms of what were called **"critical days"** (*krises*). These were days on which patients experienced the most pronounced symptoms or days on which an illness took a sharp turn (for either the worse or the better). Critical days usually segmented illnesses into uniform units of time (see fig. 18). Some scholars attribute ancient medicine's tendency to divide up the course of an illness to the common practice of observations and note-taking, which was essential to case histories (see chapter 8), while other scholars argue that the tendency was more likely the result of the intellectual impulses of antiquity (including mathematical reasoning in Assyrian numerology, Pythagorean philosophy, and ancient astrology) that seeped into medical thinking.

TEXT 5. HIPPOCRATIC CORPUS, *ON THE NATURE OF HUMANS*[1] SELECTION (1–9)

On the Nature of Humans *was attributed to* **Hippocrates,** *but as with all the texts in the Hippocratic corpus, the authorship is uncertain. The text may have been written by a certain Polybus, who was believed to be the son-in-law of Hippocrates, and it likely dates to the later part of the*

---

1. This text has traditionally been translated with the title *On the Nature of Man,* but because the original Greek word translated as "man" is gender-inclusive we have chosen a title that more accurately reflects the word's meaning.

*fifth century BCE. The author seems to have been a physician and a debater, since some sections of the text show signs of oral delivery for an audience of other physicians and philosophers. The author responded to claims that human beings consisted of only a single substance (or **humor**), but rejected the single-substance theory and instead offered evidence in favor of the theory that the human body is made up of the four humors. (The author does not use the Greek word "humor" to describe these substances, and the humoral theory of health appears still to be in development in the fifth century BCE, when* On the Nature of Humans *was written.) The author explains the relationship between the four humors and the four seasons of the year, maintaining that sickness was a result of an imbalance of the humors. And the author suggests that medical treatment should follow the principle of opposites, in order to produce equal proportions of the humors, and thus restore health.*

SOURCE: Translation by Robert Nau based on the Greek text from Jacques Jouanna, *Hippocratis De natura hominis*, 2nd ed., Corpus Medicorum Graecorum 1.1.3 (Berlin: Akademie Verlag, 2002).

Chapter 1. Those who customarily listen to people speaking about the nature of humans beyond its connections to medicine will not find this account useful. For I do not claim at all that a human is air, fire, water, earth, or anything else that is not visibly present in a human. I yield these claims to people who want to make them. It seems to me, however, that those who say these things do not understand correctly, for they all hold the same opinion, but they do not say the same things. They draw the same conclusion from their opinion—for they say that what exists (whatever it is) is a single thing and that this is the one and the all—but they do not agree on its name. One of them, when he speaks, declares that air is this single thing and the all, another water, another fire, another earth, and each supplements his account with evidence and proofs that are worthless. When they all hold the same opinion and do not say the same things, clearly they know nothing. Someone present when they debate may easily observe this by what happens. For when the same men debate one another in the presence of the same audience never does the same man win three times straight, but at one time this man prevails, at another time that man and at another time the man who happens to speak in the most flowing style before the crowd. Yet it is right that the one who claims to have correct knowledge of the facts will always provide his as the winning argument, if indeed he understands how things really are and makes the case correctly. But I think that people such as these, through lack of understanding, refute themselves with what they say and uphold the theory of **Melissus**.[2]

Chapter 2. I think that I have said enough about these people. Some physicians say that a human is blood, but others claim that a human is bile, and some say phlegm. They also reach the same conclusion that a human is a single thing (calling this what each wants) and that this thing changes its form and property—to become sweet, sharp, white, black or whatever

2. The theory of the philosopher Melissus held that what exists is unchanging, eternal, and a single unity, much like the suggestions of the unnamed philosophers mentioned here about earth, water, air, and fire.

else—when forced by the heat and the cold. But it seems to me that these claims are incorrect. Most people hold opinions of this sort, or extremely close to them. But I say that if a human were a single thing, they would never suffer pain, for there would be nothing that could cause a single thing to suffer pain. Even if a human did suffer pain, any healing agent would also have to be a single thing. As it is there are many cures, for there are many elements in the body that generate sicknesses when they are warmed, cooled, dried, and moistened by one another against their natural state. There are consequently many forms of sicknesses and many remedies. I require that the person who claims that a human is blood only and nothing else to demonstrate that its form does not change or become all kinds of things, and to show the time of year or period of a human's life when only blood visibly exists inside a human. For there is likely to be a single time in which what exists appears on its own in its proper form. My demands are the same for one who claims that a human is phlegm and for one who claims that a human is bile. For I shall prove that my definition of a human is always consistently the same, according to convention and nature, regardless of whether the person is young or old, and whether the season is cold or hot. I shall also provide proofs—and demonstrate the necessary causes—why each element in the body increases and decreases.

Chapter 3. First, birth necessarily does not arise from a single thing. For how could what is really a single thing generate anything unless it has united with another? Secondly, there is no birth if the species copulating are not of the same kind and do not have the same property, nor would this result in any offspring. And again, birth would not occur, if the hot is not equal and in proper proportion to the cold and likewise the dry to the moist, but there is much more of one than the other, and the stronger element dominates the weaker. How then is it likely for something to be generated from a single thing, since they will also need luck on their side for the copulation to lead to offspring? Therefore, since this is the nature of all other things, including humankind, a human is necessarily not a single thing, but each of the things contributed to birth continues to have the property contributed in the body. Indeed, each necessarily reverts again to its own nature when the body of a human being dies: moist to moist, dry to dry, warm to warm, and cold to cold. This is also the nature of animals and all other things. All things are born in the same way and all things die in the same way. For their nature is formed from all the things that have been mentioned and die in accordance with what has been said: each thing returns to the same state from which it was composed.

Chapter 4. The human body has in itself blood, phlegm, yellow bile, and black bile. These make up the nature of the body and through these it suffers or is healthy. The body is very healthy when these are in appropriate proportion to each other in strength and amount and when they have been completely mixed together. But the body suffers when an excessive or deficient amount of one of these is concentrated in the body and not mingled with all the rest. For, necessarily, when any of these is concentrated and stands by itself, not only does the place from where it is separated become unhealthy, but the place where it is now located and has overfilled causes pain and distress, since there is more than there should be. For when more of an element flows out from the body than is required to expel the abundance, the depletion causes suffering. Conversely, if the depletion, relocation, and separation from the other elements happen inside the body, according to what has been said, it must inevitably cause a double pain to the body, both from where the element has left and where it has collected in excess.

Chapter 5. I promised to prove that what I claim are a human's elements are always the same, according to convention and nature. I say that they are blood, phlegm, yellow bile, and black bile. First, I say that, according to convention, their names are distinct and that none share the same name. Second, I say that, according to their nature, their forms are recognizably different. Phlegm is nothing like blood, nor blood like bile, nor bile like phlegm. For how could these be similar to each other, since their colors do not seem alike when they are seen, nor do they seem to be alike to the touch of a hand? They are not warm, cold, dry, nor moist to the same degree. Well then, given that there is such great difference between each in form and property, these are necessarily not a single thing, if indeed fire and water are not a single thing. You can see by the following proofs that all these elements are not one, but each has its own property and nature. Should you give a person a **drug** that expels phlegm, you will have phlegm vomited, and if you give a drug that expels bile, you will have bile vomited. Likewise, if you give a drug that expels black bile, black bile will be purged. And if you damage someone's body enough to leave a wound, that person's blood will flow. And you will find that all these things happen every day and night, both during winter and summer, so long as one has strength to draw breath [*pneuma*] and expel it again, or until one is deprived of one of these congenital elements. The things that I have mentioned are congenital, for how could they not be? In the first place, a person clearly has in oneself all these elements, though unseen, for as long as one lives. Secondly, a person is born from a human who has all these elements and is nursed in a human who has them all, namely the elements I am talking about and proving.

Chapter 6. It seems to me that people who say that a human is a single thing follow the same reasoning. They have seen people who drink drugs die from excessive purges, some vomiting bile and some of them phlegm, so they believed that the person was composed only of one of these elements, the element they saw being purged, which led to the person's death. Those claiming that a human is blood use the same reasoning. They see blood flowing from the body when people are cut, so they believe that this is the person's soul. They use these proofs in their theories. But, first, no one has yet died through excessive purges by vomiting only bile. But, whenever someone drinks a drug that expels bile, first the person vomits bile and then also phlegm. After these, people then vomit black bile and, when they die, vomit pure blood. People suffer the same things under the drugs that expel phlegm. For first, they vomit phlegm, then yellow bile, then black bile, and towards the end pure blood. At that point they die. For when the drug enters the body, it first expels the bodily element that best matches its character, and then draws and purges the rest. For, just as things that grow and are sown in the earth each draw to themselves what is in accordance with their own nature: the acidic, the bitter, the sweet, the salty, and so on. At first it draws to itself most of whatever best matches its character, and then also draws the rest. In such a way, drugs also act in the body. A drug that expels bile first would purge the most unmixed bile, then the mixed. Drugs for phlegm first expel the most unmixed phlegm and then the mixed. And the blood of people cut first flows warmest and reddest, and then it flows mixed with phlegm and bile.

Chapter 7. Phlegm increases in a human during the winter, for this is the coldest of the body's elements, and is very much in accordance with winter's nature. Here is proof that phlegm is coldest: if you want to touch phlegm, bile, and blood, you will find that phlegm is coldest. And yet it is very viscous and, after black bile, takes the most force to expel. Things that move because they are forced become warmer under the force. But, despite these factors, phlegm appears the coldest because of its own nature. That winter fills the body with phlegm you can see by the following: the discharges that people spit up and blow from their noses contain the most phlegm during the winter, and during this season especially swellings become white and sicknesses are generally characterized by phlegm. During the spring phlegm is still strong in the body even as blood increases. For the cold subsides, rains come, and blood is increased by the showers and warm days. These aspects of the year are very much in accordance with blood's nature, for it is wet and warm. You can see this by the following: during the spring and the summer people are especially troubled by dysenteries and blood flows from their noses and they are very hot and red. During the summer, the blood is still strong, and bile rises in the body and extends into autumn. In autumn, the blood decreases, for autumn is the opposite of blood's nature. Bile dominates the body during the summer and autumn. You can see this by the following: during this season, people vomit bile on their own and when drinking drugs the vomit purged is filled with bile. This is also made clear by people's fevers and complexions. But during the summer phlegm is at its absolute weakest, for the season, which is dry and hot, is opposite to its nature. In autumn, people have the least blood, for autumn is dry and already begins to chill a person. During autumn there is the most black bile and it is the most powerful. When winter takes hold, the bile is chilled and decreases, and the phlegm increases again by the abundance of rains and the length of the nights.

And so the human body always has all these elements, and they increase and decrease as the year progresses each in turn and according to its nature. Indeed, every year shares in every element—the warm, the cold, the dry, and the wet—for none of the elements could remain for any time without all the things that exist in this universe. But if any one of the elements ceased to exist, all would vanish, for from the same necessity all things have been constructed and are nourished by one another. Thus, if any of these congenital elements of a human were to cease to exist, a human could not live. In the year sometimes the winter is very powerful, sometimes spring, sometimes summer, and sometimes autumn. So too in a human sometimes phlegm is powerful, sometimes blood, sometimes bile, first yellow and then that called black. There is a very clear sign of this: if you want to give the same drug to the same man four times during the year, he will vomit for you matter full of phlegm in the winter, matter full of moisture during the spring, matter full of bile during the summer, and the blackest matter during autumn.

Chapter 8. And so, this being the case, the sicknesses that increase in winter must wane in the summer. Sicknesses that increase in summer must cease during the winter, except those that do not change in a period of days; I will speak about the period of days later. One must expect the sicknesses that occur in spring to wane in the autumn. Those autumn sicknesses must wane during the spring. One must know that whatever sickness outlives the span of these seasons will remain for a year. When confronting sicknesses, the physician must hold the conviction that each of them has strength in the body in accordance with its particular season, especially as the season aligns with its nature.

Chapter 9. In addition to those points, one must know the following: sicknesses caused by being full are healed by depletion, and sicknesses caused by depletion are healed by being full. Sicknesses that arise through exercise are healed by rest, and those that inactivity produces are healed by exercise. In sum, the physician must counter the prevailing sicknesses, constitutions, seasons, and ages, and relax the things that tighten up and tighten up the things relaxed. Whatever is sick can in this way most be relieved, and I think that this is what healing is.

Some sicknesses arise from regimen and some from the air [*pneuma*] we inhale and live by. One must distinguish between the two causes in this way: when many people are troubled at the same time by a single sickness, the cause must be attributed to what is most common, and what we make the most use of, namely what we breathe in. For indeed it is clear that the regimen of each of us is not the cause when sickness touches all one after the other, the young and the old, women and men, people who are drunk and people who drink water, people who eat barley cake and people who dine on bread, and people who exercise a lot and people who exercise little. And so, when people living every manner of life are troubled by the same sickness, regimen could not be the cause. But when all sorts of sicknesses happen at the same time, in each case regimen clearly causes each sickness and one must treat them by countering the cause of the illness, just as I have said elsewhere, and by changing their regimen. For it is clear that the person's customary regimen does not suit them, either entirely, for the most part, or in some single aspect of their practices. When these features are observed, one must change them, after examining the person's age and constitution, the season of the year, and the manner of the sickness. One must provide treatment by adding some things and removing others, just as I have also said earlier. And one must make a change in treatment and regimen accounting for particulars of age, season, appearance, and sickness. But when an epidemic of one sickness has established itself, regimen is clearly not the cause, but what we breathe is, and the air clearly causes problems from having an unhealthy emission. During this time people should be advised as follows. They should not change their regimen, since this is not the cause of the sickness, but, by progressively reducing the amount they usually eat and drink, see to it that their body is very thin and very weak. For if one changes regimen quickly, there is danger that the change will cause something worse to happen in the body. Rather, regimen must be used in such a way that it obviously does not harm the person. Then one must take care to inhale into the body the purest air [*pneuma*] and as little of it as possible and the most pure air [*pneuma*] by removing oneself as far as possible from the regions where sickness has established itself, and by making the body thin, for in this way people avoid the need to breathe deeply and frequently.

SEVEN

Diagnosis

When ancient physicians visited a patient at the onset of an illness, they followed a relatively standard diagnostic protocol. First, the physician looked for bodily "signs" that would provide clues as to what might be going wrong in the body. These signs included the patient's manner of breathing; manner of talk (loud or quiet, talkativeness or silence, evidence of lucidity or delusion); the quality of their evacuations (stool, urine, sputa, vomit, sweat, blood); coughing, sneezing, belching, crying, flatulence; the nature of the patient's face (complexion, eyes, ears, nose, and tongue), hair, and nails; pulse; pain; sleep or sleeplessness; mood (hope, despair, misery, fear, optimism); disruptions of the body's normal functioning; the patient's overall state (restless, listless, weak), and the state of the specific parts of the body where the illness manifested.

Even when bodily signs could be observed with the eye, physicians used their full range of senses in diagnosis. They *touched* the body, feeling the skin to take the patient's temperature (fever or chill) and to note dampness or dryness. They palpated the body to feel for the swelling of internal organs, lumps, and tumors, or to better discern where pain was concentrated (see fig. 19). They *listened* for abnormal respiration, the rumbling of the stomach, sounds that accompanied defecation, and the vocal irregularities and confused mutterings of patients. They *smelled* the odors of the skin, breath, ears, sores, and their patients' sweat, urine, stool, pus, vomit, and sputum, paying attention to minute differences of foul, sour, and sweet smells. Sometimes they even *tasted* skin, sweat, tears, ear wax, and **humors** in order to detect saltiness, bitterness, or metallic flavors. And, when necessary, physicians used medical instruments as extensions of their senses—for instance, to "feel" inside the body by probing wounds, internal organs, and bones.

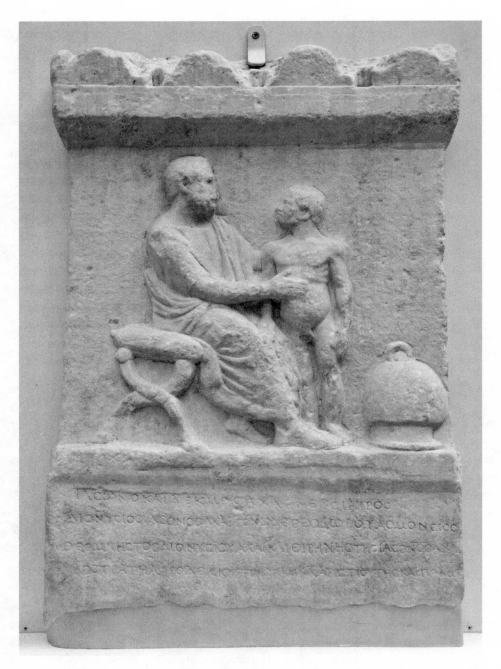

FIGURE 19 Second-century CE marble funerary monument for an Athenian physician named Jason. His appearance, bearded and clothed in a draped garment, resembles that of a philosopher, possibly a way to elevate his status. The scene depicts him palpating the stomach of his patient. On the bottom right is a cupping vessel (the scale exaggerates its ordinary size), which was used to extract blood or pus from a wound, or to relax a part of the body. British Museum (1865,0103.3). Photo credit: Carole Raddato (CC BY-SA 2.0).

Then physicians had to sift through all the bodily signs they collected during the physical examination to discern which were most pertinent to their patient's illness. Physicians called to mind their training about normal anatomy and physiology, hoping to zero in on what precisely in their patient's body was deviating from the norm. But this inference was complicated by the fact that every individual's body was different, and what was abnormal for one person could be normal for another. Thus, physicians had to calibrate what they had learned in school to the unique baseline of each individual patient. Furthermore, physicians had to determine when to exclude bodily signs that derived not from illness, but from other aspects of the patient's constitution or context. For example, women were thought to be colder than men, and young people were thought to be hotter than older people. Moreover, some bodily changes could derive from the waters, winds, soil, or climate characteristic of the place, or the season of the year.

Another challenge of diagnosis was that not all ailments produced visible signs on the surface of the body, and thus not all internal ailments were directly perceptible to physicians. The Hippocratic author of *On the Art of Medicine* (Text 3, Chapter 11) warns: "It is impossible for a person who sees only with his eyes" to learn anything about internal ailments. Some might resort to opening up their patients' bodies, though this was risky and should be avoided. Instead physicians were advised to use the "eyes of the mind" to imagine what might be going on internally. They could also interpret the qualities of their patients' urine or pulse as proxies.[1]

With respect to urine, physicians observed the flow and frequency of their patients' urination, and they closely inspected urine collected in flasks. As we see in the selection from **Pliny the Elder's** *Natural History* (Text 7), the color of urine was particularly meaningful. Physicians gauged their patients' urine against a color scale (see fig. 20), which indicated the deficiency or overabundance of certain humors. For example, red urine was understood to result from an abundance of blood, whereas ocher urine resulted from an excess of yellow bile. Other qualities of the urine—including its thickness/thinness, cloudiness, bubbles, odor, and the presence of sediment—also provided clues about humoral imbalances, as well as digestive ailments (for instance, thin, white urine was understood to result from under-concocted food), and problems with the organs (especially the liver, the organ thought to be in charge of converting food into blood and waste products).

As with urine, physicians attempted to gather useful information about the internal bodily state of their patients by taking their pulse. They attempted to sense various qualities of the pulse, including its size, speed, vigor, and evenness; the rate of (or interval between the beats of) the pulse; and the smoothness or hardness of the artery through which the pulse beat. Because even subtle differences were a clue regarding what was going on inside the body, physicians devised sophisticated measurement techniques. For example, **Herophilus**

1. For a discussion of other diagnostic proxies, see Celsus's use of blood, pus, and serous fluid (Text 12).

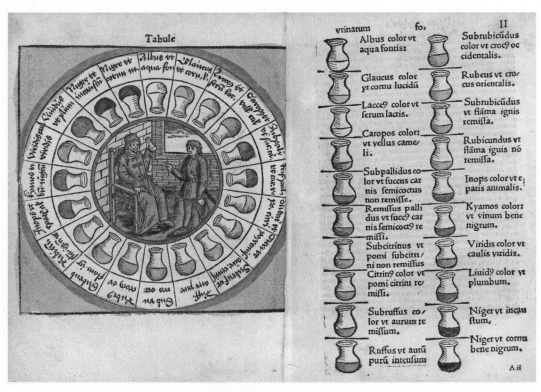

FIGURE 20 Illustrations from the 1506 CE manuscript *Epiphaniae medicorum,* depicting urine colors that would aid physicians in uroscopic analysis and diagnosis. The painted vessels illustrate the various colors of urine, with labels that provide even more detail. For example, the labels compare various urine colors to camel's wool, the juice of meat, saffron, dark wine, and ink. The labels also indicate the urine color's intensity. Folger Library Digital Image Collection (CC BY-SA 4.0).

used a water clock to detect deviations from normal pulse rates. (For Herophilus, such irregularities in pulse helped physicians anticipate fevers.)

But **Galen** asserted that pulse diagnosis should be reserved for advanced practitioners given that it required the physician to have developed an acute sensitivity to the multidimensional sensations they felt. According to Galen, pulse diagnosis also required the physician to keep in mind the "feel" of every individual patient's *unique* pulse rhythm, and then to detect subtle changes or deviations therefrom. Once mastered, Galen argued, pulse diagnosis could be an effective way to discriminate between physical and mental/emotional ailments that produced the same bodily signs. Galen explained that, because the pulse originated in the heart, it was the principal sign from which to detect passions such as love, anxiety, fear, worry, and stress. These passions manifested in physical symptoms, but ailments of the soul and mind were to be treated differently than ailments of the body that produced the same physical symptoms.

Some information salient to diagnosis could only be learned by questioning the patient directly. Thus the medical writer **Rufus of Ephesus** appealed to his fellow physicians not to overlook this crucial step of diagnosis (Text 6). According to Rufus, physicians should ask a variety of questions to extract the patient's medical history to discern if the sickness was recurring or out of the ordinary; to determine the course of the illness (including its onset, **critical days,** relapse, etc.); to identify any changes in diet, activity levels, or unusual events that correlated with the beginning of the illness; to get information on symptoms only the patient could relay (such as the content of their dreams, the quality of their pain, etc.); and to learn about remedies that worked for the patient in the past, including especially local remedies unknown to physicians who were new to the region. Moreover, because every patient's baseline was different, the physician must come to understand from patients what bodily signs they considered normal and abnormal. Finally, the manner in which patients answered the questions—their mood, aspects of their speech, etc.—could provide additional clues about their illness.

Although information gathered from patients could be quite valuable in diagnosis, it was not always easy for patients to describe their bodily experiences. A prime example was pain. Patients might find it easy to explain the location (e.g., localized, diffuse), frequency (e.g., intermittent, continuous), and duration of their pain (e.g., temporary, chronic), but patients used a wide array of terms to characterize the *nature* of their pain—such as "throbbing," "twisting," "stabbing," "biting," "tearing," "shooting," "numbing," "sharp," "dull," "heavy," "itching," and "nausea." Additionally, different patients might use the same term to describe different sensations, or different terms for the same sensations; some descriptors—such as "sweet," "salty," or "rough"—were hard to decrypt with regard to pain; and there was no easy or agreed-upon way to measure the intensity of pain. Patients might also be incapable of providing clear information because of their physical or mental distress, lapses of memory, language barriers, or age (children and the elderly were thought to have a compromised ability to communicate). In these cases, physicians were urged to consult with members of the patient's household, such as friends who had been sitting bedside, and with other physicians who previously treated the patient.

Skilled physicians sought not only to arrive at a diagnosis, but also to forecast the course and probable outcome of the illness (i.e., **prognosis**). For example, one Hippocratic text explained that the quality of pus should be studied to determine whether a patient would recover or not: "A sign whether the person is going to escape: if the pus is white and clean, and contains streaks of blood, the person generally recovers; but if it flows out on the first day yolk-colored, or on the following day thick, slightly yellow-green, and stinking, when it has flowed out the person dies" (*Diseases* 2.47). (**Celsus** follows similar reasoning in Text 12.) Prognoses were instrumental in guiding the physician's decisions about when and how to provide treatment, but just as important, a correct prognosis also bolstered their credibility. When illnesses took the course predicted by physicians, it inspired patients' confidence, in turn incentivizing them to follow their physician's instructions (as well as attracting new clients). When the prognosis was bad, it could free physicians from responsibility and blame that they had done something wrong.

TEXT 6. RUFUS OF EPHESUS, *ON THE IMPORTANCE OF QUESTIONING THE SICK PERSON*[2]

Rufus of Ephesus *(late first century CE) was one of the more influential physicians of the Roman Empire. Rufus wrote around 100 medical texts, of which only four authentic treatises survive completely in the original Greek, with a considerable quantity of fragmentary material in Arabic, Syriac, or Latin translation. Rufus's* On the Importance of Questioning the Sick Person *insists that physicians seek information directly from the sick people they treat, information that is essential to accurate diagnoses.*

SOURCE: Translation by Melinda Letts based on the Greek text from Hans Gärtner, *Rufi Ephesii Quaestiones medicinales* (Leipzig: Teubner, 1970).

1. You must ask the sick person questions, from which anything connected with the sickness can be more accurately identified and better treated. 2. That is my first principle: put your inquiries to the sick person himself. I say this because from this you can learn not just how healthy or unwell the person is in his mind, as well as his physical strength or weakness, but also what type of sickness he has been laboring under and its location. If he answers coherently, appropriately and with good recall, with no slips of the tongue or the mind, and in a way that corresponds to his own natural inclination—mildly and moderately if he is otherwise moderate, or again boldly if he is naturally bold or fearfully if he is naturally timid—then you should consider his mind, at least, to be in good order. But if you ask one question and he answers another, if he loses his train of thought in the middle of speaking, if his speech is tremulous and unclear and there are shifts from the original temper to the opposite, all these are signs of mental disturbance. Deafness in the sufferer, too, is indicated in this way. 3. If he does not hear, one must additionally ask those with him if he was already hard of hearing or has become so because of the present sickness; for this has a great bearing on identifying the problem. 4. You can perceive the sufferer's physical strength or weakness from how he tells you what has happened: one person speaking audibly and coherently, and another with frequent pauses and in a thin voice. [You can similarly identify] the type of disorder [and its location, if he speaks rapidly, lisps, stammers from inability to control his tongue, and suffers the usual symptoms of **melancholy** or,][3] if there is no melancholy, suffers hoarseness or paralysis of the tongue or some of the things that tend to arise in the chest and lungs. For the melancholy state is clearly indicated by over-boldness and unwarranted sad-

---

2. This text has traditionally been translated with the title *Medical Questions*, but translator Melinda Letts prefers *On the Importance of Questioning the Sick Person* because this title more accurately reflects the text's content, and also remains close to the text's opening phrase: "You must ask the sick person questions."

3. The section in square brackets represents a gap in Rufus's text as it has been transmitted. This is the translator's conjecture regarding the missing text, based on analysis of the manuscript and comparison with his text *On Melancholy*.

ness, and a person reveals his brashness or depression particularly in the things he says; he reveals them in other ways too, but if this empirical test is added, the sickness will then be clearly identified. 5. An imminent attack of lethargy is evident if, when responding to questions, a person forgets what he is saying and speaks indistinctly. 6. That is certainly so when there is a fever; but where there is none, you must expect convulsions and seizures. In sum, everything that proceeds from a mentally disturbed temper can be perceived more easily through questioning than otherwise. 7. Chest complaints can be perceived from both sharpness and roughness of the voice. If the person has the **wasting ailment** and can breathe only in an upright posture, the voice is sharp, but in someone with an abscess, hoarseness or severe catarrh it is rougher. 8. As for those with paralysis of the tongue, they have no voice at all.

9. First, as has been said, you must question the sick person himself, whoever he is, about the things you need to know; but then, if there are impediments to learning from the sick person, you must question those with him as well. 10. By impediments I mean when someone is very mentally disturbed, or has had a stroke, or is suffering from lethargy, catalepsy or speechlessness, or is otherwise simple-minded or physically completely debilitated, or will benefit from keeping speaking to a minimum, for example in a case of bleeding from the lung. Questioning someone else is also necessary on behalf of a child or a very old person, and in the case of someone who does not speak one's language one must question someone who does.

11. The first thing to ask is the point in time when the person began to be unwell. This is useful not just for the remedy but also for identifying **critical days**, since it will be sufficient for observation of their cycles of recurrence. 12. In fact knowing when it began is a great help for the full identification of the sickness, since the same ***sumptōmata***[4] have different meanings when they appear at times that are not fixed. Thus jaundice manifesting before the sixth or seventh day is bad in a fever, but after that it means a **crisis** is underway; urine and feces that are watery and crude are less bad at the beginning but more suspicious in advanced cases; and nosebleeds at four-day intervals are difficult if they are slight, and if violent mean an unfavorable crisis, even though they bring the crisis later. 13. All these things you will learn about by asking what the first day was on which the person began to be unwell, and about the acuteness and severity of the sickness, i.e. if some of the ill effects appeared rapidly and at once, after breaking out suddenly, and others slowly over time. Similarly, from the cycle of recurrence you will also learn whether the sickness is intensifying in a straightforwardly regular manner, or began chaotically but is subsequently settling into some kind of order. From this too you will learn about remission from three-day fever, and changes in and recovery from certain other disorders. 14. That is how useful I say

4. We have left the Greek word *sumptōma* (plural: *sumptōmata*) untranslated because it lacks an exact equivalent in English. A *sumptōma* is something that happens, sometimes, but not always, with the implication that what has happened is bad or undesirable. See the word's glossary entry for more details.

it is to ask about the beginning of the sickness, the point at which the person began to be unwell.[5]

15. The next thing to ask is whether or not the present attack is among the disorders from which the person commonly suffers, and whether it has happened before. This is because many people on the whole succumb to the same things, suffer the same effects, and are treated in the same way, and the physician might be worried by something on the grounds that it is difficult to resist and not susceptible to treatment when in fact it is not difficult in this person's case, at least, or not unsuitable for treatment in the present episode of sickness. In all cases habituation is most important both for the endurance of the ill effects and for remedying them. 16. So I think that one will do well to ask about every aspect of every person's constitution too. For we are not all constituted the same, but are completely different from each other in every respect whatsoever. So, if you want to examine the state of the digestion, for example, you will find that different things are easy or hard for different people to digest. Again, **drugs** that people drink for laxative or diuretic purposes have different effects on different people: purgatives can also encourage vomiting, and **emetics** can also have an effect down below. In short, none of these things is fixed so as to end in a single meaning for the physician. 17. This is why one must also learn from the sufferer how he responds to each item of drink and food; nor must one overlook any obvious experience he may have of a drug, for in this respect one will very often hit the mark by asking the sufferer also about events that are unusual for him.

18. In sum, we must ask if he has a good appetite or is off his food, if he is thirsty or doesn't want to drink, and what his habits are in relation to every single thing; for this too is important: to be no less acquainted with his habits than with his constitution. People consume familiar food, prepared in the quantity and style in which they customarily take it, with less discomfort than that which might otherwise seem to be best. 19. Besides, familiar things are always better, whether a person is sick or healthy. 20. We can give a more accurate prognosis, too, by knowing the person's habits with respect to power of judgment, manner of conversation, state of relaxation, and any other function whatsoever. For things that are habitual in a healthy person do not constitute signs when he is unwell.

21. In these matters too there is nothing that the physician will be able to learn by himself, without inquiring of either the sick person or someone else who is with him. So for my part I am amazed by the physician **Callimachus**, who alone of earlier physicians—or at least of those one can take seriously—denied the need to ask questions about sicknesses, including injuries, especially head injuries, on the grounds that just the signs in every single case were enough to indicate the condition and its cause, which were the basis of both full prognosis and better treatment. Asking questions was unnecessary, he said, even about the

5. In this section, Rufus uses well-known aspects of Hippocratic doctrine merely as examples, assuming that his readers will be familiar with them. His purpose in this treatise is not to teach medical doctrine but to persuade physicians to question the people they treat, rather than rely on doctrine alone.

antecedent causes of sickness—such as the regimen being followed, and other habits, and whether the person was tired or cold when he became unwell—on the grounds that the physician had no need to learn any of these things if he gave careful and accurate consideration to the signs that afflict people along with their sicknesses. 22. But what I think is that, although one can indeed discover many of the things related to sicknesses on one's own, one can do it better and more clearly in the course of questioning, for if the answers correspond with the *sumptōmata* it is easier to know what is going on. Thus if a sick person suffering what we would expect in a case of satiety says that he has exceeded his previous regimen by taking in more food and drink, we can come to know clearly that the sickness is satiety and, moreover, discover the entire remedy. Or take someone who says he has been working very hard: if he is suffering what we would expect in a case of working hard, it will be easier to tell that the sickness is fatigue and apply the treatment appropriate to fatigue. 23. The *sumptōmata* in such cases can also provide some indication for forming a judgment;[6] but as to the timing of the sickness, and the person's habits in relation to every single thing, and the singular constitution of each individual, these are things that one cannot, in my view, know without asking questions, while knowing them is more critical than anything else to the medical art.

24. The identification of disorders varies depending on whether the attack arises from inside or outside, and the identification of internal ones is somehow harder, I think, than that of external ones. If the person is shivering, for example, it is less alarming if it is due to cold or fear but more difficult if it has arisen from some internal cause. Again, if someone is out of his mind, it is easier to remedy if caused by strong drink or a drug that causes mental disturbance, but more difficult if due to another cause. 25. Thus you will find that the method of treatment also differs in all cases. Some cases of fatigue, for example, are due to much hard work and others to satiety; the former cases benefit from rest, sleep, soft massage, and warm baths, the latter from exertion, wakefulness, and every other kind of depletion. 26. This is how much difference it makes to the physician to ask about the causes as well, and it is not possible to know them without asking questions. This means that one must ask questions even when there are signs: if there is a bluish-gray color, whether it is because of a blow or the person's age or the time of the year (for otherwise a bluish-gray color in fever signifies death); if the tongue is dry, whether the person has been thirsty or has had a major evacuation, and, if it is black, whether he has eaten something black; things like that would not constitute cause for suspicion.

27. Similarly one must also ask questions about excretions during sicknesses: urine, feces, and saliva; for here too it is very important to know, in relation to their quantity, consistency, and color, how much food the person has had, of what kind, and exactly when it was given.

6. The Greek word *endeixis* translated here as "indication" is a technical term used in ancient medical debates about the relative value of theory vs. experience in forming a diagnosis. Rufus's view is that good diagnosis calls for a combination of theory, experience, and the sick person's knowledge of their own body and circumstances.

28. One must ask questions about sleep, too: whether he has slept or not, and what his normal habits are regarding sleep and sleeplessness, and if he is having any visions or dreams, since the physician can draw conclusions from these too. 29. I cannot deal with dreams comprehensively, but just enough to point out the subject in my discourse and remind the physician not to overlook any of these kinds of things. Myron of Ephesus, a wrestler, when seemingly healthy, had a dream of the following kind: all night long he thought he was in a black marsh of drinkable water. When he got up he told this to his trainer, who thought nothing of the dream and set Myron to his exertions. Before Myron was halfway through, he was attacked by breathlessness, weakness and palpitation of the entire chest, immediately after which he lost the use of his hands and feet, and then the power of speech. Shortly thereafter he dies.[7] 30. He would not, I think, have died if he had happened to find a wise trainer and had had himself fully bled before his exertions. 31. Another man who was acutely feverish kept being visited in his sleep by an Ethiopian man who seemed to be wrestling with him and strangling him. This man told his physician the dream, but the physician did not himself give much thought to what it meant, until the sickness was brought to a crisis by a violent nosebleed. 32. There was also the man who thought he was swimming in the Cayster River,[8] whose sickness became chronic and culminated in **dropsy**. 33. I am quite convinced that, in accordance with the body's humors, dream-visions arise that indicate things for the person, both good and bad, and that there is no other way of apprehending these if one does not hear about them.

34. And what of congenital disorders? I ask you, is it possible to know about them in any other way than by asking questions about them too? And nobody could say that this was a trivial question, unless it is also a trivial matter to identify a disorder that is easier to deal with and one that is harder; for it is a correct assumption that all congenital sickness is harder to treat than that which is not congenital.

35. Furthermore, any cycle of recurrence there has been, and relocation of the sickness, and all the *sumptōmata* that have previously afflicted the person—these things too one must inquire about to know; and if they are taken into consideration they are of no small help to both prognosis and treatment.

36. One must also ask questions about the type of regimen the sick person has observed while unwell—not the one he follows when he is healthy, about which this has already been said, but his current one: what regimen he has been following during his sickness, whether any drugs have been administered, the whole treatment he has been given, and what condition he manifests in relation to every single thing. Such things are useful to know, whether for adjusting present arrangements, avoiding disturbance of previous arrangements, or discovering if he has neglected anything essential.

37. We must also ask if the person has taken food or not. Even this, I say, the physician cannot come to know by himself; though the common people find it a most absurd question

7. Rufus switches to the present tense here, a narrative technique with vivid effect that has been retained in the translation.
8. A river to the north of Ephesus, where Rufus was born.

if one does not know that a sick person has eaten as soon as one touches him,[9] but inquires of someone else. 38. But in my view this is another example of what you cannot identify without asking questions—just as with the timing, type, and quantity of food consumed.[10] Someone who conjectures about this on the basis of the person's strength and weakness will be frequently deceived on many counts. For sometimes a person who has eaten a sufficient amount is not sufficiently strengthened, while another person is strengthened by not eating, especially if it is surfeit that has caused the debilitation.

39. We must ask too what food tastes best to the person. Somehow this brings even more benefit than the most excellent food, since it is digested more easily than what is disagreeable. For if someone gulps it down without chewing, disagreeable food offers him the effect of each thing only weakly, but if he digests and distributes it, it can offer him a different effect.

40. We must ask, as well, what is easily excreted, what has a diuretic effect, what provokes acidity, and what is harmful in any other way. For these are things that are specific to the individual and do not apply across the board. So I would also praise the physician meeting the sick person for the first time who does not work out the treatment by himself alone, but summons for consultation someone who knows the sufferer as well—preferably a physician, but if not, even a layman. In this way he will not make a mistake about what is beneficial.

41. The amount of pain occurring with sicknesses is another area for questioning. One can conjecture that someone is in pain from other signs as well: from groans and cries and thrashing about, distress, the way the body is lying, the complexion, thinness, and the touch of the hands—whether it is you that wishes to touch him or [. . .];[11] for the painful part is immediately obvious. Also, the sufferer himself presses the painful areas in particular, so that even when it comes to the pains of people who cannot speak you will not be mistaken if you draw your conclusions from such things. It is possible to identify pains in sick people from their cries, but thorough inquiry is necessary as well; yet not even that is quite sufficient for complete identification, since weakness and delicateness make many people act out pain as elaborately, one might say, as tragic actors groaning on the stage. 42. One must give careful consideration to the other factors too: whether the person is of sound mind, and courageous, and self-controlled; such a person, at least, would not dissemble at all about his sickness. 43. Since pain on the whole has cycles of recurrence, we must ask questions about this too. For we cannot say that it is essential to inquire about the exact timing of other acute attacks while overlooking those of pain.

44. There is also some value in asking about the state of the person's bowels—whether or not defecation is easy; and the same applies to the other discharges. 45. For sweating, urinating and vomiting come easily to some and with more difficulty to others.

9. Rufus here alludes to pulse theory, which held that the pulse was affected by the quantity of food consumed.

10. Rufus refers here to the questioning recommended at §27.

11. A section of the Greek text appears to be missing here. The grammar of the part that remains suggests that it may have said something like "he that invites you to do so."

46. So in the case of general sicknesses, and especially feverish ones, these and similar things are the areas for questioning.

When it comes to wounds, if the wound was inflicted by a dog, we must ask whether the dog happened to be rabid, for it makes a great difference. If it was not, a hemostatic drug or a sponge soaked in vinegar suffices, but if it was rabid then we must **cauterize**, no matter how small the wound is, and apply pungent drugs, leave the wound open for a long time,[12] and administer a drink of wormwood, birthwort, buckthorn, boiled river-crabs, garlic, parsley, and the root called gentian. It is also a great help if from time to time you wash it with hellebore. Unless you do all this, there is a danger of the person developing convulsions, going out of his mind, becoming afraid of water,[13] and dying. 47. For example, I know a man who was bitten by a mad dog and did not take the wound seriously, despite much encouragement from physicians as well as from his family. 48. He died not much later, having suffered what people suffer in that sickness. His wife, who had had intercourse with him when he already had the wound, and was three months pregnant, developed a fear of water herself, with the result that in my view she would have perished in the same manner if we had not quickly told her to abort the embryo. 49. Bites and blows inflicted by other beasts will also do best if we inquire carefully about them. For if we devise what is suitable for each case before the *sumptōmata* attack, we will treat it more easily. In these cases too, judgment from signs is still possible, even if the person who has been bitten does not speak. In the case of the dog this is not possible before the affection comes.

50. When men are wounded in war by arrows or spears, weapons that stick out or are lodged in the **flesh** are obvious to the sight and touch. As for those that were hidden inside, if someone happens to have pulled the weapon out of the person, we must ask if he pulled it out complete with its tip or only got the shaft. 51. For a buried tip can escape the notice of even a very experienced person. This is why physicians are right to advise soldiers to let arrows stay lodged in their flesh, so that they can be sure of extracting them themselves, in order that nothing is left in the wound and so that they can do the extraction skillfully. 52. It is necessary, I suggest, before treating it, to inquire about ointment on the arrow. For many people have discovered drugs with which they smear their arrows, allowing even a small injury to be fatal. 53. If we know of this beforehand, we have a chance of providing some antidote for the individual drug. 54. This is a question for some prisoner of war or deserter rather than for the injured man.

55. We must ask about injuries in the head in the following way, especially if, in the absence of any obvious damage to the bone, the man who was struck becomes unable to speak, vomits first food or phlegm, then bile, and subsequently develops an acute fever with mental disturbance. There is a risk that the bone is broken, either at the site of the wound

12. A reference to the practice of keeping the wound from a rabid dog's bite open for as long as possible to prevent scarring and to allow the poison to be evacuated.

13. Rufus here refers to the fact that people infected with rabies develop excruciating spasms in the throat when drinking, and eventually even when thinking about drinking.

itself or elsewhere. 56. In other cases there is no wound at all, but the bone is broken beneath the skin, and the person suffers as described. 57. This is how it went in the case of the Samian, for example.[14] They were holding their local festival in which they stand apart and throw stones at each other. This man was struck during that activity, and had no obvious injury, but becomes speechless and dizzy.[15] A little later he seemed well, but on the 20th day afterwards he begins to be out of his mind. So when I was called in and saw that he was constantly touching his head, and was trembling and mentally disturbed, I asked if he had ever been struck on the head. When they said that he had, I said confidently that his bone had been broken. 58. Then we made a large cut through the part which he kept particularly touching with his hands, and found a very long fracture of the bone, which we subsequently treated as one treats fractures of the skull. This is what happened in that case.

59. So, as I was saying: if someone is injured in the head, we must ask questions about the shape and size of the weapon, and how hard it was. For, from similar throws, objects that are round, large, and solid are likely to cause fractures, while those that are sharp are more likely to cause injury. 60. You must ask, too, about the strength of the man who threw it, and how vigorously he aimed the blow, and whether the weapon that caused the injury came from above or was ricocheting. You will find all this very helpful, or in some way important, with regard to both obvious and hidden fractures. 61. Slingshot projectiles have more force than those thrown by hand, while catapulted ones are the most forceful; so you must not reject even these questions. 62. Finally you must also ask about the aforementioned[16] post-blow signs. For if any of them happens, you absolutely must believe there to be some damage to the bone.

63. These, then, and others very like them, are the questions for the sick person and those with him. Concerning groups of people, they are different. For example, if you go to a foreign place you must inquire what the waters are like and if they have any special powers, such as are frequently found, some purging the belly, some encouraging urination, some bad for the digestion, some harmful to the liver and spleen, some also causing kidney- or gall-stones, and others with other effects, some bad, some good. So for example the water at Leontini in Sicily kills those who drink it, as does the water of Pheneus, in Arcadia, which is called Stygian.[17] As for the water of Clitor in Arcadia, anyone who washes in it is unable to bear even the smell of wine. The water of Lyncestis causes intoxication;[18] 64. that of the Arethusa, in Chalcis, induces gout.[19] All the different characteristics that are found in the waters, food crops, and climate among individual groups of people, and that do not resemble

---

14. "Samian" refers to a man from the island of Samos, located in the Mediterranean just southwest of Rufus's birthplace of Ephesus.

15. Here and in the next sentence, Rufus again switches to the present tense for vivid effect.

16. See §55.

17. Arcadia was a region in central Greece.

18. Lyncestis was a region in northern Greece.

19. The Arethusa was a spring in the town of Chalcis, which is located on the Greek island of Euboea.

the characteristics that generally exist, one must know either by inquiring of local inhabitants or by testing them over time. There is no other accurate means of identification, given that local disorders also cannot be known in any other way; for there is much in them that is incalculable, area by area. 65. So, for example, in the land of the Arabs we find a disorder called "Ophis,"[20] which in Greek is called "sinew." 66. It is as thick as a lyre-string, and moves and turns in the flesh in a reptilian manner, particularly in the thighs and lower legs but also elsewhere in the body. 67. I myself, for example, saw an Arab man in Egypt with this sickness. Whenever it was about to emerge, he developed pain and fever, and a swelling appeared, like an abscess, until the worm came through the skin, turned clammy, and putrefied. 68. He had it on his lower leg, but his serving girl had it in her navel, and another woman in the groin. 69. When I inquired if the sickness was common among the Arabs, they said that not only do Arabs become unwell in this way but also many foreigners who come to the country are affected by it if they drink the water, which they said was the principal cause.

70. You could discover thousands of other things like this to explore, if you were only keen to discover also the remedies that are specific to each group of people; thus the Egyptians use voiding and vomiting and enemas, while others use bloodletting, and others again use hellebore purges.

71. So now, I think, my idea is clear, [whatever point it wants to arrive at].[21] A discourse is not, of course, sufficient on its own, nor is there enough time for explaining or discovering everything. But the essence of my thinking, once found and adopted by the physician, would have everything he needs.

72. And if anyone should say that my thinking is opposed to that of **Hippocrates,** who as you know said he had discovered an art enabling a physician, on arrival at a city with which he is not familiar, to know about the waters, the seasons, the condition of the inhabitants' bowels, whether they enjoy drinking and whether they eat a lot, what sort of disorders are endemic there, how the women experience childbirth, and everything else that Hippocrates professed to learn by means of the art, on his own, without asking the inhabitants any questions; if anyone, citing this, finds fault with me for disagreeing with the greatest of physicians about the most important matters, this is my reply: I mean no disrespect to any of Hippocrates' precepts, but while some things certainly do get found by his method—things to do with the state of the seasons and the natural state of the body and types of regimen, as well as the general advantages and disadvantages of the waters and the general type of disorders—there are other things that cannot be clearly identified without making inquiries among the inhabitants, especially anything unusual or strange in them individually. 73. I admire the man unreservedly for the cleverness of his method, by which he has made

20. "Ophis" may be identified with the Medina or Guinea worm; a small gap in the text here probably represents the ancient local word for "worm."

21. The meaning of the text at this point is not at all clear. The phrase in square brackets translates the Greek as it has been transmitted.

good discoveries in many cases, but I urge anyone whose intention is the acquisition of full and accurate knowledge not to refrain from asking questions.

TEXT 7. PLINY, *NATURAL HISTORY* SELECTION (28.68–69)

The Natural History *by **Pliny the Elder** (c. 23 or 24–79 CE) is an encyclopedic text that covers a range of topics, including geography, botany, agriculture, horticulture, zoology, mineralogy, and medicine. The* Natural History *records information Pliny drew from reading widely, and from observations picked up during his administrative work and travels throughout the Roman Empire. In the selection below Pliny discusses the use of urine in medical diagnoses.*

SOURCE: Translation by Molly Jones-Lewis based on the Latin text from Alfred Ernout, *Pline l'Ancien, Histoire naturelle, Livre XXVIII* (Paris: Les Belles Lettres, 1962).

Book 28. 68. Predictions of health are given from urine.[22] If it is bright white in the morning, then becomes ruddy-brown, the first situation means that digestion is happening, and the second that digestion has finished. Red urine is a bad sign, but the worst is black urine, and bubbly urine is also bad. Thick urine in which some white matter sinks down means that there is going to be pain around the joints or the gut. Green urine means illness of the gut, pale urine means bile, and urine that goes red means blood. It is also a bad sign if bran-like particles and little clouds appear in the urine.

69. Watery and white urine is defective, but that which is thick with a strong odor indicates death, as is thin and watery urine in boys. The Magi forbid undressing to urinate facing the sun and the moon, or to splash the shadow of any object with urine.[23] **Hesiod** suggests that one should urinate up against an obstruction so that the nudity not offend any god.[24] **Ostanes** promises that one's own morning urine sprinkled on the foot helps against all poisonous **drugs**.

22. See figure 20.

23. "The Magi" refers to a group of priests from Persia, but the term came to be used more widely to describe a range of religious experts and magicians.

24. See Hesiod, *Works and Days* 727. The cover would keep a person from accidentally exposing their genitals to a god.

EIGHT

Case Histories

The Hippocratic collection *On Epidemics* (Text 8) is our most comprehensive collection of case histories from the ancient Mediterranean. Although this genre—sometimes called case notes, clinical notes, patient charts—has become a mainstay in medicine today, we see here some of the earliest recorded attempts to systematically observe and document the full course of a patient's illness.

Case histories are a treasure trove of information about medical practice. They reveal the level of detail involved in physicians' physical examinations. They also reveal the kinds of details physicians deemed important to diagnosis. For example, physicians noted a consistent set of bodily signs, including the quality and quantity of patients' evacuations (e.g., stool, urine, sweat, phlegm, sputa, vomit, flatulence); the nature of their breathing and of their pulse; the color and temperature of their skin; their appetite or thirst; their mental state (expressed in their mood, silence or talkativeness, and coherence or incoherence); their sleep patterns and dreams; coughing, sneezing, hiccups; and the rigor or looseness of body parts or functions (on diagnostic protocols, see chapter 7). Physicians also recorded the progress of an illness, including **critical days**, relapses, complications, and the ultimate outcome of the illness, whether recovery or death. Physicians also took notes on the external influences that may have contributed to illness—such as the season or the position of the sun, moon, or stars, as well as the patient's diet, exercise, and bathing habits at the onset of their illness—indicating the physician's view that environment and regimen influenced individuals' bodily condition (on environmental theories, see chapters 4 and 6; on regimen, see chapter 10). Finally, physicians documented the gender and age of the patient, which also might influence their interpretation of bodily signs (on the bodily state of women, see chapter 9; on bodily states linked to various life stages, see chapter 14).

Compilations of physicians' case histories enable us to see the range of illnesses physicians confronted as they traveled from city to city: from common illnesses they encountered regularly to local or regionally specific illnesses that were new to them. Compilations of case histories also reveal a range of physicians' notation styles. Some took notes several times per day for the full course of a patient's illness, while others wrote only a sentence or two for the whole case.[1] Some organized their notes by individual patient cases; whereas others organized their notes by day, combining their description of several patients into a single entry. In the selections below we include case histories of individuals only, though there are also extant case histories of community-wide illnesses wherein the symptoms of whole communities were synthesized in the case notes.

Case histories appear to have been primarily useful in documenting symptoms in order to arrive at a diagnosis. While physicians documented the *evidence* that went into their deliberation, they often did not record *their precise reasoning* about how they used such evidence to arrive at a diagnosis and treatment plan. We occasionally find some shorthand principles like "opposites cure opposites" or "purge after **crisis**," but, otherwise, we are forced to infer physicians' medical reasoning through the kinds of information they recorded (for example, whether they paid attention to **humors** or bodily constriction suggests their theoretical approach). That said, case notes are sometimes also places where physicians worked out thorny diagnoses, mulling questions that befuddled them (for example, "Question: Is it easier always to make full with food or with drink?" and "How can one recognize very serious pains?"). And just as physicians' medical reasoning is largely absent from case notes, neither do they always document the treatment applied.

After a case concluded, case histories remained useful as reference works or teaching tools. For instance, when faced with a similar illness, a physician might refer back to a similar case to determine what to do (see, for example, the comparison of symptoms of Olympiodorus's daughter with those of Hipponax's wife and Aristeus's servant in Text 8, Hippocratic Corpus, *On Epidemics* 4.33). Cases were incorporated into lectures to illustrate medical theories or principles, and these scenarios were given to physicians-in-training so they could practice what they might do if they were to encounter similar cases. Taking notes was also sometimes a central feature of training: when apprentices were charged with keeping an eye on patients and recording notes on their symptoms, this act of note-taking served the useful purpose of honing their skills of observation and habituating them to perceive the most salient signs of illness.

Beyond providing information about physicians' practices and training, case histories also offer a window into the broader social context of healing in antiquity. From case notes, we gather information about the gender, age, status, and occupations of those who consulted

1. The varying level of detail may be related to the amount of time spent with patients: physicians who could post an apprentice in the home to document the course of the illness (even when they were absent) may explain longer notes, whereas shorter notes could be indicative of physicians who could visit only periodically. (On the use of apprentices, see chapter 11.)

physicians. We also get glimpses into the environments in which healing took place, learning about the kinds of beds where patients convalesced, the people who cared for patients, and the mundane routines of caring for the sick. And we sometimes see the presence of multiple physicians, suggesting that the client might hire more than one physician, to get a second opinion, or a physician might call in colleagues to consult on a particularly challenging case.

Beyond physicians' case notes, we also hear about individual cases from a few other sources. Difficult cases were invoked when physicians wanted to prove their medical chops. For example, **Galen, Erasistratus,** and **Rufus** wrote about disagreements they had with other physicians and about how their view ultimately prevailed. Additionally, we learn from the Greek orator **Aelius Aristides** (117–after 181 CE) that some people kept their own personal medical records. Aristides, for instance, reports that he kept a diary recording details of the illnesses he experienced.

TEXT 8. HIPPOCRATIC CORPUS, *ON EPIDEMICS* SELECTIONS (CASES FROM BOOKS 1, 2, 4, AND 5)

*On Epidemics was attributed to **Hippocrates**, but as with all the texts in the Hippocratic corpus, the authorship is uncertain. The seven books that make up this text appear to have been written by different authors (for example, Book 1 was likely written around 410 BCE, but perhaps as early as the 470s or 460s, Books 2 and 4 around 400 BCE, and Book 5 around the middle of the fourth century BCE). The different books were eventually combined into the single compilation we have today. The standard English title,* On Epidemics, *can be somewhat misleading in that, in this context, it does not refer to a mass disease event that strikes a whole community. Instead, "epidemics" is a translation of the Greek word* epidemiai, *which could have two different meanings. One meaning refers most literally to the "visits" that traveling or itinerant physicians would make to different communities. The other meaning refers to the existence of illness in a community. Both senses of the word may be implied in the title of this text.* On Epidemics *provides something like the case notes or case histories that physicians took when they saw patients. As such, the cases collected in* On Epidemics *show Hippocratic physicians at work, providing insight into the value they placed on making careful and detailed observations of their patients' bodies and of the course or stages of an illness, observations that proved useful in diagnosis and in gaining experience.*

SOURCE: Translation by Robert Nau based on the Greek text from W. H. S. Jones, *Hippocrates,* vol. 1, Loeb Classical Library 147 (Cambridge, Mass.: Harvard University Press, 1923) and W. D. Smith, *Hippocrates,* vol. 7, Loeb Classical Library 477 (Cambridge, Mass.: Harvard University Press, 1994).

Book 1, Case 2. Silenus lived on flat land near the house of Eualcidas. A fever took hold from fatigue, drinking, and ill-timed exercises. He started to suffer pain in his loins. There was heaviness of head and tenseness in the neck.

On the first day, unmixed, foamy, and deep-colored discharges filled with bile passed from his **cavity.** Urine was black with black sediment. He was thirsty. His tongue was dry. He did not fall asleep during the night.

On the second day, there was acute fever. Excrement, thinner and frothy, was in greater quantity. Urine was black. The night was difficult. He was a little delirious.

On the third day, everything worsened. There was an oblong tightness of the upper abdominal region, soft underneath, from both sides to the navel. Excrement was thin and blackish. Urine was cloudy and blackish. He did not fall asleep during the night. There was much talking, laughter, and song. He could not control himself.

On the fourth day, it was the same.

On the fifth day, excrement was filled with bile, oily, and smooth. Urine was thin and translucent. He had brief periods of lucidity.

On the sixth day, there was slight sweating about the head. Extremities were cold and bluish gray. There was much restlessness. Nothing passed from the cavity. Urination ceased. Fever was acute.

On the seventh day, there was loss of speech. Extremities would no longer warm up. He did not urinate at all. There was acute fever.

On the eighth day, cold sweats everywhere. After sweats, small red spherical pustules, like acne, remained and did not abate. After slight stimulus, much thin stool, as if undigested, passed painfully from the cavity. Urination was painful and pungent. Extremities warmed a little. There was light sleep. He was lethargic. There was loss of speech. Urine was thin and translucent.

On the ninth day, it was the same.

On the tenth day, he did not take drinks. He was lethargic. There was light sleep. Stool remained the same. Urine was abundant and thick and had a white, grainy sediment when left to sit. Extremities were again cold.

On the eleventh day, he died. In this case, from the start through to the end, breathing [*pneuma*] was thin and deep. There was constant throbbing of the upper abdominal region. He was about twenty years old.

Book 1, Case 4. In Thasos,[2] the wife of Philinus gave birth to a daughter and had normal discharge and in other respects was doing well. Fourteen days after childbirth, a fever with cold shivers seized her. She felt pain, starting with the heart and the right side of the upper abdominal region. There was genital pain. The discharge ceased. These troubles were alleviated by a **pessary,** but pains of the head, neck, and loins remained. She did not sleep. Her extremities were cold. She was thirsty. Her cavity was inflamed. Little excrement passed. Urine was thin and at first colorless.

On the sixth day, at night she was greatly out of her senses but returned to her right mind.

On the seventh, she was thirsty. Excrement was slight, filled with bile, and deeply colored.

2. Thasos is an island in the northern Aegean Sea.

On the eighth day, she had cold shivers. There was acute fever. There were many convulsions accompanied by pain. She raved greatly. The use of a suppository caused her to get up to defecate and much excrement passed along with a discharge of fluid. She did not sleep.

On the ninth day, there were convulsions.

On the tenth, she came to her senses for short periods.

On the eleventh day, she slept. She remembered everything, but she again quickly lost her senses. With people only occasionally reminding her, she urinated. This was accompanied by spasms and there was much thick and white urine, like urine that was agitated after it had deposited sediment. But, in this case, the urine did not deposit sediment, though it was left sitting for a long time. Its color and thickness were like that of cattle's urine. I myself saw what her urine was like.

About the fourteenth day, there was throbbing throughout the whole body. She spoke a lot, but she quickly again lost her senses.

Around the seventeenth day, she became speechless.

On the twentieth day, she died.

Book 1, Case 14. Violent pain of the head, neck, and chest started to trouble Melidia, who lay sick by the temple of Hera.[3] At once an acute fever took hold. Slight menstrual bleeding appeared. Pains of all these parts were continuous.

On the sixth day, she was lethargic, nauseated, and shivering. Cheeks were red. She was slightly delirious.

On the seventh day, she sweated. Fever left. Her pains remained. She relapsed. There were short periods of sleep. Throughout, urine was a good color, but thin. Excrement passed that was thin, filled with bile, pungent, small, black, and foul-smelling. Sediment in the urine was white and smooth. She sweated.

On the eleventh day, she reached a perfect **crisis.**

Book 2, Case 2.8. The girl whose right hand and left leg were paralyzed after coughs, which lasted a short time and are not important, did not change otherwise—or certainly not much—in countenance or in mind. She started to get better around the twentieth day. It occurred around when her menses broke forth, which perhaps also happened then for the first time, for she had come of age.

Book 2, Case 3.11. Scopas had followed a poor regimen following discharges filled with bile and inflammation of the throat. And then his cavity was obstructed. There was an unbroken fever, his tongue was bright colored, and he did not sleep. There was distension of the abdomen, strongly, evenly, and eventually on the bottom right side. Breathing [*pneuma*] was somewhat quick. While he breathed or turned there was pain in the upper abdominal region. Without a cough, he spat up fairly thick matter.

3. Hera was the wife of Zeus, and a goddess associated with women and childbirth.

On the eighth day, the wartweed given expelled matter from the upper abdominal region, but this did not result in defecation.

On the next day, although two suppositories were given, no fecal matter appeared, but there was thick and cloudy urine with a uniform, consistent, and stable cloudiness. Then the belly was softer and the spleen was elevated and inclined downwards. For drink he had vinegar and honey.

On the tenth day, a little watery blood came from the left nostril, then not so little or weak. And urine passed that had sediment and, additionally, beneath the sediment, left smooth and whitish matter on the vessel, neither like nor unlike sperm in appearance. It dispersed in a short time.

On the next day, he reached a crisis. He was without fever.

On the eleventh day, he passed a somewhat sticky discharge and the accompanying fluid was filled with bile. There was a substantial purging of urine in quantity and with sediment. Before he started to drink some wine [the sediment was white, then][4] like scum.

On the eleventh day, though in small quantities, there passed sticky and cloudy matter like feces. Does this type of excrement point to a crisis of the sort of Antigenes?

Book 2, Case 4.5. The house servant of Stymarges, who did not bleed when she bore a daughter, had the mouth of her womb[5] turned back and there was pain in her hip joint and leg. After a vein was opened at the ankle, she recovered. Also, though, trembling seized her whole body. But one must approach the cause, and the source of the cause.

Book 4, Case 8. Around the setting of the Pleiades,[6] the wife of blind Maeandrias started to spit up matter that was sometimes green and sometimes like pus.

Around the sixth day, there was swelling of the liver and a little discharge of stool below. Above, there was purulent **flesh**. She spat up a small quantity of flat white matter. She did not eat. She died near the twentieth day.

Book 4, Case 14. In Crannon,[7] the wife of Nicostratus, who had had a seizure, suddenly experienced on the fourteenth day loss of control of the neck and of other parts. Food was locked up inside until the tenth day.[8] Breathing [*pneuma*] was frequent and short. There was loss of

---

4. The section in brackets is missing in the Greek text but can be reconstructed from a later commentary by **Galen** that directly quotes this case.

5. The mouth refers to the opening of the womb (see fig. 21). We believe that most ancient authors identified the mouth with what we now call the cervix, though some might have identified the mouth as the vaginal opening.

6. The Pleiades are a group of stars in the constellation Taurus. The rising of the Pleiades marked the beginning of summer, while the setting of the Pleiades marked the beginning of winter.

7. Crannon was a city in Thessaly, a region in central Greece.

8. The expression "food was locked up inside" likely means that she was constipated.

control. She groped about with her fingers, raved, and there were bouts of sweat. Neck was drawn towards the right, likewise mouth, eye, nose. Some sediment in her urine was white and like vetch seed, some was white and similar to filings, and some was yellowish and yolk-like. Sometimes there is fatty matter on the urine. This is concentrated, not spread out, like the separated, suspended matter of the sort that settles and then passes out in urine. Some of the urine was like this and some of it was stable. At another time, a little of it was dispersed in a flat region and at another time it was diffused. At another time, the suspended matter was like a darkish cloud and seemed to have substance, but was unsubstantial. At another time, it was thin. At another time, the suspended matter was thin. At another time, it was like horse urine. At another time, it was like darkish matter.[9]

Book 4, Case 20e. After the setting of the Pleiades, there were attacks of shivering and nose-bleeds. One man, the shoemaker, who had suffered very badly, reached a crisis on the seventh day. There was a break in the illness for one day and then it struck again for one day. He reached a crisis on the fourth day.

Another man of the household of Leocydes reached a crisis on the seventh day. Another man reached a crisis on the fourth day.

Moschus bled violently on the ninth day from the left nostril and slightly from the right. Towards the fourteenth day he reached a crisis, just as was necessary. It started and grew worse. There were errors in diet on the seventeenth day. To the right of the ear there was something hard inside and small, spongy, and painful outside. On the nineteenth day, during the night, it went away.

Book 4, Case 33. Olympiodorus' little girl bled from the right nostril. Around the twentieth day, she reached a crisis, like those suffering from fever. Her feces were like what is common there during the summer. On the eighth day, she suffered in the same way as Hipponax's wife and Aristeus' servant had.

Book 4, Case 36. The children suffered from an upset stomach and dry cough. During the later course of the cough, sometimes suppuration occurs on the shoulder. The fuller[10] suffered this on his head and neck. On the seventh day, his hand numbed and on the ninth day his leg. Numbness and cough ceased.

As for the woman with the twisted jaw, in the fifth month of her pregnancy, it was drawn to the left.

---

9. Some manuscripts include another sentence at the end of this paragraph, expressing surprise at the varieties of urine: "How many there were!" This sentence may belong to the original author or a later scribe copying the text.

10. A fuller is someone who cleans and mills cloth.

Book 4, Case 51. The slave in Muris' household did not seem to be in a sick state because, though she was delirious, she did not have a fever. Then she entered a state marked by trembling of the whole body, emaciation, loss of hunger, and thirst. She became cold.

Book 5, Case 9. In Athens, a man had itching over his whole body but especially on his testicles and forehead. He suffered terribly from this and the skin over his whole body was thick and looked like white scales. Nowhere could any of the skin be removed because of its thickness. No one could help this man. After he came to Melos,[11] where there are warm baths, he found relief from his itching and thick skin. But he contracted **dropsy** and died.

Book 5, Case 10. In Athens, an intestinal ailment seized a man and he suffered from vomiting, diarrhea, and pain. Neither the vomiting nor diarrhea could be stopped. He lost his voice and was unable to move from his bed. His eyes were misty and sunken. There were spasms from the intestine like hiccupping. There was by far more diarrhea than vomit. This man drank hellebore in lentil broth and also drank as much as he could of additional lentil broth. Then he vomited it out and was compelled to do it again. Both vomiting and diarrhea ceased. He became cold. He bathed his lower body up to the genitals in a lot of water until his upper body warmed. And he lived. On the next day he drank thin barley in water.

Book 5, Case 16. In Larisa,[12] Hippocomus, the eleven-year-old son of Palamedes, was struck on the forehead above the right eye by a horse. The bone did not seem healthy and a little blood spurted from it. This boy was **trepanned** extensively to the diploe.[13] Despite the state of his bone, which was previously festering, he was healed. On the twentieth day, a swelling began by the ear, and fever and shivering. During the day there was more swelling and it was painful. He had a fever that began with shivering. His eyes swelled and his face swelled. He suffered from these swellings more on the right side of the head, but the swelling also spread to the left. Really, this was not at all harmful. When the fever was coming to an end it became less continuous. These things lasted until the eighth day. After being **cauterized,** he lived, purging the swelling by drinking medicine, and by having it **plastered.** The wound was not at all the cause of his problems.

Book 5, Case 25. In Larisa, the servant of Dyseris in her youth suffered very severe pain whenever she had intercourse, but otherwise was free of pain. She never became pregnant. At the age of sixty, she suffered pain starting from midday, as though in stubborn labor. Before midday she had eaten many leeks. When pain seized her, very severe compared with earlier pains, she stood up and could feel something rough in the opening of her womb. Then, once she had fainted, another woman inserted her hand and squeezed out

---

11. Melos is an island in the southern Aegean Sea.

12. Larisa was a city in Thessaly, a region in central Greece.

13. "Trepanned to the diploe" means that a hole was bored to the spongy material between the outer and inner part of the skull.

a rough stone about the size of a spindle weight. Then at once and afterwards she was healthy.

Book 5, Case 26. The man from Malia:[14] a wagon ran over him and its weight passed over his ribs and broke some of them apart. Over time pus settled beneath the ribs. He was cauterized below the spleen and the wound was packed. He then carried on for ten months. After the skin was cut away, an opening in the peritoneum was visible that went in two directions, running in a putrid state to the kidneys and the bones. The state of his body was filled with bile, but no one noticed. In the body and in the unhealthy matter there was much putrefaction of the peritoneum and other flesh, which at once had to be evacuated, if one could, with a drying **drug,** while the man had some strength. For he did not improve at all from the moistening drugs, but his flesh putrefied. Since moisture was held by the packing, shivering took hold and a fever attacked and his flesh putrefied more. Rather dark, putrid, foul-smelling matter flowed out and before one endeavored to treat him, a lot of which escaped each day, but it did not have a healthy flow. It was recognized that the nature of the illness went deeper than just below the skin. If he had undergone all these treatments correctly, it nevertheless seems that he might not have been saved. Also, diarrhea afflicted him.

Book 5, Case 69. Melisander, whose gums became diseased, caused pain, and swelled severely, had a vein opened in his arm. Egyptian alum initially reduces swelling.

Book 5, Case 73. After the Dog Star,[15] fevers were accompanied by sweat and these did not cool down entirely after the sweat. Rather, they grew warmer again, were relatively long, did not reach a crisis, and were not accompanied by excessive thirst. In a few cases they ceased in seven days and nine days and reached a crisis on the eleventh, fourteenth, seventeenth, and twentieth. Polycrates' fever and the nature of his sweat were as described here. After a drug, purging below occurred and the characteristics of the fever were mild. Again, towards the evening there was sweating of the temples and around the neck and then over his whole body. The fever grew hotter again. The fever reached a pitch on the twelfth and fourteenth days. There were slight discharges of feces. After the purge, he took servings of gruel. Around the fifteenth day there was belly pain at the spleen and left side. Hot remedies helped less than cold. Through the use of a soft enema, his pain decreased.

Book 5, Case 83. The case of Phoenix: it seemed to him that many lights like lightning flashed from his right eye. After a short time a terrible pain developed in the right temple, then in his whole head and in his neck, where the head is joined to the vertebra behind. There was rigidity and hardness around the teeth. Straining, he would attempt to open them fully. His vomiting, whenever it happened, averted the aforementioned pains and made

---

14. Malia was a city in Thessaly, a region in central Greece.

15. The rising of the "Dog Star" (Sirius) was associated with the hottest summer days (whence the modern expression "dog days of summer").

them less harsh. Bloodletting helped and hellebore drinks expelled all sorts of matter, often the color of leeks.

Book 5, Case 100. In Cardia,[16] the son of Metrodorus suffered tooth pain, gangrene of the jaw, and a growth of flesh over his gums. Festering was moderate. His molars fell out and his jaw collapsed.

16. Cardia was a city in Thrace, a region to the north of Greece.

NINE

Common Complaints

The most common complaints we hear about in ancient sources have several things to teach us about the ancient Mediterranean world. First, common complaints reveal connections between ancient people's living and working conditions and the illnesses and ailments that troubled them. For example, they complain about health problems resulting from crowded and unhygienic living conditions (such as digestive and intestinal ailments, and epidemics), as well as injuries linked to dangerous workplace conditions (such as wounds and fractures). They also grumble about nuisances of the natural environment, including animal and arachnid bites and stings.

Second, common complaints provide a window into the physical and mental experiences of ancient people, giving us a glimpse of the illnesses and ailments that caused the most distress. In other words, common complaints reveal the health problems that were the most painful, caused the most fright and worry, and were considered most troublesome in terms of impairing functions necessary to daily routines or making a living. For example, our sources spend considerable time discussing ophthalmological problems (from sight impairments to injuries to the eye) and various forms of mental afflictions, both of which would have been disruptive to daily life. Other complaints signal the most pressing concerns for society as a whole. For example, a set of ailments categorized as "women's illnesses" relate almost exclusively to reproduction, revealing the societal concern to maintain a stable population in the face of a perennial demographic crisis. Likewise, the amount of attention given to the treatment of wounds incurred on the battlefield demonstrates the concern to maintain a healthy military.

In each section of this chapter, we describe a distinct ailment or set of related ailments that were common complaints for people in the ancient Mediterranean. We summarize the medical views on their causes and treatments, and situate the ailment(s) within the material and societal conditions of the time. When possible, we also address how these complaints show up in nonmedical sources.

WOMEN'S ILLNESSES

According to ancient medical writers, everyone experienced certain ailments, such as imbalances of **humors** or a body's overlaxity and overconstriction. Many medical writers also identified a set of illnesses experienced only by girls and women, a medical category called "gynecology" (deriving from the Greek word *gunē*, meaning "woman," and *logos*, meaning "explanation" or "theory").[1] Because these ailments related to reproduction they threatened not only the well-being of individual women but also that of society as a whole.

Ancient medical writers theorized that gynecological ailments stemmed from women's inferior anatomy and physiology, malformations that started in utero. All babies, they observed, had similar anatomical structures. That is, the penis, vas deferens, and testes in boys were equivalent to the vagina, Fallopian tubes, and ovaries in girls. Yet, they noticed, some of these anatomical parts protruded in male bodies, whereas they were located internally in female bodies. A wide range of thinkers, from philosophers like **Aristotle** to medical writers in the Hippocratic corpus and **Galen,** explained this internal/external difference in terms of the amount of heat present in the womb. More specifically, they regarded male bodies to be fully "cooked," and thus their genitalia to be fully developed and externalized; whereas female bodies were thought to be "undercooked," and thus their genitalia remained underdeveloped and were retained inside their bodies.

Moreover, medical writers assumed that the temperature of the womb in which a fetus developed influenced the temperature of their body throughout their lifetime, with men's bodies remaining hotter and women's bodies remaining colder throughout their lives. Body temperature was understood to have an impact on not only the anatomical development of genitalia, but also physiological functioning, such as digestion. As discussed later in this chapter (see the section on digestive and intestinal ailments), ancient medical writers described digestion as a **concoction** process in which food was cooked and mixed in the stomach. In a properly functioning body, digested food would be converted into blood that circulated, distributing nourishment throughout the body before being expelled in the form of urine, feces, sweat, and semen. Because women were colder, medical writers reasoned, they lacked the innate heat to digest their food as completely as men, resulting in a thicker, unrefined blood by-product that was difficult to expel. Additionally, because women's **flesh** was thought to be more loosely woven, porous, and spongy, women's bodies absorbed and

---

1. **Asclepiades of Bithynia**, on the contrary, did not believe there were any conditions that afflicted only women. He argued that since men and women were both made up of the same components, they were both susceptible to the same illnesses, and their bodies responded to the same set of treatments.

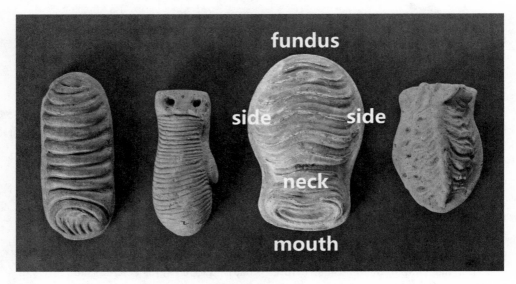

FIGURE 21 Collection of terracotta votives from Italy (dating 200 BCE–200 CE) in the shape of uteruses. Anatomical votives like these—clay and stone objects shaped to resemble body parts—were offered to the gods along with petitions for healing those parts. Labeled here are the parts of the uterus discussed in Texts 9, 10, 44, and 45. Science Museum (object no. A636075). © Science Museum Group.

retained more moisture than men's bodies, becoming saturated with the "wet" humors like blood.

Women's bodies ultimately had a way to expel their thick blood through a periodic discharge (the Latin term *mensis,* meaning "month," denoted the frequency of this periodic purge of blood), but it was regarded as less efficient than men's expulsion of digested food and also made women vulnerable to various ailments that did not afflict men. As enumerated in the Hippocratic text *Diseases of Women* (Text 9), for example, a woman's vagina might not be wide enough for the thick blood to pass through, the "mouth" (opening; see fig. 21) of the uterus might be closed or folded over such that the exit out of the body was blocked, the "mouth" of the uterus might be dislodged from the vagina such that the blood flowed to another part of the body rather than out the exit; the uterus might lack the strength to roll and coil sufficiently to push out the blood; or the menstrual fluid might be too thick to pass. For any of these reasons, menstrual blood that could not be evacuated backed up inside a woman's body. Backed-up blood was thought to cause pain wherever it amassed. And it was thought to be most harrowing when the blood collected around the organs, disrupting their proper functioning. For instance, blood collecting around the lungs could compromise breathing, and blood collecting around the heart—where some ancient philosophers and medical writers thought the rational mind was located—could cause mental and emotional distress.

The Hippocratic author of *Diseases of Women* also posits that women were susceptible to ailments related to "uterine suffocation" (what has come to be known as the "wandering womb"). As the womb was forced to work hard to evacuate thick menstrual blood, the Hippocratic author reasoned, it became overheated and dry. When this happened, the womb detached from its proper place, roamed around the body, and attached to organs from which it could soak up moisture. Like the problems associated with backed-up blood surrounding organs, so too the womb was thought to disrupt the functioning of organs to which it attached, crowding or blocking passages of respiration, for example, when attaching to the lungs, or causing mental and emotional distress when attaching to the heart. Moreover, because the opening of a wandering womb became misaligned from the vaginal exit, menstrual blood could not be evacuated, in turn triggering the myriad ailments related to backed-up blood.

A number of treatments were prescribed for these gynecological ailments. For backed-up blood, some physicians administered purgatives (ingested or delivered through suppositories) that would provoke the expulsion of the overabundant humor, either by thinning the blood or by relaxing the body. In the case of a womb that had roamed to the upper regions of a woman's body, physicians attempted to repel the womb downward by having the woman inhale foul smells (such as smoke produced by burning the horns of goats or deer, sulfur, and pitch), by inserting into her nostrils wool soaked in acrid mixtures, or by having her ingest a repulsive drink (such as castoreum, bitumen, and burnt pitch or burnt hair). Conversely, to lure a roaming womb back into place, physicians recommended **fumigating** a woman's vagina with sweet-smelling fragrances (such as cardamom, cumin, anise, fennel, and rose) or inserting pleasant-smelling **pessaries** into her vagina. **Aretaeus of Cappadocia** (second century CE) explained why these treatments worked: because the womb is an "animal within an animal [woman]" that "delights in fragrant smells and advances toward them; and has an aversion to foul smells and it flees from them" (*On the Causes and Symptoms of Acute Illnesses* 2.11). Still other treatments included **cupping**, bloodletting, bathing, herbal douches, massage (including digital palpation of the vagina), and binding the woman's midsection.

According to many ancient medical writers, however, the most effective treatments for women's illnesses were sexual intercourse, pregnancy, and childbirth. Intercourse and childbirth widened the vessels throughout the body (including the vagina), so that a woman's blood circulated more freely to the womb and purged more easily during her monthly evacuation. Still more, they reasoned, semen from intercourse heated and thinned the menstrual blood in the womb, making it easier to purge; semen also moistened the womb, so that it did not need to seek moisture elsewhere in the body. And once a woman was impregnated, the fetus weighed down her womb, anchoring it in place, and accustomed the woman's body to being "full," so that backed-up blood caused fewer health problems in the future.

Historians have noticed how ancient gynecology buttressed the interests of elite men and the state. First, it entrenched men's superior status by grounding a gender hierarchy in anatomical distinctions. Second, the dominant treatments for women's illnesses—especially pregnancy and childbirth—ultimately served the reproductive interests of elite households (who wanted to pass on their family name and wealth to heirs), while also serving the reproductive interests of the state (which was continually dealing with population shortages).

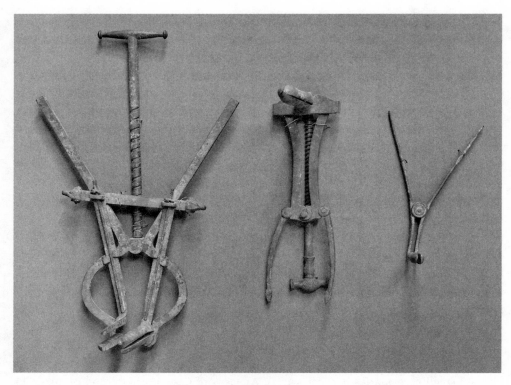

FIGURE 22 Collection of Roman specula, 50 CE. When physicians/obstetricians needed to dilate an opening of the body—such as the anus, vagina, cervix, and sometimes a wound—they used various kinds of specula (singular: speculum). These dilators allowed them to see more clearly during physical inspections; to have more space to perform surgeries, such as repairing fistula; to access the uterus during examinations or childbirth; and to insert medications, such as pessaries. Specula could have four, three, or two blades (quadrivalve, trivalve, and bivalve, *left to right*), and they could open via a screw mechanism (*left and middle*) or manually by squeezing together the handles (*right*). Moreover, the blades varied in length to match the depth of the canal into which they were inserted. Aëtius warned physicians to be careful using a device of the incorrect size because it might perforate internal parts. To make the procedure less uncomfortable, Aëtius also suggests that padding be placed between the device and the patient's skin, and Muscio recommends that the device be lubricated with oil and warmed. Wellcome Collection. Attribution 4.0 International (CC BY 4.0).

Even though societal assumptions about women's inferiority remained in place across ancient gynecological sources, explanations of women's illnesses did develop over time. In his dissections **Herophilus** observed the ligaments and vessels that fastened the uterus in place, and thus by the second century CE many medical writers no longer believed the womb roamed around the body. Replacing the earlier theory, Galen instead explained that women's ailments stemmed from the blood and (female) semen that were trapped in the uterus, where they rotted. The decay poisoned the womb, which either swelled to interfere with neighboring organs or spread to other parts of the body. Galen also suggested that the blood vessels that fed the uterus could become congested and enlarged, causing it to tense and contract. Such uterine contractions, Galen explained, might make it *appear* as if the uterus were on the move.[2]

Soranus of Ephesus (second century CE) seemed to be the most dramatic outlier in terms of rethinking women's health. Soranus did not assume that a lack of menstruation was a sign of ill health; in fact, he noted that menses became irregular or ceased altogether in older women, pregnant women, and women with "manly" lifestyles (i.e., those engaged in heavy labor or athletic activity), and yet these women remained healthy. He concluded that treatments prescribed for women's illnesses, thus, were not always necessary, and could even be dangerous. For example, he warned that suppositories and fumigations could cause inflammation and ulcers in the uterus, or could inadvertently induce abortions. Additionally, Soranus noted that at the young age (around fourteen years old) when a girl began menstruating and when physicians began to prescribe sex, pregnancy, and childbirth as medical treatments, her uterus was too underdeveloped and her vagina was too narrow to endure such treatments; thus they endangered her life. (A contemporary of Soranus, **Rufus of Ephesus**, agreed and advised that pregnancy should wait until girls reached the age of eighteen.) Finally, for girls and women of all ages, Soranus observed that pregnancy and childbirth were far from healthful, but rather drained the body, and sometimes resulted in death.[3]

One of our most interesting gynecological sources of late antiquity was authored by a woman who went by the name of **Metrodora**, which in Greek means "gifts of the uterus." In this source (Text 10), Metrodora largely adopts the Hippocratic view that most of women's illnesses relate to problems with the womb. That said, she describes ailments beyond backed-up blood and the wandering womb, discussing also inflammation, abscesses, hemorrhages, and prolapse of the womb. Moreover, she combines traditional gynecological theory with humoral theories (or theories of hot/cold, wet/dry). And finally she asserts that not all symptoms women present arise from uterine troubles.

Although these ancient gynecological ideas might sound strange to modern readers, some of them remained influential until very recently. For example, the medieval and early modern condition of "hysteria"—a term that derives from the Greek word for "uterus" and that combined the symptoms of several ancient ailments into a single malady—is rooted in the ancient ideas about women's emotional and mental instability being related to ailments of their reproductive organs.

2. Around the time the theory of the roaming womb was losing favor, we find a proliferation of amulets inscribed with wombs and magical formulas, suggesting that the women who bought and wore the amulets found other ways to understand and deal with their troubling wombs. We also have numerous extant votives that would have been offered to the gods along with petitions for protection or healing for gynecological conditions (see fig. 21).

3. Although Soranus concluded that lifelong virginity was most healthful for women, he was still steeped in a culture that prized reproduction; thus he understood it to be women's primary role.

TEXT 9. HIPPOCRATIC CORPUS, *DISEASES OF WOMEN* SELECTIONS (1.1–2, 4–7)

Diseases of Women *was attributed to* **Hippocrates,** *but as with all the texts in the Hippocratic corpus, the authorship is uncertain. The author appears to have been a specialist in the reproductive health of women, compiling three texts that discuss this subject from several perspectives. The work of compilation likely happened in the late fifth or early fourth century BCE. The focus of much of Book 1, selections from which are presented below, is on issues relating to menstruation, with an emphasis on how to ensure that women are capable of becoming pregnant and that they bear healthy children. The author also makes clear the importance of regular sexual activity for the good health of women.*

In the translation, the notation sc. *(an abbreviation of the Latin* scilicet, *which means "certainly") appears where the translator is supplying a word or idea that is not explicitly spelled out in the Greek text.*

SOURCE: Translated by Paul Potter based on the Greek text from Paul Potter, *Hippocrates, Diseases of Women 1–2,* Loeb Classical Library 538 (Cambridge, Mass.: Harvard University Press, 2018). Copyright ©2018 by the President and Fellows of Harvard College. Loeb Classical Library ® is a registered trademark of the President and Fellows of Harvard College.

Book 1, Chapter 1. Concerning diseases of women: I assert that a woman who has not borne children becomes ill from her menses more seriously and sooner than one who has borne children. For when a woman has given birth, her small vessels allow a freer flow for her menses, since the lochial cleaning makes them fluent. Also, if there has been an involution of her body, it is the parts nearest to the **cavity** and breasts that involute, although the rest of the body involutes too—why this occurs I have explained in *Nature of the Child in Childbirth.* As the body involutes, the vessels are forced to dilate more and to allow a freer flow for the menses: the uterus too must dilate more, as the child moving through it causes straining and stretching. These things being so, a woman will clean out her menses with less difficulty once she has experienced the lochia. Also, if some condition that prevents the menses from being cleaned befalls a woman who has previously borne children, she will bear the trouble more easily than if she had not borne children, since her uterus and the rest of her body are accustomed to being full, just as they are in a woman who is pregnant, and at the same time there is more open space for blood in her body after she has given birth, since her body has involuted, so that the blood, being in an open space, will be less troublesome, as long as the vessels do not overfill and overstretch.

Since in a woman who has not given birth the body is not accustomed to being filled up (sc. with blood), but is robust, solider and denser than if she had experienced the lochia, and her uterus has not been dilated, her menstrual flow will be accompanied by more pain, and more troubles will be present: i.e., her menses will be obstructed when she has not given birth. This is so for the reason I first indicated when I contended that a woman is more porous and softer than a man; this being so, a woman's body draws what is being exhaled from her cavity more quickly and in a greater amount than does a man's.

Thus, if someone sets both some clean flocks of wool and a clean densely woven carpet of exactly the same weight as the flocks over water or a moist location for two days and two nights, on removing them he will discover, on weighing them, that the flocks have become much heavier than the carpet. This happens because (sc. moisture) always moves up away from water present in a wide-necked vessel, and flocks, being porous and soft, take up a greater quantity of what is moving away, while a carpet, being compact and densely woven, becomes saturated without accepting much of what is moving toward it.

In the same way, a woman, being more porous, will draw into her body more of what is being exhaled from her cavity, and more quickly, than a man does. Also, because a woman's **flesh** is softer, when her body fills up with blood, unless the blood is then discharged from her body, the filling and warming of her tissues that ensue will provoke pain: for a woman has hotter blood, and for this reason she herself is hotter than a man;[4] if, however, most of the blood that was added is subsequently discharged, no pain will arise from it. A man, having solider flesh than a woman, will never overfill with so much blood that, unless some of it is discharged each month, he feels pain, and besides he takes in only as much (sc. blood) as is necessary for the nourishment of his body, and his body—lacking softness as it does— is never overstretched or heated by fullness as a woman's is. A great amount of this is also due, in a man, to his exerting himself physically more than a woman, which consumes a part of the exhalation (sc. rising from his food).

Chapter 2. Now when, in a woman who has not given birth, the menses fail to appear and cannot find their way out, a disease arises, and this happens if the mouth[5] of the uterus is closed or folded over, or some part of the vagina has become constricted; for if any of these things happens, the menses will be unable to find their way out until the uterus returns to a natural healthy state. This disease generally occurs in women whose uterus has a narrow mouth or its neck[6] lying further forward into the vagina. For if either of these be the case, and the woman does not have intercourse with her husband, and her cavity is more empty than it should be as the result of some disease, the uterus turns aside. For it has no moistness of its own, since the woman is not having intercourse, and there is an open space for it since the cavity is too empty, so that it turns aside because it is drier and lighter than it should be. And sometimes as it turns aside its mouth becomes displaced too far to one side

4. The author takes an unusual position here, opposite from the view of most ancient medical writers that women were colder than men.

5. The mouth referred to the opening of the uterus (see fig. 21). We believe that most ancient authors had in mind what we now call the cervix, though some might have identified the mouth as the vaginal opening.

6. The neck referred to the area just behind the mouth (i.e., the opening of the uterus; see fig. 21). If the author understood the mouth to be the cervix, then the neck would be the area directly behind the cervix. If the author understood the mouth to be the vaginal opening, then the neck would be the vaginal canal.

because its neck is lying too far into the vagina. For if the uterus is moist as the result of intercourse and the cavity is not empty, it is not likely to turn aside. This is why the uterus closes as the result of a woman not having intercourse.

. . .

Chapter 4. If a woman's menses flow, but less than they should, due to the mouth of her uterus being slightly inclined away from her vagina, or closed although still having a gap, so that although they flow they are obstructed from these things † . . . and the passages which penetrate through . . . †[7] for when they have come down into the uterus, since exactly the middling amount of blood is always pressing on the mouth, they flow a little at a time. Then, when the days arrive on which she has been accustomed to be cleaned, and blood is left behind enclosed in her uterus, and additional menses coming down on top of this do not expel the blood that is closed in, but this gradually weighs the woman down, it is still possible that she will not perceive this very much for the first two or three months. But as months pass by, her suffering will continually increase, and she will not become pregnant as long as this persists; fever will seize her, especially on the days when she was accustomed to be cleaned, although of a mild sort. It is likely in the intervening times, too, for her to have fever, chills, and heartburn, and to suffer pain generally in her body at various times of the day, especially in her loins, back and groins; in the joints of her arms and legs she will also suffer pain. These things the patient does not suffer all at one time, but now and then, in whichever part the blood that is being excreted weighs her down since it cannot enter her uterus. Wherever blood becomes fixed in the body, edema occasionally forms, together with violent spasms of the body's joints; also, some of the other signs described above appear in the woman at one time or another.

If this patient is treated in the proper way, she will recover, but if not, the disease will continue for seven months or longer, and she will die or become lame, or lose command over some of her limbs, if, as the result of chilling or her failure to eat, the blood, wherever it happens to go, congeals around the cords. This disease occurs more often in unmarried women: if on the other hand the diseases which have been, or are about to be described befall women who have borne children, they will be of longer duration but less troublesome. The same signs and outcomes pertain both to a woman who has not borne children and to one who has experienced the lochia, if they go untreated. Treatment must be applied immediately: if not, the diseases will become manifest.

Chapter 5. If the menses flow more than they should and thicker, due to the woman's body being by nature wide open and the orifice of her uterus lying near her vagina, and besides she has frequent intercourse with her husband, and she then at some time overindulges herself (sc. at table), a great volume of menses will descend, and through their pressure forcefully widen the mouth of her uterus even more. And if no emptying of the vessels supervenes, but a further great flux occurs and widens the mouth yet more, and the patient's body—as the result of her overindulgence and having intercourse with her husband—has

7. Some words from the Greek text are missing here.

passages open to the uterus so that a massive flux occurs, she will remain pale as long as this state persists; and if later some disease or affection emaciates her body, her uterus will continue in its usual widemouthed state, and her body will remain fluent with it.

After this, fever will set in, the woman will fail to eat, she will be distressed, she will become thin and feeble from her menses, and she will suffer pain in her lower back; with time, unless treatment is applied, her pains will increase in the time between the menses, she will run the risk of becoming barren and emaciated due to the disease and its chronicity, and if some other disease befalls her in addition, she will perish from it.

Chapter 6. The menses flow thickest and in the greatest amount on the days in their middle, in less quantity and thinner when they are beginning and ending. In every healthy woman the amount of the menstrual flux to pass is equal to two Attic **cotyles,** or a little more or less—this over two or three days if the time is more or less than this, it indicates disease and barrenness. You must gather evidence by inspecting the patient's body and asking her how her previous menses were in comparison, and whether or not they were unhealthy. For if they pass for more or less days than they are used to, or in a greater or less quantity, this indicates malignancy, unless the woman is by nature diseased or barren.

If the case is such, and then there is a change in the direction of better health, it will be better. If a woman is healthy, her menstrual blood will pass like that of a sacrificial animal, and it will quickly congeal. But women who are naturally cleaned for more than four days and who pass very copious menses will become thin and have fetuses that are thin and weak. Those in whom the cleaning occurs for less than three days or in a small amount will be stout, of a good color, and manly, but not prolific or likely to become pregnant.

Chapter 7. If suffocation suddenly occurs, this happens mainly in women that are not having intercourse with men, and more in older women than in younger ones: for their uterus is lighter. Generally it comes about as follows: When a woman has empty vessels and exerts herself more than she is used to as her uterus is warmed by the exertion, it turns to the side because it is empty and light: for there is open space into which it can turn, seeing that the cavity is empty. In turning to the side (sc. the uterus) falls against the liver and comes into contact with it, and then it falls against the hypochondria. For it moves rapidly upward toward the moisture, since it has been excessively dried by the exertion, and the liver is full of moisture. On falling against the liver, the uterus immediately produces suffocation by occupying the air space around the cavity. Sometimes, simultaneously with the uterus' first contact with the liver, phlegm also flows down from the head into the hypochondria as a result of the woman's suffocation, so that sometimes with this simultaneous defluxion of phlegm, the uterus moves away from the liver back to its own location and the suffocation ceases. The uterus moves back down in this way on filling with moisture and becoming heavy, and a gurgling sound arises from it when it returns to its natural location. After it arrives there, sometimes the belly is moister than it was before; for the head has already released phlegm into the cavity. When the uterus is lying against the liver and the hypochondrium, and thereby provoking suffocation, the patient turns the whites of her eyes up, and becomes cold; some immediately turn livid. She may also grind her teeth, salivate in her mouth, and take on the appearance of people suffering from Hercules' disease (epilepsy). If a woman's uterus stays against her liver and hypochondria for a longer time, she chokes to death.

Sometimes, when a woman has empty vessels and she exerts herself, her uterus turns away and falls against the orifice of her bladder, bringing on strangury; but there is no further trouble, and on being treated she will quickly recover—sometimes even spontaneously. In some women, as the result of their exerting themselves and going without food, (sc. the uterus) falls against the loin or hips and causes pain.

TEXT 10. METRODORA, *ON THE CONDITIONS OF THE WOMB* SELECTION (1–19)

*On the Conditions of the Womb, authored by **Metrodora** (first to sixth century CE), discusses a variety of gynecological conditions and treatments. This text is especially significant because it is the only medical text attributed to a woman author to survive from Greco-Roman antiquity. (The name Metrodora means "gifts of the uterus" in Greek, so there is a chance that this was not the author's real name but rather a moniker related to her area of expertise.) Many of the gynecological ideas and treatments in this text draw from the Hippocratic tradition, but the text also provides content and recipes for cures that appear in no other ancient text. The first nineteen sections of the text, focusing on conditions that might affect the womb, are presented below. The remainder of the text discusses additional ailments of the womb, as well as conception and contraception, childbirth, conditions of the breasts, and the beautification of the body.*

SOURCE: Translation by Tara Mulder based on the Greek text from G. Del Guerra, *Il libro di Metrodora: Sulla malattie delle donne e il ricettario di cosmetica e terapia* (Milan: Ceschina, 1953).

Chapter 1. Female conditions are many and varied, but all, so to speak, concern the womb. It is thus necessary to write down the ***sumptōmata***[8] that accompany the conditions of the womb. For some of these conditions are difficult to treat and others are entirely incurable, and we identify each of these through examination. Let us start with uterine suffocation.

Since generally uterine suffocation arises in most women, let us start with it. Whenever the uterus is disturbed it attacks itself, from which strong pains overcome the woman. Unless these pains are quickly relieved, the uterus gradually festers with time in these places. Thus whenever the uterus attacks the upper abdominal regions it causes suffocation, just as from hellebore. And immediately sharp heart pains arise. Women vomit as soon as

---

8. We have left the Greek word *sumptōma* (plural: *sumptōmata*) untranslated because it lacks an exact equivalent in English. A *sumptōma* is something that happens, sometimes, but not always, with the implication that what has happened is bad or undesirable. See the word's glossary entry for more details.

the mouth fills up with a great quantity of wet saliva and numbness grips the head and tongue. You may comprehend that these sorts of women are speechless and that they have clenched teeth. Give them to apply to the uterus a ball of wool dipped in myrtle oil, or in marjoram, or in white lily, or in some other sweet-smelling oil. Apply to the nostrils a **fumigation** of bitumen or of the horn of a black goat or black cumin or castor. Coat the nostrils. Make sure that the application of the wool is continuous, so that the condition does not return again. But if the uterus occupies the space underneath, a groin swelling arises. Sharp pain occurs in the urethra, and numbness in the legs; sometimes it blocks up the urethra. One must therefore treat these things.

Apply to the nostrils everything sweet-smelling: a stick of cinnamon, a leaf of ginger, and all the sweet-smelling things you have. And apply to the uterus a fumigation of wild mint and use this same method until it returns to its place. Among widows in their prime or virgins, who have passed the right age for marriage, and who because of the lack [of intercourse] suffer in the uterus because their natural desire is dormant, a number of conditions arise: sharp heart pain, vomiting, and salivating. Also, the legs grow cold, the head and tongue grow numb, and simply put, all conditions associated with uterine suffocation arise. They must therefore be treated in this way: first of all, if the condition is sudden, know how to use all the things I have said were appropriate for uterine suffocation. Among these women it is the womb, in its displacement, which provokes these *sumptōmata*. Also, especially among widows, and virgins use wax salves made beforehand with dill and cardamom. Grinding them all and making them into a **plaster,** apply it to the vagina. It provokes the expulsion of watery matter and puts a stop to the condition.

Chapter 2. Odors for Mute Women
Throw the fumigation materials on the coals, to bring together and urge the women to ingest the fumigations with every inhalation. For example: jet stone, goat horn, castor, milt waste, softened yellow rue to apply to the nostrils, or apply ground brimstone, white hellebore, or ostrich root.

Chapter 3. Drink for Uterine Suffocation
Make her drink castor with wine, add rue ground up with honey. Alternatively, infuse pig dung in rose oil and apply in a **pessary.** Wet excrement, mix it with wine until smooth, heat it with honey and apply.

Chapter 4. For Inflammation of the Womb
We have first laid out uterine suffocation, the arising *sumptōmata* and the remedies. So now let us turn to womb inflammations, indicating clearly the relief for each part.

When the whole uterus is inflamed, intense heat occurs around the lower abdomen and hardness and pain of the loins and shaking and swelling of the stomach. There is vomiting of mucus, acid, and bile. There is also difficulty urinating, stoppage of the **cavity,** lack of appetite, and thirst. The tongue is rough and darkened, as though tinted with something black.

There is pain in the neck and a spreading chill. So then, if you put your finger on the vagina, you will feel a lot of heat and dryness and closing and throbbing of the mouth[9] of the womb.

How it must be treated: make a pessary for the inflamed womb and add Indian spikenard. Apply a **clyster** of butter and deer marrow mixed together. Apply in a pessary and **poultice** fresh marshmallow leaves and fenugreek and crushed flaxseed and goose fat with black antimony. These remedies all pertain to inflammation of the womb.

Let us turn to inflammation of the uterus by parts. When the fundus[10] of the womb is affected, fever, vomiting, nausea and secretions and pains of the stomach and headaches often accompany it. If you apply your finger and touch the mouth of the womb, since parts of the affected organ are cold, the mouth of the womb is cold. If the inflammation is in front, pains and hardness and a mass accompany it, a strong discomfort in the whole lower abdomen, strangury, a pain of the loins, constipation, and especially when the neck[11] of the uterus is inflamed. All these things are combined and as many as were laid out above.

In the case of inflammation in the front of the womb, it takes hold of the mouth, which is ulcerated because of the ulceration of the inflamed parts. This is called torsion. In inflammation of the back of the womb, torsion is in the back part. When the sides are affected, the torsion of the mouth of the womb happens on the sides. Among these women, therefore, the leg on the inflamed side is painful and swollen and there is pain in the sides and the flanks. These same signs occur both when the whole womb is inflamed and when only a part of it is. Apply the remedies accordingly, as I have said: butter and deer marrow and goose or bird fat. Apply them mixed together and with a pessary made from wool. Women who have intercourse with a man and who suffer from the womb during sex have a face with large veins rather than the clear one they had at first.[12] But when the condition persists they grow pale due to inflammation in the mouth of the womb, or rather the womb is pushed out from inside. A sign among these women is that the corners of their eyes are in pain. Therefore treat these manifestations of the condition in the following way: take the milk of a woman who has borne a male child and heat it, then make it into a pessary and apply it to the mouth of the womb. Or take the yoke of an egg along with rose oil and make it into a pessary, then apply it. Another remedy: two ounces of frankincense, two ounces of goose fat, two ounces of butter, and a sufficient quantity of honey. Make a pessary and apply it. Another fragrant

9. The mouth referred to the opening of the womb (see fig. 21). We believe that most ancient authors had in mind what we now call the "cervix," though some might have identified the mouth as the vaginal opening.

10. The fundus referred to the bottom of the womb (see fig. 21).

11. The neck referred to the area just behind the mouth (i.e., the opening of the womb; see fig. 21). If the author understood the mouth to be the cervix, then the neck would be the area directly behind the cervix. If the author understood the mouth to be the vaginal opening, then the neck would be the vaginal canal.

12. Metrodora seems to be referring here to the belief, common in the Greco-Roman world, that a woman would undergo significant physical changes, including to her face and complexion, when she first had vaginal intercourse.

pessary: two ounces of rush blossom and balsam wood, two ounces of costus root, two ounces of ginger and saffron, six grams of aromatic reed, and honey in sufficient quantity. Another pessary: sixteen ounces of turpentine and sixteen ounces of dried grapes with seeds removed. Chop up and apply.

Chapter 5. For Pains of the Lower Belly and for Women Bitten by a Snake
Crush celery with kohl and goose fat and apply in a pessary. Alternatively, take equal parts balsam tree sap, spikenard, and turpentine with three ounces of beeswax, three ounces of deer marrow, two ounces of hyssop, two ounces of saffron, four ounces of turpentine, two ounces of duck fat, four ounces of egg yolk, and a sufficient amount of rose oil. Alternatively, crush and apply honey, butter, Cyprian olive oil, and turpentine.

Chapter 6. For Abscesses of the Womb
Among those who have an abscess of the womb, at first the breasts of the woman swell and become hard and fever and chill occur and a hot discharge runs out from the vagina. Such women cannot bear to be touched until the abscess is broken and the pus flows out. Then the throbbing pain stops for a little while. These same women belch up dense, acidic, and somewhat bitter things. These sorts of women lack an appetite for food. Most of them therefore remain anxious. Therefore, treat in the following way: twigs of myrtle and cypress, spikenard, and corn. Boil these together in water, add honey, natron, warm it and wash the womb with it. After this, wash it again with wine. And smear on butter or deer marrow and goose or bird fat.

Chapter 7. For Hardening Conditions of the Womb
Among those women who have hard conditions of the uterus there occur fever, chills, thickening of the skin, and swelling in the lower abdomen and it remains like stone and numb. Some have called this *skleros* ("the hard thing"), others call it a *mulos* ("millstone") because it is found to be hard like a stone. Pains arise in the bladder and rectum and what was mentioned before for abscesses. Therefore treat in the following way: to soften the hardness of the ulcer, apply cerates made with wax, from resin, from butter, and all the things I have mentioned for abscesses.

Chapter 8. For Crab-Like Afflictions of the Uterus[13]
Among those women who have crab-like conditions in the uterus, the following *sumptōmata* occur: pain of the bladder and the rectum as if the mouth of the womb contained a piece of wood and a splinter. There is sometimes also discharge of blood with urine, with the result that it seems necessary to treat them in this way. Apply a preparation of wild beet, alum, and

13. The English word "cancer" derives from a Greek word originally meaning "crab-like." This was a reference to the swollen veins that might surround a tumor, leading some ancient observers to think this looked like a crab. References in ancient Greek texts to "crab-like conditions" might match up with modern diagnoses of cancer, but ancient physicians also applied this label to a variety of other conditions that modern physicians would not identify as cancer.

Greek sodium carbonate to soften the hardness of the ulcer. Crush these things and make a plaster for all afflictions and crab-like ulcers in the womb and in the whole body. After this apply in a pessary the juice of a nightshade with goose fat in equal quantities.

Chapter 9. On Red and White Womanly Flux

The womanly flux is a perceptible and prolonged discharge that comes from the uterus, that can be distinguished mainly by watery, or red, bloody, or even black **humor**, without pain, sometimes also with pain and labored breathing, swelling of the feet, and pain around the eyes. The woman has a greenish color in the corner of her eye, her head is a little hot, and there is a persistent fever within her whole body, which occurs in an irregular fashion. Therefore treat in the following way: take a very old cork out of a jar, burn it completely on a branch of wood, crush it and give two seeds' worth mixed with a ladle of sour wine mixed with water, morning and evening, with woman's milk. Place it in her genitals in a pessary.

Chapter 10. For Hemorrhages That Occur at the Mouth of the Womb

Hemorrhages can occur around the mouth of the womb, when the period stops and blood accumulates from the intertwining of veins and nerves and produces a protrusion of **flesh.** It is therefore necessary to use a speculum to know the place affected and to inject the remedies there. Therefore treat in the following way: take thorn tips, chop and make a powder, sprinkle it over the area and it will be dried up.

Chapter 11. For a Womb That Has Fallen Out

When the uterus falls to the outside, have the woman lie on an inclined bed, pour hot butter into the womb, then [. . .] of rose oil.[14] [. . .] apply castor oil with butter to the uterus, raise the legs so it does not come out. In order to reach the womb, inject gall nut and alum with a *mētrengchutēs*.[15] Inject warmed dark wine mixed with sea water in sufficient quantity. When the womb has been washed on the inside, cross the feet of the woman and bind with a simple knot. Let her rest, lying on the inclined bed, the feet at the top and the head at the bottom, until the womb returns to its place.

Chapter 12. For the Uterus Which Hangs Out Because of Prolapse, and Swells for This Reason

Whenever the uterus has fallen out of the body and stays outside for a long time and swells up and is full of serous fluid, foment it with a decoction of beet, and, after the douche, pour a pungent vinegar over the uterus and after the pouring of the vinegar, sprinkle fine salt on it. After the salt is dissolved, wash clean with a decoction of beet and draw up in the aforementioned manner, along with a vapor bath. And take care of the intestines and the diet so that they are not thrown into confusion. And introduce sneeze inducers for those who are in good health and the most fragrant incense.

14. Some words from the Greek text are missing here.
15. A *mētrengchutēs* was a special syringe used for making injections into the womb.

Chapter 13. For the Womb That Falls Out

With a decoction of beet or fenugreek or flax or some other sort of washing plant, anoint the womb itself with cedar oil or with myrtle or with old urine or with urine sediments. Alternatively, crush and apply in a pessary eight **drachmas** of beeswax, sixteen drachmas of bone marrow, one drachma of opium, one drachma of saffron, and a sufficient quantity of rose oil.

Chapter 14. For the Womb Filled with Worms

Whenever worms in the intestines press on the uterus, there arises in these women a pain around the womb and an itch around the genitals and the stomach and a moistness around the vagina, to the point that it seems to be afflicted by discharge. Treat in the following way: mix iris root and the heated juice of sweet sumac and administer in a wash whenever the woman urinates. Repeat frequently until she is healed.

Chapter 15. For Chills of the Womb

For those women who have caught a chill and who suffer from strangury because of the cold, and for other conditions arising in the womb because of the cold. Treat in the following way: about one drachma each of turpentine and nard, six drachmas of catmint, and one drachma of vinegar. Chop the dry ingredients, add them to the wet and apply in a pessary to the mouth of the womb.

Chapter 16. For Winds in the Mouth of the Womb

All the women who have pain in the uterus, in the small part of the cavity, in the loin and groin, as well as the jaw, for these women a wind [*pneuma*] has arisen and occupies the cavity, from which the pain comes, and it is trapped. Treat these women in the following way: mix equal quantities of butter and deer marrow with the yolk of a cooked egg. Crush and mix well with rose oil, making it like honey in consistency. Put the mixture on a wool pessary and apply to the mouth of the womb.

Chapter 17. For Dropsy of the Womb

Whenever mucus from the nostril area passes through to the womb, and women have sickly eyes and they are hot in this part of the body, for these women dropsy arises in the womb. Treat in the following way: crush up and mix cumin, raisins, and a little bit of salt, insert it into a pessary of wool and apply it.

Chapter 18. For Wombs Filled with Humors

All the women whose wombs are filled with viscous humors have a vagina that becomes moist. But the front part of the head and the corners of the eye especially become bloodshot and there arise continuous fevers without an obvious cause. Treat in the following way: chop up together three parts of boiled mandrake root, one part of bitter cucumber, one part of wool stuffing, mix with the milk of a woman, make elongated sticks, and apply them having previously bathed the area in hot water.

Chapter 19. For Very Wet Uteruses

All the women who have very wet uteruses have very cold vaginas, incapable of adapting to the heat of a man for conception. In fact, a cold liquid flows from her vagina. Therefore, it is treated in the following way: chop equal parts of pine bark and quince, make into a powder, and give to be applied. Then let her wash in a decoction of rushes, myrtle, and wine. I also use this remedy for making incisions and for women who have miscarried.

DIGESTIVE AND INTESTINAL AILMENTS

According to ancient medical writers, digestion began in the mouth, where the teeth and saliva began to break down food. Next, food was further disintegrated by being mixed and "cooked" in the stomach ("**concoction**" using the body's innate heat), though others thought that food was further digested by being ground up or by rotting in the stomach. The digested food was then carried to the liver, where some of it was converted into blood, which then circulated throughout the body, bringing nourishment to all of its parts. Eventually, the hot, fluid parts of the blood evaporated and were expelled in the form of sweat, urine, and semen, while the "earthy" parts of blood cooled and conjoined with the **flesh**, organs, tissue, bones, nails, and skin.

Yet, according to ancient medical thinkers, there were numerous ways digestion could go wrong. If the body lacked sufficient heat to transform food fully into blood, it could remain in a thick state that was difficult to evacuate (such as, for example, the women's ailment described above) or it could mutate into a **humor** other than blood, leading to imbalance in the body. If the veins were underdilated or became blocked, the blood in the veins backed up, in turn causing food to back up in the stomach, leading to nausea and indigestion. Moreover, when the veins were underdilated or blocked, the nutrients could not reach the body, causing weakness. If the stomach became weak—from, for instance, seasickness, overeating or overdrinking, ingesting food the stomach was not used to, overly seasoned food, or something harmful (such as bad water or a poison)—the stomach could not properly perform its digestive functions. And, finally, if the body was too constricted, it retained food so long that it backed up in the stomach or intestines and sometimes rotted there. Or if the body was too relaxed it discharged the food too quickly, before it was fully digested.

Caelius Aurelianus's *Chronic Conditions* catalogs the variety of digestive and intestinal ailments people in the ancient Mediterranean experienced, describing their symptoms and recommending treatments (Text 11). As Caelius taught physicians to discriminate between a range of conditions, he urged physicians to take careful observations of their patients' evacuations (such as the colors of their stool, its odor, and the sounds the body made during defecation), as well as the condition of the body that accompanied the ailments (such as fever, distention, cramps, flatulence, weakness, pallor, swelling, lack of appetite, etc.). Caelius's guide was particularly useful to physicians attempting to distinguish between ailments with similar symptoms. For example, Caelius notes several conditions that all cause loose stool: including *koiliakos* (an ailment that gets its name from the Greek word *koilia*, meaning "the belly" or, more literally, "the hollow **cavity** of the abdomen where the person experienced distress"), diarrhea,[16] and dysentery.[17] Caelius aimed to teach readers how to distinguish between these ailments by paying attention to the degree and quality of the discharge, the duration of the illness, whether pain and cramping accompanied the discharge, and from which end fluid was discharged (i.e., vomiting from the mouth, loose stool from the anus, or both).

Caelius also discussed varieties of worm infestations. In agreement with most medical writers, he believed that rotting food in the stomach or intestines gave rise to worms. We imagine that theories like this were devised by analogy: ancient people imagined what was happening inside their bodies based on what they saw in the world around them. And just as they observed "worms"—what we call maggots—in rotting corpses or food, so too the worms inside their bodies must have been generated from rotting material. Using similar reasoning, one Hippocratic author asserted that worms were most prevalent in pregnant women, explaining that when the fetus defecated in utero and when that feces rotted, it gave rise to worms. Worms were also thought to be more prevalent among people who ate too much; their digestion presumably could not keep up with the volume, hence the food rotted in the stomach and produced worms.

When treating ailments of the stomach and intestines, Caelius and other medical writers commonly turned to a handful of remedies. Sometimes they recommended reducing one's food intake or fasting in order to reduce the burden placed on the digestive system, giving it time to reset. Sometimes they recommended eating food that was more easily digestible, requiring the body to do less work and thus to recover proper functioning more quickly; and sometimes they recommended specific foods thought to aid digestion (for example, in his first-century CE cookbook, Apicius provided a recipe for *garum*, a fermented fish sauce that was thought to help with digestion[18]). Sometimes they prescribed specific food, drink, and **drugs** that possessed other properties, such as diuretics, purgatives, **astringents**, or those that heated or cooled the interior parts. Sometimes they used a **clyster** to inject water, sometimes mixed with medicine, into the anus (figs. 23, 24). Sometimes they recommended binding or **plastering** the midsection of the body to encourage constriction of loosely digested matter inside. Other times they recommended **cupping** to relax internal organs that were overly constricted (see figs. 31, 48). And finally sometimes they recommended that patients rest, lying on their back with their midsection and feet raised.

Digestive and intestinal ailments are among the most commonly addressed illnesses in our medical sources, indicating how widespread and distressing they were. It is not surprising then that we regularly find vivid descriptions of intestinal ailments in stories depicting torture and punishment in the afterlife. For example, in the tour of hell depicted in the second-century CE Christian text the *Apocalypse of Peter*, sinners were tortured by

16. The term "diarrhea" derives from the root words "flow" (*rhoea*) and "through" (*dia*).

17. The term "dysentery" derives from the root words "bad" (*dus-*) and "bowels" (*entera*).

18. In fact, we have come to learn that ingredients in recipes like these indeed have antibacterial or antihelminthic (antiparasitic) properties, and thus would have been successful in alleviating distress.

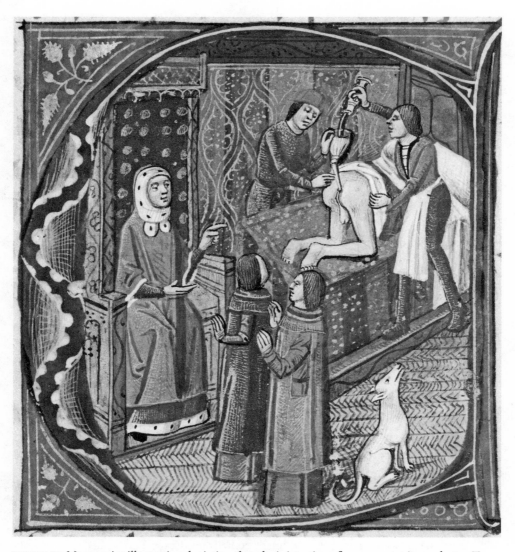

FIGURE 23 Manuscript illustration depicting the administration of an enema using a clyster. To perform this procedure, physicians filled a pouch (often made out of animal skin or organs) with fluid or medication, attached it to a tube that was inserted into the patient's body, and then squeezed the pouch to force the fluid or medication into the body. Sometimes physicians were reported to have used a device like a blacksmith's bellows to inflate the bodily opening first before inserting the clyster. Photo credit: Sächsische Landesbibliothek, Staats- und Universitätsbibliothek, Dresden; http://digital.slub-dresden.de/id337794197/150; Mscr.Dresd.Db 93, fol. 392v.

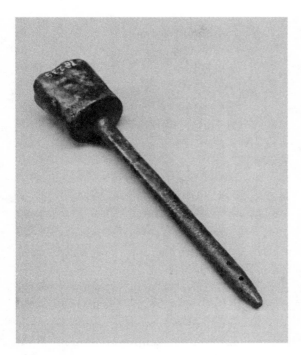

FIGURE 24 Clyster from the Casa del Medico Nuovo (II), Pompeii. A clyster was a narrow tube, closed but with perforated holes at one end and a cup on the other end. After the perforated end was inserted into the body, a pouch filled with fluid or medication would be attached to the cup. When the pouch was squeezed, it forced the fluid or medication into the body. Another type of clyster used a plunger method to force the fluid or medication through the tube. Clysters were used either to clean out a body part or to dispense medications into the body. For example, a clyster could be inserted into the rectum to wash out waste that accumulated from a fistula or into the ear to flush out wax buildup; clysters were also used to inject medications into the mouths of resisting children. Naples Archaeological Museum (inv. no. 78235). Photo credit: Kristi Upson-Saia.

wallowing in a lake of their own defecation, which dripped down their legs and exuded an unbearable stench; others had their entrails devoured by unrelenting worms. Even more gruesome, the third- or fourth-century CE Christian text the *Apocalypse of Paul* describes sinners being devoured by worms (with an extreme close-up of one man spewing worms out of his mouth and nostrils) and a terrifyingly giant two-headed worm that never slept. Scholars read these scenes of bodily torture as indications of ancient people's most acute fears and anxieties about their current lives that are being projected into a future dystopia, all the more terrifying because they would be experienced for an eternity.

Recently, scientific methods known as paleoparasitology have enabled scholars to verify just how widespread digestive and intestinal ailments were, and to glean more precise information about the specific kinds of ailments ancient people experienced. Paleoparasitologists collect evidence from archaeological sites—coprolites (fossilized human feces; fig. 25) and soils from toilets, sewers, trash pits, and burial sites into which feces have leached—in order to detect remnants of parasites, such as adult parasites we can observe with the naked eye, parasite eggs visible through microscopy, or DNA and proteins produced by parasites detectable through the use of biomolecular methods. Using these methods, researchers have found the presence of two kinds of parasites in sites across the Mediterranean: protozoa (single-celled organisms, such as *Giardia duodenalis,* malaria, and the lancet liver fluke) and helminths (worms, such as roundworms, tapeworms, and whipworms). As we identify the kinds of parasites that troubled ancient people, we come to understand better the symptoms

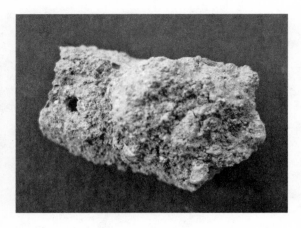

FIGURE 25 Eight-thousand-year-old human coprolite (fossilized human feces) from Çatalhöyük, Türkiye. Fecal material at archaeological sites provides information about health, such as evidence of parasites that would have caused digestive and intestinal ailments. Photo credit: Dr. Lisa-Marie Shillito.

they would have experienced, as well as to glean more information about their lifestyles. For instance, when we find evidence of fish- or animal-borne parasites in human feces, we deduce that they likely contracted the parasite by eating meat that was raw, underpreserved, or undercooked. When we find evidence of fecal-oral parasitic infections—caused by the ingestion of infected fecal matter—we deduce that the spread was caused by unhygienic practices (such as preparing food with hands that had not been washed after defecation), or by consuming food that had been fertilized with human feces, or by ingesting water from a contaminated source (such as at the public baths, where Romans were sometimes known to eat).

TEXT 11. CAELIUS AURELIANUS, *CHRONIC CONDITIONS*[19] SELECTIONS (4.3, 4.8)

Caelius Aurelianus *(fifth century CE) was a physician from Roman North Africa, and subscribed to the Methodist school of medicine. His two surviving texts,* Acute Conditions *and* Chronic Conditions, *are translations of Greek texts written by the physician* **Soranus of Ephesus** *(second century CE). A comparison of the few surviving pieces of Soranus's texts shows that for the most part Caelius offered a literal translation, but that he sometimes chose to adapt and paraphrase the Greek of Soranus.* Acute Conditions *and* Chronic Conditions *present a lengthy catalog of ailments and the treatments recommended by earlier physicians. The selections below offer advice about how to treat people who have stomachaches and intestinal worms. The passages reveal some of the basic elements of Methodist theories of illness, which held that all illnesses were caused by one of three bodily states: (1) being too dry and tense; (2) being too wet and loose; (3) combined features of both states 1 and 2.*

SOURCE: Translation by Jessica Wright based on the Latin text from Gerhard Bendz, *Caelii Aureliani Celerum passionum libri III, Tardarum passionum libri V*, Corpus Medicorum Latinorum 6.1 (Berlin: Akademie Verlag, 1990).

19. This text has traditionally been translated with the title *On Chronic Diseases*. In chapter 1 we explain our rationale for avoiding the English translation "disease."

Book 4, Chapter 3. On stomach aches, which the Greeks call *koiliakos,* and other discharges

19. Stomach ache, which the Greeks call *koiliakos,* receives its name from the part of the body that suffers.[20] It is brought about by recurring indigestion that precedes it, severe swelling, or dysentery. For those afflicted by this condition, evacuation of stools of various kinds and colors follows—sometimes thin and watery, sometimes rough and uneven or compact, sometimes white, sometimes similar to camel urine, sometimes reddish-yellow and frothy, sometimes green, bluish-gray, black, purulent, or bloody. 20. The feces have a heavy odor, and there is intestinal rumbling, which the Greeks call *borborygmos.* During the discharge, and after the evacuation has taken place, there is a noise like a little bladder erupting with excrement. This occurs sometimes night and day without pause, and sometimes in large quantities but at intervals, for example, once or twice a day, or with an interval of one, two, or more days in between; it is sometimes characterized by distention, flatulence, anguish, pain, hiccups, the sinking and drawing together of the skin that stretches around the belly, thirst, violent heat in the stomach itself, and a light, cold numbness in the inner parts. 21. Sleepless nights also follow, together with loss of appetite for food and a tremendous appetite for other things, deterioration of strength, a whitish pallor, and sometimes fevers—because of which the body odor is extremely foul, so that whatever they have touched with their own hands also putrefies and can hardly be freed of the odor it has absorbed—and, finally, swelling of the face and feet. For some people, dysentery comes about simultaneously, since the intestines are easily ulcerated by the pungency of the matter that flows out.

It is, then, a condition of looseness that sometimes also includes tightness, since indeed some of its features seem to be combined, as may be concluded from what is written above. But it is distinguished from a general flux of the stomach, since indeed there are many discharges in this condition, but they are not differentiated by the combinations of features described above.

22. Therefore, when the condition is still new or emerging, or has been present for a very long time but is disposed in an attack (which the Greeks call *epitasis*), at this time the sick person will need to be put in an **astringent** position,[21] as we have often taught, and it is necessary to prescribe rest and, as strength permits, fasting. For, in this situation, the stomach is suffering and does not tolerate the food that has been consumed and that must be distributed and appropriated to the body, just as suffering eyes are disturbed in the task of seeing. Prescribe much sleep and dehydration, and cover the stomach lightly with soft wool that is moistened in advance in Spanish oil, quince oil, rose oil, myrtle oil, or mastic oil.

23. If the sick persons have also been affected by flatulence or pain, then, during the period of remission, dip wool in sweet olive oil, anoint with green olive oil also, and wash the face in advance with lukewarm water. Next, provide food such as spelt that has been

20. The word *koiliakos* comes from the Greek word *koilia,* which referred to the **cavity** of the abdomen, or sometimes the organs within the cavity.

21. An astringent treatment was meant to help a patient to become drier and tenser.

prepared in cold water in such a manner that removes its digestive difficulty, as happens by roasting the grain or by serving it with a decoction of Theban dates. Offer bread also, either on its own or with a soft-boiled egg, and likewise porridge made from rice, spelt groats, spelt meal, millet, prepared with a little Spanish olive oil and a few grains of salt. Or, if pain makes it necessary, a **cupping** glass must be applied [. . .][22] for a longer time, however, make sure that, if the sponge has absorbed anything solid, there should be no compromise in gentleness.

24. Then, with the **clyster** bulb squeezed lightly so that the liquid might be expelled, it is necessary to test to make sure that the mouth of the clyster is not closed. Then a tube must be inserted into the anus using the right hand, all the way to the joint that the Greeks call the "little shield"[23] with gentle pressure and without either being directed straight against the parts opposite or a sudden or strong force from above, since swellings and abscesses are formed in this way. Gradually, therefore, and with the direction angled a little downward, make an insertion toward the part where the sacrum is located, which the Greeks also call the "sacred bone,"[24] for in that place, the space within the rectum is wider.

25. Then, once the application has been completed, it is necessary to withdraw the finger by which the opening has been obstructed, to hold the tube very still with the left hand, and to squeeze the clyster bulb with the right—gently and moderately, whenever the lower intestines are known to be ulcerated. Next, procure a short tube with quite a broad mouth that is able to transmit the drug to the suffering part in an unobstructed flow, to avoid the **drug** being kept from the parts that suffer and so not only bringing no advantage, but even hurting the healthy parts that it rushes upon. But for those whose upper intestine has become ulcerated, it is necessary to exert stronger pressure on the clyster bulb and for a longer tube to be procured, so that the liquid of the drug might be able to reach there. 26. And the sick person is to be encouraged to prevent the drug from being pushed out by holding their breath. And if there is a great deal of putrefaction, which the Greeks call *nomē*, it is not inappropriate to hollow out the tube of a clyster on each end, making what the Greeks call an *amphitrētos*, through which it is possible for the liquid of the drugs to reach the sides of the intestines through both ends.

Then, when the entire clyster bag has been emptied and folded together, or drained by manual pressure, so that we may infer that the drugs have reached their destination, the tube is to be removed with a cautious hand, and, with the sick person's legs spread apart, sponges are to be put into the anus, after being wrung out from a decoction of hot liquid in which pomegranates have been cooked in advance. 27. With the parts of the rectum squeezed together by the herbs' astringent power, which the Greeks call *stypsis,* and by heat of their application, the injected drugs are held in. Then, when a short interval of time has passed,

22. Some words from the Latin text are missing here. The meaning of the rest of the sentence is uncertain.

23. In Greek, *aspidiskos.*

24. In Greek, *hieron osteon.*

the items which have been set beneath the buttocks must be withdrawn. If the sick person feels the urge to defecate and there is ulceration in the lower intestines, even more so if ulceration has been observed in the rectum, he must be encouraged to resist for a short time and to retain the injected drugs, with us touching those parts which are known to be affected, as often as we see the sick person feel forced to void the drug. But if the ulcers are in the upper intestines, sick persons must be permitted to defecate whenever they want. 28. For the drug, quickly running back and flowing down into the lower intestine, ulcerates the healthy rectum by affecting it with its harmful power. For, when the foul, dead matter is drawn down, the parts that have not been ulcerated are injured and consumed when it has been brought near to the body and lingers there too long. After a sufficient interval of time, therefore, when mucous fluids, shreds of matter, and various intestinal fluxes have been thrust out, together with the drug, we understand that the drug has been successfully administered.

. . .

30. Then, after the discharge is complete, the anus must be wiped clean with sponges; if nothing has been discharged, after the interval of one hour and once he has been anointed, refresh the sick person with appropriate food most suitable for the stomach, 31. such as lettuce stem, endive with vinegar that has been prepared with myrtle, or olives either crushed or steeped, which the Greeks call *kolymbades,* and soft-boiled eggs and the birds recently mentioned, which have been nourished with astringents, such as myrtle, rose, or mastic. For thus their fat disappears and their **flesh** is made astringent, more so in their breasts, of which the parts neighboring the bones are considered more suitable, for they are more tender than the rest. Some cooked, astringent fruits and vegetables must also be given, of which we have spoken above and also in writing about other maladies. 32. We give cold water to drink. But if the sick person tolerates it very poorly, we will provide very hot water from the cistern. And if the sick person is without fever, we will give wine with a little more stimulating power, as we taught above. For wholly inciting or encouraging appetite, which the Greeks call *orexis,* we need to guard the strength of the stomach, unless the belly is loosened and accompanied with nausea. Moreover, it is appropriate to take care that we do not give a very large amount of food or drink, nor that the sick people believe it is necessary to drink before they should have consumed solid food. 33. For it is unsuitable to keep the intestines either burdened or moist.

Book 4, Chapter 8. On Intestinal Worms

106. [. . .][25] And for some people, indeed, diarrhea is brought about without the expulsion of the intestinal worms, sometimes accompanied by loss of appetite, weakness, and pallor with the wasting away of the body, and sometimes by a smooth, dry cough that is provoked now and then, other times by the weakness and collapse of body and consciousness, which they call *leipothumia.* Children, however, are affected by disturbance of the limbs while they are sleeping, accompanied by groaning, agitation, and teeth-grinding. Often, contrary to

25. Something is missing from the Latin text at the start of the chapter.

usual custom, they lie prone, and then call out without obvious reason, jumping up with their cries. 107. But for other people, the attack occurs suddenly, so that they are over-whelmed and become mute, having never before been affected in this way. Sometimes, like-wise, they are seized by the convulsion or contraction of the limbs, and some become silent at intervals and are weighed down in a fever by a sinking feeling similar to that of lethargy. Further, they appear changed, with loss of color that gradually spreads beyond measure across their whole face, sometimes also with coldness of the joints, and it can be difficult to get a response when asking a question. They toss and turn with hands raised high, also sweating. In children, the worms often turn around or knot themselves together, so that the part of the intestines which is thinnest feels hard to the touch. 108. Then, finally, patients are killed by the expulsion of these worms. The pulse, moreover, as **Themison** writes in the ninth book of his *Letters,* is uneven and frequently interrupted.

The worms are expelled sometimes through the bowels, sometimes through the esopha-gus and mouth or nostrils. Sometimes they are expelled in a mass that is joined together spontaneously in the likeness of a sphere, a large quantity of them bound together by mutual embrace. Sometimes they are expelled individually. Likewise, they might be expelled cov-ered in blood or bile, or with feces or **bilious humor** through the anus, living or dead, full or empty, and all or in part white or reddish-yellow. Sick people may be affected by very many other effects, by which we must categorize those mentioned above. Sometimes the effects are minimal, while at other times they are quite significant, depending on the number and shape of the animals. 109. Or, again, sometimes they cause the most possible damage, sometimes the least. The specific locations vary, since they sometimes ascend to the esopha-gus and sometimes remain in the intestines. The sick person is sometimes weakened, but at other times remains strong, and is sometimes with fevers, sometimes without.

. . .

123. Food and drink necessarily affect the worms that are in the stomach more quickly than drugs, but for those in the intestines, drugs are injected through an enema. For these animals often retreat from the stomach to the intestines and again from the intestines to the stomach. It will be more conducive to health, therefore, if, once we realize that there is an abundance of worms, we first make use of appropriate food and drink, similarly keeping in mind the use of **poultices** and **plasters**, then an enema.

. . .

129. If the worms are broad, vomiting must be induced with oil, not radishes, and on the next day an enema should be used, mixing in a portion of niter or salt. In addition, saltwater must be given for drinking, or a decoction of licorice root, or, equally, uncooked juice of licorice root. But some have recommended three **drachmas** of licorice root with niter, others three **obols** of scammony juice with two drachmas of the herb polypody, others a drug made from feathers. 130. But, when the situation allows, one should always attempt to use those drugs that minimally affect the stomach. Then, when the sick people have felt the sensation that indicates the creatures' imminent departure, as if forewarned by the distur-bance of the belly, hot water must be injected as an enema, so that the parts might be relaxed

and the animals rush out, rather than retreating after being struck by the cold. Care must be taken, furthermore, that these animals not be reborn in great numbers, and that we fortify bodies by regular treatment, with an expert present, and with the application of cyclical restoration of the body, which is achieved by vomiting induced with radishes, eating acrid food, by pitch-plaster and mustard-plaster, by heat, and by things similar to these in effect.

WOUNDS AND FRACTURES

We need only recall the conditions of the ancient Mediterranean to understand why reports of wounds, bone fractures, and complications that arose from wounds and fractures—such as inflammation, suppuration (pus formation), necrosis, and gangrene—were so common. Scholars estimate that 80–90 percent of people in the ancient Mediterranean were involved in some form of manual labor or craft work, much of which was dangerous and caused injuries we hear about in our medical case histories. For example, we hear of a boat skipper whose hand was crushed by an anchor; a cobbler who stabbed his own thigh with an awl while repairing a shoe; and a man whose chest was crushed when he was run over by a cart. We also hear about animals used to plow fields, to carry trade goods, or slaughtered for food who behaved unpredictably, causing grave harm. Additionally, we hear about many men who sustained wounds and injuries during military training or in battle. A man who visited the **Asclepius** shrine at Epidaurus, for example, sought assistance removing an arrowhead that had been lodged in his lung for a year and a half. Our study of human remains from the period corroborates the injuries discussed in our ancient sources. We find numerous healed bone fractures, suggesting that many people lived with the lingering effects of these injuries, experiencing limited function and chronic pain.

Thus it should not be surprising that some of the earliest medical writings we have, such as the Edwin Smith Papyrus from Egypt (1600 BCE), are interested in the treatment of wounds and fractures, and that a good deal of attention is paid to wounds and fractures in many of the medical texts from the period. Many ancient treatments appear to have been effective. Despite the fact that this was a world that did not know about the existence of bacteria, medical writers made recommendations for wound care that, if followed carefully, would have done a remarkable job at limiting inflammation and necrosis. For instance, they prescribed the careful cleaning of wounds, sometimes with vinegar or myrrh, which we now know to have antimicrobial properties.

Although ancient medical thinkers recognized the importance of keeping wounds clean and free from foreign matter, their explanation for inflammation, swelling, suppuration, and necrosis of a wound was quite different than today. When a wound became inflamed, swollen, hot and red, when it suppurated or, in the worst case, when the **flesh** around it began to turn black, lose sensation, and eventually die, ancient medical thinkers assumed it was due to an imbalance (i.e., an excess) of a substance of the body, a substance that was rotting or putrefying inside the wound. These substances included clotted blood, bits of flesh, dirt, cloth, and foreign objects, such as wood splinters (for instance, from tools) and weapons (arrowheads or spearheads).

According to ancient medical thinkers, the body itself tried to expel these excess and putrid substances and restore balance by transforming substances in the wound—by **concocting** them—into certain kinds of healthy pus. In fact, physicians studied the kinds of pus found in wounds to determine whether the body was on a good path toward healing or whether the injury was taking a turn for the worse (see the discussion in Text 12, **Celsus**, *On Medicine* 20A-F). Good pus was white, pure, and clean-looking, and odorless. This kind of pus was a sign that the wound was healing properly. If, on the contrary, the pus was thick, foul-smelling, and green or the color of an egg yolk, it was considered a bad sign.

Ancient medical writers, including Celsus, developed a careful and complex taxonomy of types of wounds based on a wound's severity and a physician's ability to treat it. Celsus connected the seriousness of wounds to where they occurred on or in the body. He observed that the wounds that are generally mortal (i.e., those that lead to death), and thus untreatable, included injuries to the brain stem, spinal marrow, heart, entrance to the liver, middle of the lung, large blood vessels in the neck, and so forth. Celsus next discussed wounds that were difficult to heal because they are located in places that inhibited healing, but were nonetheless not without some hope of treatment. For example, he observed that flesh wounds were far more likely to heal than wounds in a finger joint, the armpit, or other "hollow" spaces. This is likely based on the fact that these latter kinds of wounds were more difficult to keep clean and free from putrefying material, and hence more prone to inflammation and necrosis. Finally, Celsus commented on how the shape of a wound affected the healing process. For example, a jagged-edged wound or a mangled and contused wound were harder to heal than a clean cut, likely because of the potential for the crushed flesh in the wound to putrefy.

If determined to be treatable, there was a standard process for wound care. First, it was important to staunch excessive hemorrhaging from an injury in order to prevent the patient from dying of blood loss. Some physicians recommended using cold water and sponges. In extreme cases, wounds were **cauterized** using either hot iron implements (see fig. 26) or chemical compounds, such as lye. Other physicians recommended using a tourniquet to reduce blood flow to the limb on which the wound was located (see fig. 27).

Once bleeding was stopped, the next concern was to clean the wound thoroughly. Sea sponges, clean water, vinegar, and sometimes wine were used for this process. This was followed by stitching, if necessary, using needles and thread or, as Celsus recommended, **fibulae** (metal pins similar to our modern safety pins; see fig. 28). If the physician was concerned about the development of rot, the wound would be covered in some kind of salve, a mixture of herbs thought to promote healing. As we discuss in the section on pharmacology (in chapter 10), recipes for these kinds of balms and salves were developed over time, and some of them became standard particularly for wound care. Given the antimicrobial ingredients in common mixtures—including vinegar, frankincense, copper, honey, and myrrh in other recipes—they must have been relatively effective at staving infection. Then, the wound would be dressed and bandaged (see fig. 57). Hippocratic texts like *On Fractures* gave detailed

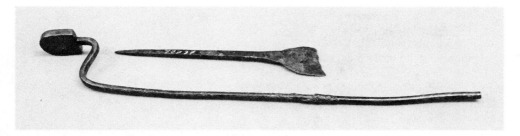

FIGURE 26 Roman tile cauteries. Cautery tools—usually made from iron because it was thought to be the most effective conductor of heat—were heated and then pressed onto a blood vessel or a wound to stop bleeding and to prevent infection. In order to minimize damage to healthy tissue nearby, cauteries came in various sizes and shapes to fit the wound or body part being treated. Many physicians may not have had a specialized tool dedicated only to cautery, but rather used other tools to cauterize, such as probes, spatulas, or spoons. Naples Archaeological Museum (inv. no. 77737). Photo credit: Kristi Upson-Saia.

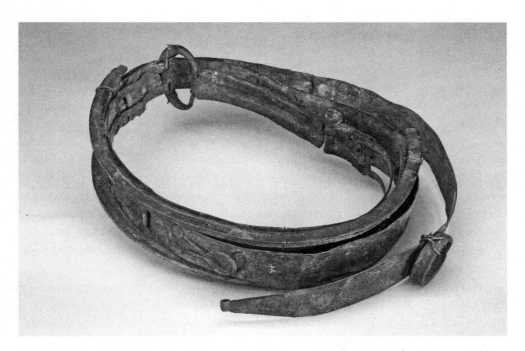

FIGURE 27 Bronze thigh tourniquet, Roman, 199 BCE–500 CE. Tourniquets for the arms and legs were used to control bleeding during bloodletting and surgical procedures on the limbs. They were also used to stop or slow the spread of toxins for those bitten by venomous snakes or rabid animals. The metal straps of the tourniquet pictured here would originally have been covered with leather to make it more comfortable when put on the patient. Science Museum, London. © Science Museum Group.

FIGURE 28 Bronze aucissa-type fibula, Roman, late 1st century BCE–mid-1st century CE. A fibula (plural: fibulae) was a metal pin, similar to a modern-day safety pin, used in the treatment of wounds, whether inserted into the flesh to hold the sides of a wound together or used to hold bandages in place. When closing a wound, Celsus recommended fibulae instead of stitching with a needle and thread when the edges of a wound were not easily drawn together or when the wound needed to remain somewhat open so that blood, pus, and fluids could drain out of it. Metropolitan Museum of Art (1991.171.26).

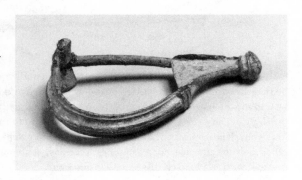

instructions on bandaging, including the width of the bandage relative to the size of the wound and the importance of not binding the wound too tightly or too loosely. Finally, wounds should be inspected and bandages changed at regular intervals. On the occasions in which wounds became necrotic and gangrenous, more extreme measures were taken, including surgical procedures (for more on these techniques, see chapter 10 and Text 29).

Scholars estimate that people in the ancient Mediterranean would have experienced at least one broken bone, though probably multiple fractures, over the course of a lifetime, often caused by dangerous occupational conditions and by malnutrition that weakened bone density. Archaeologists have discovered that the most common fractures found in ancient human remains were to the collarbone, arm bones, and wrists. After age fifty, hip and spinal fractures became very common. As in the case of wounds, ancient medical writers understood and documented distinctions between kinds of fractures based on their severity and location in the body.

Many minor fractures would have healed on their own as long as the bone was somewhat properly aligned. But often physicians had to intervene by setting bones back into place, a process called "reduction." Closed reduction—the manipulation of the bone or bone fragments without surgically opening up the area—would have been the most common practice. Some extreme fractures, where bone pierced through the skin, would have required open reduction: surgically dissecting the wound in order to reposition bone fragments. Our sources describe various forms of traction that would have been necessary for reduction. Sometimes tractioning could be accomplished through the use of leather straps and strong assistants, but physicians also devised more complicated techniques. For example, to realign a fractured humerus (the bone that runs from the shoulder to the elbow), the physician would hang a rod from the ceiling and position the patient's armpit over it, while the patient's hand would rest on a solid surface and heavy weights were affixed to the patient's elbow.

After the bone was carefully set in place, linen strips used were often stiffened with substances such as starch or cerate (a mixture of wax or resin with oil) and then wrapped around the injury to form a kind of cast. Or, alternatively, splints were used to keep the bone in place. Or, in some extreme cases, we hear of physicians resorting to external fixation, which involved drilling holes into the bone, which were then attached to a wooden rod that would immobilize the bone while it healed.

TEXT 12. CELSUS, *ON MEDICINE* SELECTION (5.26)

*On Medicine, written by Aulus Cornelius **Celsus** (c. 25 BCE–50 CE?), was originally part of an encyclopedia that covered a range of topics, including agriculture, medicine, rhetoric, philosophy, and military science. The section on medicine, the only one surviving, is organized around the three major divisions of ancient medicine: regimen, pharmacology, and surgery. Scholars debate whether Celsus was himself a practicing physician, but his text offers hints of real experience, especially in the sections on surgery. In the selection below Celsus comments on different types of wounds and how they should be treated. Because this selection is taken from his discussion of pharmacology, his focus here is on wounds that should primarily be treated with **drugs**, and only secondarily with surgery. Throughout the discussion, Celsus describes in careful detail the features of different kinds of wounds, the substances that ooze from wounds, and the signs to look out for in the days following the wounding. He displays a keen interest in infections (what Celsus calls "inflammation" and **"canker"**), as well as the rotting of **flesh** and blood he calls "gangrene."*

SOURCE: Translation by Jared Secord based on the Latin text from W. G. Spencer, *Celsus, On Medicine, Books V–VI*, Loeb Classical Library 304 (Cambridge, Mass.: Harvard University Press, 1938).

Book 5, Chapter 26. 1A. Now that I have described the properties of drugs, I will set out the kinds of injuries to the body. There are five: when something external injures the body, as in the case of wounds; when something internal has been corrupted, as in the case of a canker; when something comes into being, as in the case of a stone in the bladder; when something has grown, as in the case of a vein that swells up and is changed into a varicose vein; when there is some problem, as when some part of the body is mutilated.

1B. For some of these, drugs are more helpful. For others, the hand is more helpful.[26] I will postpone speaking about injuries that especially require the scalpel and hand and now speak about those that especially need drugs. As before, I will divide this part of treatment, and speak first about those injuries that happen in any part of the body, and then about those that attack certain parts of the body. I will begin with wounds.

26. The "hand" refers to surgery, one of the three divisions of ancient medicine, along with regimen and pharmacology.

1C. Before all else, however, a physician should know which wounds are incurable, which may have a difficult treatment, and which a quicker treatment. For, first, a sensible person would not touch what cannot be saved, and would not take on the appearance of having killed someone whom fate had put to death. Next, when there is grave fear without certain hopelessness, a sensible person would inform family members that there is little reason to hope, so that if the art is overcome by disaster, the physician does not seem to have been ignorant or mistaken. 1D. But while these things are appropriate for a sensible person, a boastful person would exaggerate something small to seem more important. It is fair to be committed with the acknowledgement of a simple case, so that the physician may examine it more carefully with the goal that a situation that is small in itself may not become larger by the negligence of the person providing treatment.

2. A person cannot be saved when the stem of the brain, the heart, the esophagus, the entrance of the liver, or the spinal marrow has been pierced. The same is true when the middle part of the lung or the jejunum or the small intestine or the stomach or the kidneys have been injured. And this is also true when the large veins or arteries around the throat have been cut.

3A. But people hardly ever achieve health when there is a wound in any part of the lung or the thick part of the liver or the membrane that encloses the brain, or the spleen or the womb or the bladder or any parts of the intestines or the diaphragm. People are in great danger who have had the point of a sword sunk into the large veins located inside the armpits or behind the knees. Wounds are also dangerous wherever the veins are larger, because profuse bleeding can drain out a person. 3B. And this happens not only in the armpits and behind the knees, but also in the veins that reach to the anus and testicles. Besides this, a wound is bad whenever it is in the armpits or thighs or hollow spaces or in the joints or between the fingers. The same is true whenever a muscle, a tendon, an artery, membrane, bone, or cartilage is injured. The safest of all wounds is one that is in the flesh.

4. And these wounds are more or less dangerous depending on their location. But, whenever a wound is large, it causes real danger.

5. There is also something of note in the type and shape of a wound. For a contused wound is worse than one that is only cut, meaning that it is more desirable to be wounded by a sharp rather than a blunt weapon. A wound is also worse when a piece has been cut out, or if the flesh is cut away from a part or hanging from another. A curved gash is worse, and one cut in a straight line is safest. Therefore a wound is worse or more tolerable if its shape is curved or straight.

6. But age, physical condition, way of life, and the time of the year also make a difference. A boy or youth recovers more easily than an old man, and a strong person better than a weak person. Someone not too thin and not too plump recovers more easily than someone who is thin or plump, and someone of sound condition more than someone of unsound condition. Someone who exercises recovers more easily than someone who is inactive, and someone who is sober and self-controlled more than someone devoted to wine and sex. And the most favorable time for treatment is the spring, or at least when it is neither hot nor cold, since too

much heat and too much cold damage wounds, especially when there is a variety of hot and cold weather. For that reason autumn is the most dangerous time.

7. Most wounds are visible to the eye. As we have demonstrated elsewhere, when we made clear the positions of the interior organs,[27] there are signs for the locations of some wounds. Because, however, some of these wounds are close to hand, and it matters if the wound is on the surface or has penetrated inside, it is necessary to point out the signs through which we can know what has happened internally. And from these signs arises either hope or despair.

8. So, when the heart is pierced, much blood is produced, the pulse fades, the color is extremely pale, cold sweats of a bad odor arise as if the body had been sprinkled with dew, the extremities are cold, and a quick death follows.

9. When the lung is pierced, there is a difficulty in breathing. Blood foams out from the mouth, red blood from the gash. At the same time, breath is drawn with a sound. Lying on the wound provides relief. Some people stand up without any reason. If they have been laid down on the wound, many people speak. If they lie on the other side, they become incapable of speech.

10. Signs that the liver is wounded are a large outpouring of blood from under the right part of the upper abdomen. The upper abdominal regions are set back to the spine. The wounded person has relief from lying on the stomach. Stabbing pains and anguish stretch up to the throat and where it is joined to the broad shoulder blades. Additionally, sometimes there is vomiting with bile.

11. When the kidneys have been pierced, pain radiates down to the sexual organs and testicles. Urine is passed with difficulty, and either it is red with blood or blood itself is produced.

12. But when the spleen is pierced, black blood rushes forth from the left side. The upper abdominal regions together with the stomach on that side become hard. A great thirst arises. Pain reaches to the throat just as when the liver is wounded.

13. But when the womb has been pierced, there is pain in the groin, hips, and thighs. Blood flows down partly through the wound and partly through the vagina. Vomiting of bile follows. Some women become incapable of speech, some are disturbed in their mind, others who are in control of themselves explain that they have pain in the tendons and eyes, and when they are dying they suffer what those wounded in the heart do.

14. But if the brain or its membrane has received a wound, blood flows out through the nostrils, and also, for some people, through the ears. Vomiting of bile generally follows. The senses of some people are deadened, and they do not notice when they are called. The facial expression of some of them is fierce. The eyes of some move from here to there as if they were detached. On the third or fifth day delirium generally comes. For many people, the tendons are also distended. Before death, however, many tear up the bandages with which their head had been bound, and expose the bare wound to the cold.

27. Celsus, *On Medicine* 4.1.1.

15. When the stomach, however, has been pierced, hiccupping and vomiting of bile follow. If any food or drink has been consumed, it is immediately brought back up. The pulse of the veins fades, thin sweats arise, and because of these the extremities become cold.

16. Signs that the small intestine and stomach have been wounded are the same. For food and drink flow out through the wound. The upper abdominal regions harden. Sometimes bile is brought back up through the mouth. In the case of the intestine only, the location of the wound is lower. Other intestinal wounds produce feces or the smell of it.

17. When the marrow that is in the spine is broken, the tendons release or are stretched. Sensation ceases. Once some time has elapsed the lower parts produce either semen or urine or even feces involuntarily.

18. But if the diaphragm has been penetrated, the upper abdominal regions are drawn upwards, the spine is painful, breathing is difficult, and foamy blood is produced.

19. A wounded bladder causes pain for the groin because what is above the genitals is stretched. Blood takes the place of urine, but from the wound itself urine flows. The esophagus is afflicted, so the injured people either vomit bile or hiccup. Coldness and, from it, death follow.

20A. Once these things are known, there are still other things to be learned pertaining to wounds and sores, about which we will speak. From wounds flows blood, serous fluid, and pus. Blood is known to everyone. Serous fluid is thinner than blood, with variations in thickness, stickiness, and color. Pus is thickest and whitest, stickier than both blood and serous fluid. Blood flows out from a recent wound or one already healing. Serous fluid flows out between these two times, and pus from a sore already becoming healthy. 20B. In turn, there are different types of both serous fluid and pus recognized in the Greek language. For there is a type of serous fluid that is called either "ichor"[28] or "honey-like."[29] There is a type of pus called "olive oil-like."[30] Ichor is thin, whitish, and flows out from a bad sore, especially when inflammation accompanies an injured tendon. Honey-like serous fluid is thicker and stickier, whitish, and somewhat similar to white honey. 20C. This is also produced from bad sores, where the tendons around the joints have been wounded, especially from the knees. The pus like olive oil is thin, whitish white, almost greasy, and in color and coarseness not unlike white oil. It appears in large sores that are healing. Blood is bad when it is either too thin or thick, when it is bluish-gray or black, when it is mixed with mucus or variegated. The best blood is hot, red, moderately thick, and not sticky. 20D. Consequently from the outset the treatment of a wound is more straightforward when good blood flows from it. Also later there is more hope for the wounds from which all the discharge is of the better type. Serous fluid, consequently, is bad when there is a lot of it, when it is too thin, bluish-gray or pale or black or sticky or bad-smelling, or when it erodes the sore itself and the skin surrounding it. Serous fluid is better when there is not a lot of it, when it is moderately thick, and reddish or whitish.

28. In Greek, *ichōr*.
29. In Greek, *melitēros*.
30. In Greek, *elaeodes*.

20E. Ichor, however, is worse when there is a lot of it, when it is thick, bluish-grayish or some-what pale, sticky, dark, hot, or bad-smelling. It is less severe when it is rather white, and has all the other features opposite to the foregoing. Honey-like serous fluid is bad when there is a lot of it and when it is very thick. It is better when it is thinner and there is less of it. Among these fluids pus is the best. But it is also worse when there is a lot of it, when it is thin, watery, and even worse if it is like this from the beginning. This is also true if its color is similar to curdled milk, if it is pale, if it is bluish-gray, if it is full of sediment. Besides these features, it is worse if it smells bad, unless it is the part of the body that causes this odor. 20F. Pus is better when there is less of it, and when it is thicker and whiter. The same is true if it is thin, if it produces no smell, and if it is uniform. But it should correspond to the size and age of the wound. For more pus is naturally produced from a larger wound, and more when the inflammation has not yet subsided. The pus like olive oil is also worse when there is a lot of it, and when it is not very greasy. It is better when there is less of it, and when it is greasier.

21A. Now that these issues have been explored, when a person has been wounded who can be saved, there are two things to be watched for right away: that neither a discharge of blood nor inflammation should kill the person. If we fear a discharge—which can be judged from the location of the wound, its size, and the strength of the rushing blood—the wound must be packed with dry linen, and a sponge, with cold water squeezed out if it, should be placed above this and pressed down with a hand above. 21B. If, in this way, the blood does not cease, the linen must be changed frequently, and if the linen does not do its job when dry, it should be moistened with vinegar. Vinegar should be effective when pressed down on bleeding. For this reason, some people pour it on a wound. But, in turn, there is another concern, that if too much bodily matter is kept in place with force it will later lead to a large inflammation. For this reason no corrosive or burning drugs are used because of the scab that they induce, although many of these drugs suppress bleeding. But if these are employed, pick those that have a gentle impact. 21C. But if these are also overcome by the flow of blood, the blood vessels that are pouring out blood should be grasped, and should be tied and severed around the area that is wounded in two places so that both collect together, and have their mouths closed just the same. Where even this is not possible, the veins can be scorched with glowing-hot iron. But when there has been a great flow of blood from a spot where there is neither tendon nor muscle, for instance in the forehead or the top of the head, it is still most suitable to apply a **cupping** glass to a different part of the body, so that the flow of blood may be diverted there.

22. Against bleeding there is help in the previous methods, but against inflammation there is help in the flow of blood itself. Inflammation is to be feared when a bone, tendon, cartilage, or a muscle is wounded, or when little blood flows out relative to the size of the wound. Therefore, whenever this happens, it is inappropriate to suppress the blood quickly, but to let it flow out as long as it will be safe. If it seems that too little blood has flowed out, one should also let blood from the arm, certainly if the body is youthful and robust and in good physical condition, and all the more if drunkenness preceded the wound. But if it seems that a muscle is wounded, it should be cut through. For a muscle that is pierced is fatal, but one that is cut through recovers health.

23A. It is by far most useful for the wound to be closed up when bleeding is suppressed, if too much flows out, or runs out, or if it flowed out too little on its own. This is possible for a wound in the skin or even in the flesh, however, if nothing else bad has happened to it. Flesh hanging from one part and clinging to another part can be closed up, if the flesh is still whole and is still being supported with a connection to the body. In these wounds that are being closed up, there are two types of treatment. For if the gash is in a soft part of the body, it should be sewn up, especially if the tip of the ear is torn, or the end of the nose, or the forehead or cheek or eyelid or lip or the skin around the throat or the belly. 23B. If the wound is in the flesh and is gaping, and the edges are not easily brought together into one, stitching is inappropriate. **Fibulae** (the Greeks call them *ancteras*[31]), which draw together the edges somewhat, must be inserted, so the scar is less wide later. From these examples one can deduce if flesh that has not yet lost sensation will stick to one part when it is hanging from another, and if this requires stitching or a fibula. But neither stitching nor a fibula should be inserted before the interior of the wound has been cleaned, so that no blood clot is left behind. 23C. For this is converted into pus, causes inflammation, and prevents the wound being glued up. Not even linen, which has been applied for the purpose of suppressing the blood, should be left behind on the wound, for this also causes inflammation. It is good not only for the skin but also some flesh, where there is some underneath the skin, to be caught up in suturing or a fibula, so that it may stick more strongly and not tear the skin. It is best with both suturing and fibulas to use soft yarn not twisted too much, so it can penetrate more gently into the body, and both should be inserted neither too far apart nor too closely. 23D. If the insertion is too far apart, it does not hold together. If it is too close, it causes much pain, because the more the needle pierces through the body, and the more places the stitching hurts, the worse is the inflammation that arises, especially in the summer. Neither stitching nor a fibula needs much force, but is useful as long as the skin—as if on its own—follows closely after the needle drawing it. In general, fibulae allow the wound to be wider, and a suture brings together the edges, which should not be linked together for the entire wound so that, if any fluid collects inside, it can flow out. 23E. If the wound is not amenable to either of these methods, it should still be cleansed. Every wound, then, should have laid upon it initially a sponge squeezed out with vinegar. If the sick person cannot put up with the strength of the vinegar, wine should be used. A slight gash is helped even if a sponge is placed on it that has been squeezed out with cold water. But whatever liquid is used, it is useful only as long as it is moist. Thus the sponge must not be allowed to dry up. 23F. And it is permitted to treat a wound without foreign, costly, and compounded drugs. But if someone lacks confidence in this, they should put on the wound a drug that has been made without suet, from the list of those that I proposed were suitable for bleeding wounds,[32] especially, if it is a flesh wound, the drug called *barbarum*. If the wound is of the tendon or cartilage or of some part of the body that sticks out, such as the ears or lips, the seal of **Poly-**

31. In Greek, *agktēr,* an instrument for closing wounds.
32. Celsus, *On Medicine* 5.19.1.

ides should be used. The green drug called Alexandrian is also suitable for tendons, and for parts that stick out, the drug that the Greeks called *rhaptusam*.[33] 23G. When a body is bruised, it is normal for the skin to be somewhat broken. When this happens, it is not inappropriate to open the skin more widely with a scalpel, unless there are muscles and tendons nearby, which should not be cut. When the skin has been sufficiently opened, the drug should be placed on it. But if the bruised skin, although opened too little, may not be opened up more because of the tendons and muscles, then methods that gently extract fluid should be used, especially those that I have explained are called "filthy."[34] 23H. In situations when the wound is serious, once something helpful has been applied, it is also not inappropriate, to put on top of this wool soaked with vinegar and oil, or a **poultice** that gently restrains the area, if it is soft, or something that softens if the area has tendons or muscles.

24A. The best bandage for binding up a wound is made from linen and should be wide enough so that, in a single wrap, it can cover not only the wound but also a little of its edges. If the flesh has receded from one side of the wound, the bandage is better gathered together on that side. If the flesh has receded the same amount on both sides, the bandage should cover the edges from side to side. Or if the type of the wound does not allow it, the middle of the bandage should be put on first, so that it may then be led to either side. 24B. The wound should be bound up in such a way that the bandage holds it together but without constricting it. When it is not secured in this way, the wound slips out. When a wound is constricted too much, it risks canker. In winter, the bandage should encircle the wound more times; in summer, as many as is necessary. Then the outer part of the bandage should be sewn to the interior parts with a needle, for a knot injures the sore, unless it is far away from it.

24C. No one should be misled so that he has to ask about the special treatment for the internal organs. I have discussed this above.[35] For an external gash should be treated either by a suture or some other form of medicine. But in the case of internal organs, nothing is to be moved, unless some piece should be cut from the liver or spleen or lungs that hang outside. Otherwise the regulation of diet and drugs will heal internal wounds, and by those methods that I have outlined in the earlier book as appropriate for each internal organ.

25A. Once these things are arranged on the first day, the sick person should be put to bed. If the wound is serious, the sick person, as much as their strength allows, should abstain from food before inflammation begins. The sick person should drink warm water until thirst is sated. Or, if it is summer and there is neither a fever nor pain, the patient should even drink cold water. 25B. There is, however, nothing universal about this advice, but the strength of the body must always be assessed, as weakness can make it necessary even to eat food immediately, though this will be light and meager, of course, only enough to sustain the sick person. Many people who are fainting from a flow of blood must be restored with wine before any treatment, something that is otherwise most harmful to a wound.

---

33. In Greek, *raptousa*, which literally means something like "stitched together."
34. In Greek, *rhypōdes*. Celsus, *On Medicine* 5.19.15 lists the ingredients.
35. See Celsus, *On Medicine* 5.26.8–19 above.

26A. A wound that becomes too swollen is dangerous, but no swelling at all is the most dangerous. Swelling is evidence of severe inflammation, and no swelling is evidence of a part of the body that has died. Immediately, if the sick person's mind remains under control, and if there is no accompanying fever, we may know that the wound will soon be healthy. And even fever should not inspire fear, if it persists in a large wound as long as there is inflammation. A fever is harmful that accompanies a minor wound, or that continues beyond the period of inflammation, or that causes delirium, or, if it does not bring an end to the stiffness or distortion of the tendons that arose from the wound. 26B. Involuntary vomiting of bile, either immediately after the sick person is struck, or for as long as the inflammation persists, is a bad sign only for those people whose tendons or the parts where there are tendons have been wounded. It is not inappropriate, however, to induce vomiting voluntarily, especially for those who have this habit. But this should not be done immediately after food, or when inflammation has begun, or when the cut is in the upper parts of the body.

27A. With the wound treated in this way for two days, it should be uncovered on the third day, and the serous fluid wiped away with cold water, and then have the same bandage put on again. By the fifth day, the amount of inflammation that will exist is apparent. On that day, when the wound is uncovered again, its color should be inspected. If it is bluish-gray or pale or varied or black, one may know that the wound is bad. And whenever this is observed, it should frighten us. It is most advantageous for the sore to be white or red. Likewise, if the skin is hard, thick, or painful, this signals danger. 27B. Good signs are when the skin is thin and soft without pain. But if the wound is closing up or swelling mildly, the same bandages that were first applied should be put on it. If the inflammation is serious and there is no hope of the wound closing up, then materials that cause pus should be applied. And now also the use of hot water is necessary, so that it may clear out the bodily matter, soften the hardness, and promote pus. The water should be warm enough that it is pleasant for a hand put into it, and it should be applied until the swelling seems to diminish and the color of the sore has returned to a more natural one. 27C. After this dressing, if the gash is not wide open, a bandage should be placed on it immediately, and, especially if the wound is large, the four-drug bandage.[36] If the wound is in the joints, fingers, or cartilage, the filthy bandage should be placed on the wound.[37] If the wound is open more widely, the same bandage should be liquefied with iris oil, and dry linen smeared with this oil should be placed over the gash. Then the bandage should be placed over this, and above it greasy wool. The bandages should be tied even less tightly than the first.

. . .

31A. Such is the procedure of successful treatment. But some dangerous situations are likely to happen. For sometimes a chronic condition takes over the sore, and it hardens, and the thickened edges around it become bluish-gray. After this, whatever drug is applied accomplishes little. This generally happens when the sore was treated carelessly. Sometimes

---

36. In Greek, *tetrapharmakon*. Celsus explains at *On Medicine* 5.19.9 that this contains wax, pitch, resin, and suet.

37. See Celsus, *On Medicine* 5.19.15 above.

a canker takes hold, either from excessive inflammation, immoderate heat, excessive coldness, or because the wound has been tied up too tightly, or because the body is old or in bad condition. 31B. This type of condition has been divided by the Greeks into different kinds, but there are no terms for it in our language.

Every canker corrupts not only what it attacks, but also spreads. Then it is distinguished by different signs. For sometimes a redness, in addition to the inflammation, surrounds the sore, and this spreads with pain (the Greeks call it *erysipelas*[38]). Sometimes the sore is black because its flesh has been corrupted, and this corruption is spread even more with putrefaction when the wound is moist, and from the black sore is produced a pale, foul-smelling liquid, and rotted little pieces of flesh.[39] 31C. Sometimes even the tendons and membranes are dissolved, and a probe inserted penetrates to the side or downwards, and this problem sometimes also impacts the bone. Sometimes there arises what the Greeks call "gangrene."[40] The former types of gangrene develop in any part of the body: in the limbs that jut out, that is, among the nails and armpits or groin, and generally in old people or in those whose bodies are in bad condition. Flesh in the wound is black or bluish-gray, but dry and shriveled. The skin nearest to it is mostly filled with dark pustules. Then the skin around these is pale or bluish-gray, generally wrinkled, without feeling. Skin further away is inflamed. 31D. All these things spread at the same time. The sore spreads into the place filled with pustules, the pustules into the place that is pale or bluish-gray, the paleness or the bluish-gray in the part that is inflamed, and the inflammation into flesh that is whole. 31E. An acute fever and a huge thirst accompany these conditions. For some people there is even delirium. Other people, although they are of sound mind, nevertheless can hardly explain what they are feeling due to their babbling. The esophagus begins to be afflicted. The breath itself takes on a foul smell. And the beginning of this disorder is treatable. But when it has firmly established itself, it is incurable. Most sick people die in a cold sweat.

32. And such are the dangers of wounds. An old wound, however, should be cut with a scalpel, its edges cut off, and likewise any parts around it that are bluish-gray should be incised. If there is a small swelling of the veins inside that is preventing the wound from healing, this should also be cut off. Then, when the blood has been let out and the wound made to look like a new one, the same treatment as that set forth for fresh wounds should be applied.[41] If anyone does not want to use the scalpel, one can heal with the bandage made from laudanum, and, when the sore has been eaten up under it, the bandage that induces a scar can be used.

33A. What I have said is called *erysipelas* not only comes with a wound but also typically arises without a wound. Sometimes this causes greater danger, especially if it establishes itself around the neck or head. It is appropriate, if strength allows, to let blood, then to apply

---

38. In Greek, *erysipelas* literally means "red skin."
39. On the use of bodily liquids in prognosis, see page 111.
40. In Greek, *gangrainam*.
41. See Celsus, *On Medicine* 5.23A above.

restraining and cooling agents at the same time, particularly white lead with the juice of nightshade, or Cimolian clay mixed with rain water, or flour kneaded with the same water and cypress wood, or, if the body is weaker, lentil meal. 33B. Whatever is applied must be covered with beet leaves and above that a bandage dripping with cold water. If cooling agents provide little benefit on their own, they must be mixed in this way: 1 **denarius** of sulfur; 12.5 denarii each of white lead and saffron; and these should be ground up with wine and the area anointed with them. Or, if the area is harder, the leaves of nightshade are crushed and mixed with the lard of pigs, spread on linen, and applied.

33C. But if there is a blackness that is not yet spreading, the substances that gently consume putrid flesh should be applied, and the sore should be re-cleansed and tended in the way of other wounds. If there is more putrefaction, and it is already advancing and spreading, there is a need for more powerful eroding agents. If even these are not successful, the area should be burnt until no fluid is produced from it. For healthy flesh, when it is burnt, is dry. 33D. After the burning of a putrid sore, substances should be placed on it that break up from the living flesh the crusts that the Greeks call "scabs."[42] When these disappear, the sore should be cleansed, especially with honey and resin. But it can also be cleansed with the other substances by which festering wounds are treated, and in the same way lead to health.[43]

34A. It is not particularly difficult to treat gangrene—at any rate in a youthful body—if it has not yet completely taken hold, but has to that time only begun. It is even easier to treat if the muscles are sound, if the tendons are not injured or minimally afflicted, and no large joint is unprotected, or if there is little flesh in the affected area, and therefore not much flesh that can putrefy, and if the problem is isolated in a single place, which can especially happen in a finger. 34B. In this instance, the first thing to do, if the sick person's strength allows, is to let blood. Then whatever is dry, and is harming what is next to it with its tightness, is cut off up to this point.[44] As long as the disorder spreads, drugs that tend to produce pus should not be applied, and therefore not even hot water should be applied. Although they restrain, heavy bandages are also inappropriate. But there is a need for those that are lightest. Cooling agents should be used on the parts that are inflamed. 34C. If the disorder is still not stopped, the part between what is damaged and what is sound should be burned. In this instance especially, help should be sought not only from drugs but also from regulation of diet. For this disorder exists only in a corrupt and spoiled body. Therefore, unless weakness forbids it, abstinence should be used first. Then should be given light food and drink that tightens the bowel and therefore also the body. Afterwards, if the problem persists, the same things should be put above the wound that were prescribed for a putrid sore. 34D. And at that time it will also be permitted to enjoy a fuller diet of foods from the middle

42. In Greek, *escharas*.

43. Celsus is here referring back to *On Medicine* 5.5, where he lists dozens of substances used to clean wounds.

44. The manuscripts here add the parenthetical phrase *sanum corpus* ("healthy tissue") to clarify that the tissue should be cut off up to the point of the healthy tissue.

type,[45] but only such foods that dry up the bowel and the body, and cold rain water. Bathing is inappropriate unless there is certainty that health has returned, since a wound softened in a bath is quickly afflicted back to the same bad state. Sometimes it happens that none of all the remedies is successful and the canker spreads nonetheless. In these instances, there is a miserable but single remedy so that the other parts of the body may be safe: to cut off the limb that is dying little by little.

BITES AND STINGS

Bites and stings are a specific subcategory of wounds—namely, those inflicted by other living creatures. These wounds are caused by creatures—venomous snakes, stinging insects, scorpions, and rabid dogs—that people in the ancient Mediterranean encountered in the course of daily life, especially if involved in agricultural labor. In the first selection below (Text 13, *On Dangerous Creatures* 1–7), the Greek poet **Nicander** (late second century BCE; fig. 5) mentions the hardworking plowman, cowherd, and woodcutter, all of whom were in danger when they came across venomous snakes in their habitats. And Nicander notes that most bites occurred to ankles and hands, the parts of workers' bodies that might inadvertently disrupt or surprise snakes. The farmer who threshed his grain by hand or the vineyard worker picking grapes, for instance, could easily startle a snake hidden in the grain or in the vines, and thus get bitten.

Counteracting the effects of venom injected by snakes and insects was of central concern for physicians, who worried about what they regarded as the cooling and hence deadening effects of venom. The cooling effect of venom was thought to be dangerous because it threatened the vital or enlivening heat of the body. Yet, medical writers also recognized that not all snake venom acted upon the body in the same way. For example, **Celsus** recorded a description of a certain snake, the venom from which did not cause cooling, but rather blood loss. Whatever the specific effect, there was a widespread understanding that snake venom posed a mortal threat to humans and thus required immediate medical attention.

The first step in treatment often involved an attempt to remove as much poison as possible from the wound by tying off the affected limb with a tourniquet, followed by **cupping** the wound (see figs. 27, 48). If cupping tools were unavailable, medical writers suggested sucking venom directly out of the wound (though Celsus recognized the dangers of doing so if the person applying this treatment had open wounds or sores in his or her mouth). Sometimes cupping would be supplemented by **cautery**, which was thought to staunch the poison in place, preventing it from spreading to the rest of the body. Celsus recommended **emetics**, baths, **plasters**, and certain food and drink to assist the body's recovery by removing dangerous residues and reestablishing vital heat.

45. Celsus divides food into three types (*On Medicine* 2.18.2–3) according to how much nourishment they provide. Food of the middle type includes the roots and bulbs of some plants, the meat of hares and all types of birds, and fish that are not salted or salted in their entirety.

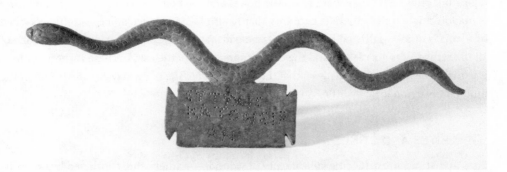

FIGURE 29 Second- to third-century CE bronze votive serpent, found at the temple of Asclepius in Pergamum (modern-day Türkiye). In addition to medical treatments, some victims of snake bites also sought help from the gods. A woman named Eutychis was instructed in a dream to dedicate this bronze votive snake after having been healed in a dream. Antikensammlung der Staatliche Museen zu Berlin (no. 31394). Photo credit: Ingrid Geske. Art Resource, NY.

While most treatments were administered after a bite, some medical authors recommend preventative measures. For instance, Nicander endorsed a recipe for a salve that would repel snakes. This salve, which one would apply to the legs, was not only useful for manual laborers, but also for those on a journey (who would be walking far distances), sleeping outdoors (an afternoon nap in the field, for instance), or threshing grain.

The most famous anti-venom **drug** was called *theriac*. Many different versions of this complicated drug were developed. According to legend, the first ruler to create this kind of drug was the Hellenistic king Mithridates IV of Pontus (his eponymous drug was called *mithridatium*). When the kingdom of Pontus eventually fell to Roman rule, so the story goes, his recipe was procured as part of the spoils of war. Yet many pharmacologists thereafter devised their own patented recipes. Some, like Nicander, included parts of dangerous animals—such as the venoms or the flesh of venomous snakes—in their recipes. As we will see in our discussion of pharmacology in chapter 10, some medicinal substances could both cure or cause harm depending on dosing, which is why the Greek word for drug, *pharmakos,* could mean both "drug" and "poison." Hence, it was crucial for these drugs to be prepared by experts. Combined with these ingredients, theriac recipes also included other botanical ingredients such as poppy juice, cinnamon, garlic, ginger, mint, licorice, and many more. By the Roman period, court physicians like **Galen** formulated theriacs intended to protect emperors from a wide range of poisoning threats beyond just bites and stings. These drugs, ingested daily, were also thought to maintain general good health or were considered a panacea, a remedy for all illnesses.

Although they are less likely to kill adults than certain species of venomous snakes, scorpions were also feared for their ability to cause serious pain and injury. A scorpion bite could cause debilitating symptoms—profuse sweating, muscle spasms, nausea and vomiting, swelling, elevated heart rate, high blood pressure, and agitation—and it was widely recognized that a large scorpion could pose mortal danger to a small child. Thus we understand why writers such as **Pliny** and Aelian (second and third centuries CE) talk about the dread and hatred invoked by these creatures, especially the largest varieties, which menaced desert travelers, and which were supposedly monstrous enough to prey upon cobras and lizards. And we better understand why the emperor Marcus Aurelius expressed relief about killing a scorpion that he found in his bedclothes before it had the chance to sting him (Text 37, Letter to **Fronto** 5.23).

We also surmise that untamed dogs, sometimes living in packs, were a common part of urban settings (where they could easily scavenge for food), so **Rufus of Ephesus** advises fellow physicians to ask patients whether they had been bitten by a dog as part of their diagnostic process (Text 6, *On the Importance of Questioning the Sick Person* 46). Ancient physicians thought people could recover from the bite of a rabid dog if treated quickly. Treatment involved cupping the wound to draw out the poison from the dog's bite and sending the patient to the baths to sweat out any remaining toxins. But many people also believed that healers tending to victims of dog bites had to be careful, since, as the Roman author Aelian warned, even a piece of cloth with the mad dog's saliva could transfer its "venom" to others.

Medical writers observed that if treatment for dog bites was delayed, victims could develop the same symptoms displayed by rabid dogs—such as "hydrophobia," fierce thirst coupled with the fear of drinking water—and eventually die from the illness. In these cases, Celsus advised caretakers to throw the suffering person into water in order to get them to drink. Those who could not swim would take in water, and thus be treated, as they began to drown. For swimmers, he suggested actually holding the patient under water at intervals to force an intake of water. We can imagine that such a violent treatment must have been born from the painful desperation of watching someone slowly die of thirst.

Given the dangers of bites and stings, it is not surprising that snakes, scorpions, and dogs were potent symbols in the ancient Mediterranean imaginary. For example, in a famous mosaic from an entrance hall of a second-century CE house in Antioch, all of these animals are depicted attacking the evil eye (see fig. 1). This mosaic was likely intended to ward off the harmful effects of the evil eye by appealing to the powers of terrifying and dangerous creatures, indicating just how much they were feared. Despite this fear, snakes were also powerful symbols in medicine as a result of their association with **Asclepius** (see fig. 4) and related healers (see fig. 50). Nonvenomous snakes lived in the temple complexes of Asclepius and were said to have participated in healing rituals. For instance, in the Epidaurian inscriptions, a snake reportedly healed a man's festering toe by licking it while he slept.

More generally, the ability of snakes to shed their skin was a symbol of shedding one's illness. Medical professionals still use a symbol of the snake winding around a staff, which resembles ancient images of Asclepius's staff with a single snake wound around it (though often has been mistakenly confused with the caduceus symbol of two snakes winding around a winged staff, an image associated with the god Hermes). Hence, it is likely that the modern medical symbol was attempting to draw its lineage from the ancient medicalized symbolism of snakes.

TEXT 13. NICANDER, *ON DANGEROUS CREATURES* SELECTIONS (1–7, 98–114, 636–655, 921–933)

Nicander *(late second century BCE) was a poet, likely a physician, and possibly a priest at a sanctuary to **Apollo** located in Ionia (modern-day western Türkiye). His poem* On Dangerous Creatures *(Theriaka in Greek) discusses snakes, spiders, and other poisonous animals, and recommends antidotes to their bites and stings. Nicander's introduction to the poem and a few sample antidotes and remedies are presented below.*

SOURCE: Translation by Molly Jones-Lewis based on the Greek text from A. S. F. Gow and A. F. Scholfield, *Nicander of Colophon: The Poems and Poetical Fragments* (Cambridge: Cambridge University Press, 1953).

Lines 1–7

I will gladly speak about the forms and dire destruction of wild creatures
Who attack out of nowhere, and the remedies for harm that are arrayed against them,
My friend Hermesianax, dearest of all my kinsmen. Then the hard-working plowman
or a cow-herd or a woodcutter would respect you, whether he is skewered
on a venomous fang in the forest or while plowing,
since you are thoroughly versed in the curing of such illnesses.
. . .

Lines 98–114

If you find two snakes mating at the crossing of three roads and,
When they have just started mating, toss them alive into a pot with certain ingredients,
You will have a defense against dire disasters.
Throw in thirty **drachmas**' worth of a newly slain deer's marrow,
Also one-third portion of rose oil, the kind that professionals grade
"first" or "middle" or "fine ground."
Then, pour in the same amount of shining oil,
And a quarter portion of wax: heat these things in a round-bellied pot,
Cooking until the **flesh** is softened around the spines and falls to pieces;
Then, take up a sturdy, well-made pestle, and grind up all the many ingredients
Mixed up with the snakes; but throw the spines far away,
Because there is a poison capable of doing harm lurking in them.
Then, rub it all over your legs whether for a journey, or sleep,

or whenever, after threshing in a dry summer, you belt your tunic up
to separate out the deep pile of grain with a pitchfork.

. . .

Lines 636–655

But now, I will go on to speak of roots that are good for repelling snakes.
First, learn about the two kinds of viper's bugloss; one of them
Has a prickly leaf that resembles alkanet
Since it is small and it stretches its small root level with the ground.
The other kind grows luxuriantly in its leaves and stems,
And is tall; it blooms purple all around with a tiny flower,
And on top grows a head like a viper, but rough and scaly.
For a remedy, of these two varieties first cut off enough for one person,
Ground fine on either a wood block or a mortar or a stone grater.
And you should grind a paste of the roots of the eryngium and
the bright-colored acanthus, and you should add a weight equal to both
of erinos which twines among the hedges;
you should also pick the drooping leaf of wild mountain basil
and the Nemean seed of evergreen celery,
In addition, let a double portion of anise lift
The scale that is dipping, weighed down by the roots;
And you should knead these, and when you have mixed them in a single vessel
You can cure the fatal bite of male vipers on one occasion, then on another
The scorpion's sting, then the bite of the venomous spider,
By crumbling three **obols**' weight into wine.

. . .

Lines 921–933

Yes, by applying a bronze **cupping** vessel to the harmful bite,
You will suck up the venom and the blood together,
Or if you pour on the milky sap of the fig-tree, or an iron
Heated deep in the heart of a hot furnace.
Sometimes the skin of a grazing goat filled with wine
Will be useful at a time when an ankle or a hand is bitten.
You will bind the affected area in the wineskin at the mid-forearm
Or the ankle, and wind the cord-ties around the groin or armpit
Until the strong power of the wine drives the pain out of the flesh.
Also, sometimes treat by feeding leeches, filling them up on the wound,
Or by dripping the juice from onions, or sometimes you should pour
Onto sheep's droppings wine-lees to mix it into a paste,
Or vinegar, then you should pack the area around the wound with fresh dung.

EYE CONDITIONS

Ophthalmological conditions were one of the most common complaints in antiquity, a time when people did not have access to corrective lenses, nor to antibiotics to deal with eye infections. Perhaps even more significant was the lack of safety regulations and equipment that led to a greater likelihood of eye injuries in the workplace. We can easily imagine the dangers to the eyes from mining, quarrying, glassblowing, woodworking, smithing, and even certain agricultural tasks, such as harvesting and processing grains to remove chaff. Given the large number of ancient men who participated in military activities, injuries to the eyes in battle or training were also a frequent occurrence. And some people would have been blinded deliberately, whether they were slaves blinded by their masters as punishment or individuals attacked by enemies seeking revenge.

The most common kinds of eye ailments we encounter in ancient sources are those we would associate with infection. We imagine most of these infections would have been the result of bacterial, viral, or fungal agents spread through the crowded and unhygienic spaces of urban settings, such as the public baths and toilets. Under such conditions, these highly contagious ailments could reach epidemic proportions.

There is plenty of evidence to suggest that visually impaired people were not necessarily stigmatized because of their ophthalmological conditions, and that they found ways of moving about their worlds with the assistance of family, friends, and—in the case of more elite classes—slaves. However, some ancient Greek myths might lead us to believe that many people in antiquity thought that blindness was punishment from the gods, in particular for moral failures of one sort or another. For instance, the seer Tiresias was blinded by Athena for spying on her while she bathed, and Oedipus blinded himself after learning of his accidental patricide and incest. On the other hand, sometimes the blind were thought to possess hypersensory powers. For instance, Tiresias was granted a different kind of sight—namely, the ability to see the future—a compensatory gift from the goddess Athena. As these examples demonstrate, sightedness and blindness had competing associations, each of which would have informed people's judgments about visually impaired members of their communities.

According to ancient scientific and medical theories, vision worked in the same way as touch. The eye was understood as a sense organ that made physical contact with the object it viewed. Proponents of the "extramission" theory thought that the eye emitted a substance (or particles) in the direction of the object to be seen. The eye sensed the object when the substance or particles bounced off the object it viewed, akin to the way one senses the ground via a cane held in one's hand. Proponents of another view—the "intromission" theory—believed that it was the objects (not the eye) that emitted something like thin films of matter, so when an eye was directed toward the object, the stream of material traveled from the surface of the object and created an impression of the object on the surface of the eye. Some theorists posited that these films were composed of a substance similar to that found in the eye itself, most often a form of the element fire or **pneuma**. Finally, still others held an optics theory that combined elements of both extramission and intromission.

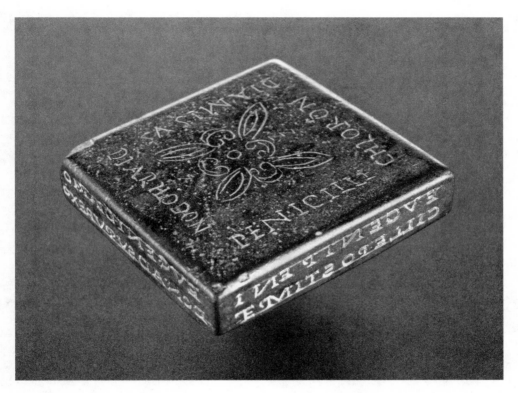

FIGURE 30 Roman *collyrium* stamp, 400 BCE–400 CE. *Collyrium* stamps or seals were impressed onto semisolid sticks of eye medicines (*collyria*), which would be dissolved for application as needed. (Note: The inscriptions are cut in reverse so they could be read correctly once an impression was created.) The stamps identified the pharmacologist who made the medication (and sometimes also the ophthalmologist), the name of the remedy and its ingredients, and the eye conditions for which the medication was useful. This information served as a guarantee of quality and proof that the medication was not a fake. The stone stamp pictured here has inscriptions on each side, one naming the oculist, "Eugenius"; the others are labels for different eye salves. These included "Chloron," a green salve made from egg whites, and "Diarhodon," a salve used to treat inflammation of the eye. Science Museum, London (A629428). Wellcome Collection. Attribution 4.0 International (CC BY 4.0).

When we understand these physical theories of sight, we are better able to discern why people in the ancient Mediterranean thought that a gaze had the power to transmit more than just images. Many believed that the envious gaze of one person directed at another—which they called the "evil eye"—could negatively affect the gaze's recipient by "drying up" his or her good fortune or health, like a kind of visual poison. The gaze, in this sense, was understood to penetrate the body of its victim. Hence apotropaic images and artifacts—objects that were thought to protect from the evil eye—sometimes depicted an eye being pierced by other powerful penetrating objects such as the teeth/fangs, claws, weapons, erect phalluses, and stingers of dangerous animals and insects (see fig. 1).

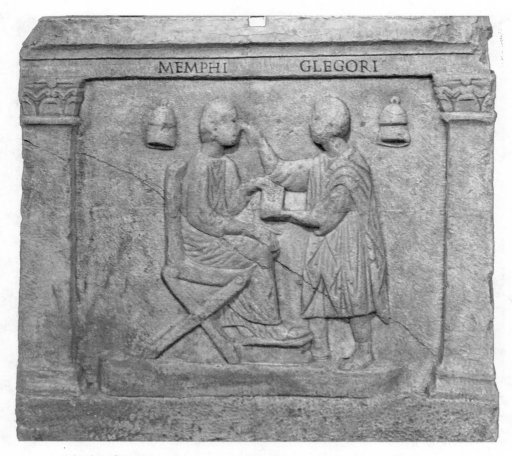

FIGURE 31 Third- to fourth-century CE sarcophagus depicting a physician conducting an ophthalmological examination or applying an eye medication to a woman's eye(s). In the upper corners are cupping vessels, which were used to extract blood or pus from a wound, or to relax a part of the body. Sosia family sarcophagus from Ravenna, Italy. Wikimedia Commons, Creative Commons Attribution 4.0.

The prevalence of eye conditions is attested not only in medical texts, but also in the archaeological record. Archaeologists have unearthed hundreds of oculist stamps or *collyrium* stamps (see fig. 30). These stamps were impressed on semisolid sticks of eye medicines (*collyria*). The stamps often identify the pharmacist who made the salve (sometimes also the ophthalmologist), the name of the remedy and its ingredients, and the eye conditions for which the medication was useful. These extant stamps give us a sense of the prevalence of various kinds of eye ailments: for example, approximately half of these stamps labeled remedies for eye inflammations, while other stamps labeled salves for corneal scarring, suppurations, and dimness or blurriness of vision.

Salves used to treat ophthalmological conditions were made from various herbs, metals, and other healing ingredients ground up and held together by gum resin, then shaped into

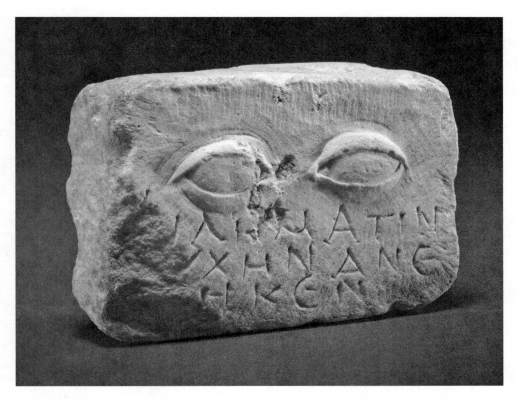

FIGURE 32 Second- to third-century CE marble votive relief with eyes, found near Pnyx, Greece. In addition to medical treatments, some people suffering from ophthalmological conditions also sought help from the gods. A man named Philomation dedicated this marble votive with eyes and an inscription petitioning Zeus. British Museum (object ref. 1816,0610.214). © The Trustees of the British Museum. All rights reserved.

the form of sticks. The physician would have broken off a portion of this stick; mixed it with water, milk, vinegar, wine, or egg albumen; and then spread it on the eyes. (This application of an ophthalmological treatment may be what is depicted in figure 31.) It is very likely that these treatments were effective given that the most common ingredients in salves—nard, poppy tears, myrrh, white lead, and lycium—have antibiotic, antiseptic, analgesic, **astringent,** and even caustic properties.

In the early Christian text the Gospel of John, we find another treatment for an eye ailment: saliva. The holy man Jesus heals a blind man by applying a paste of his own spit mixed with mud to the man's eyes and instructing the man to wash them in the Pool of Siloam. Given ancient ideas about the healing properties of spit (as enumerated by Pliny in Text 28, *Natural History* 28.35–38), it is hard to disentangle the degree to which Jesus's healing was thought to be enacted through medical or religious means, or some combination of both.

In addition to salves, some physicians prescribed dietetic remedies, as we see in the selections below from **Paul of Aegina** (Text 15). Paul describes the physician's treatment in terms of addressing imbalance in the patient's entire body. Again, such treatments may have been effective, since we now know that seasonal or nutritional blindness is often due to a shortage of food containing vitamin A, foods that are harder to procure at certain times of the year. Those experiencing vitamin A deficiencies may have regained their sight when their diet or the seasons changed. For the same reason, those who went to shrines seeking healing from the gods may have recovered when they ate sacrificial meat that was high in vitamin A (though they would have credited their healing to the petitions and votives they gifted the gods, like fig. 32).

Although most eye conditions would have been treated through topical drugs and regimen, there were occasions when one might resort to surgery. **Galen,** for instance, described the surgical treatment of various eye conditions, including ingrown eyelashes, new growth of tissue around the eye, growths on the cornea, and adhesion of the eyelids. Cataract surgery, in particular, seemed to have been relatively common and was more highly developed than we might expect. Ancient medical writers like **Celsus** thought that cataracts were an opaque, condensed fluid spreading across the area of the eyeball, which they assumed was hollow. The physician or surgeon used a needle or a thorn with a tip that was fine enough to penetrate the eye but round enough to guide the cataract below the pupil and out of the area of vision (see Text 29, Celsus, *On Medicine* 7.7.14C-F). Although we now know that this procedure caused some damage to the lens, ancient sources report that partial vision was often restored, explaining why this method continued to be used to treat cataracts for approximately 2,000 years.

Physicians' success in treating eye conditions stemmed in part from the sophisticated work of medical thinkers from Alexandria, Egypt, in mapping the anatomy and physiology of the eye. **Herophilus,** for instance, reportedly traced the optic nerves from the eye to the brain. Galen's discussion of ophthalmological ailments in the selection below demonstrates the ways medical writers benefited from the discoveries made by these Alexandrian experts (Text 14).

TEXT 14. GALEN, *ON THE AFFECTED PARTS* SELECTION (4.2)

In On the Affected Parts, *Galen (c. 129–c. 216 CE) offered an in-depth discussion of the anatomical aspects of internal illnesses. The text begins with a general discussion of pathology, focusing on how a physician should diagnose symptoms and different types of pain in the body. The remainder of the text focuses on different parts of the body, beginning with the head and spinal cord, then the abdomen and reproductive systems. In the selection below, taken from the chapter on afflictions of the eyes, Galen describes injuries to the structures of the eye (muscles, nerves, channels, and lens; see fig. 33), as well as injuries to other parts of the body (such as the stomach or brain) that manifest as eye conditions. Galen teaches his readers how to diagnose based on features that are visible to observation and features that must be detected indirectly.*

SOURCE: Translation by Jessica Wright based on the Greek text from C. G. Kühn, *Galeni Opera omnia,* vol. 8 (Leipzig: Cnoblochii, 1819–33).

Book 4, Chapter 2. In the present section, fourth of the treatise as a whole, let me now discuss the parts that lie deep beneath the face, taking as my starting point the eyes. Sometimes one or the other and sometimes both of the eyes lose either motor or sensory faculties, or both. And sometimes only one eyelid suffers by itself. But there are times when the eye itself, properly speaking, suffers damage in perception or movement. When it happens that visual sensation is destroyed with no obvious harm to the eye, responsibility lies with the nerve that travels from the brain to the eye. In these cases, the nerve has been injured by inflammation or hardening, or else by some influx of **humors,** or, alternatively, because the channel within the nerve has become blocked. Some of these things necessarily impact the eye as an instrumental part, while others impact it as a homogeneous part, according to the eight kinds of imbalance.[46] Besides these, there are also cases where either the luminous *pneuma* is not sent down from the brain at all, or only in very small quantities. In situations where the movement of just one eye is lost, the second pair of nerves growing out of the brain has necessarily suffered injury, as I explained just now with regard to the first pair.

As we learned through dissections, there are six muscles that move the eye itself, and others that encompass the root of the channel that goes to it—for anatomists call the first pair of [cranial] nerves a "channel," because there is a clear perforation through it alone. It often happens that the eye itself is not injured, but that one of the muscles or the nerve's own substance suffers harm, as I have just said, or that the nerve that descends to the eye is damaged. Part of the nerve growing from the second pair enters into each of these muscles, just as it also does in the muscles surrounding the channel. It makes no difference to the present discussion whether we must say that there are two muscles or three or one, given that we recognize the work of these muscles is to draw the eye upward and at the same time to fix it firmly, so that the soft nerve, which is called the optic nerve or the channel, is not twisted about by any turn in its journey. While there are six muscles that move the eye, if the one that draws it upward is injured, then the whole eye seems to be dragged down. But if injury occurs to the muscle that draws the eye down, it is dragged up. If the muscle that draws the eye to the smaller corner is damaged, then it is dragged to the bigger corner, and vice versa. Finally, if either of the two muscles that rotate the eye are paralyzed, then the eye as a whole will be twisted into a squint.[47]

Since there are other muscles, as I have said, surrounding the soft nerve, we must understand that their paralysis makes the whole eye fall forward. Most people with this condition see without impediment, if the soft nerve is stretched out gently and not harmed. But in circumstances when it is harmed, people suffering this have worse vision. If the condition happens to become more serious, it is clear that they are no longer able to see at all.

46. "The eight kinds of imbalance" is a reference to different types of imbalances of hot, cold, wet, and dry.

47. The Greek word translated here and below as "squint" is *diastrophē,* which literally implies twisting or distortion. From the context, it is unclear if Galen is referring to conditions that are now called "strabismus" or "lazy eye."

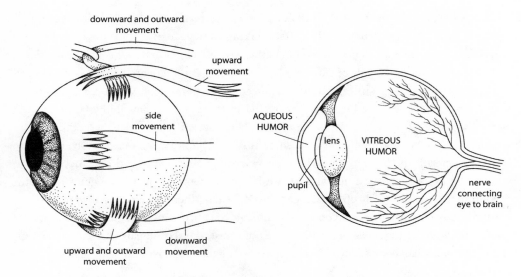

FIGURE 33 Illustrator's rendering of the anatomy of the eye, depicting the nerves, muscle, humors, and other parts Galen discussed in Text 14, *On the Affected Parts* 4.2. Created by Gina Tibbott.

In the case of a squint, if the eye turns aside to either corner, then the capacity for normal vision is preserved. But if it is turned upward or downward, as in the case of a slant, then this makes everything that is seen appear double. Since the muscles that move the upper eyelid—for the lower eyelid is immobile—are extremely small, such that they can hardly be observed even in large animals with any clarity, naturally the insertion of the nerves into these muscles is also difficult to see. But they necessarily react in the same way as the aforementioned muscles. Often these muscles suffer a condition that we know is specific to muscles, and sometimes the nerves that are inserted into these muscles are also in some way damaged.

If the muscle that draws up the eyelid becomes paralyzed, it slackens the eyelid, so that it is not possible to open the eye. If the muscles that lower the eyelid become paralyzed, meanwhile, it is not possible to close the eye. If only one of these two muscles suffers, then the eyelid is drawn across to the opposite muscle, such that it appears to be broken in the midline, toward the edge. The part that is associated with the damaged muscle is drawn upward, while the other part, which corresponds to the uninjured muscle, is drawn down. These are the conditions that are specific to parts of the eye, and in which the affected site is not visible.

Other conditions from other parts of the body attack through sympathy. These seem similar to the hallucinations of people suffering cataracts, yet arise not from the primary affection of the eye, but rather by sympathy with the mouth of the **cavity** or with the brain. But one must distinguish these conditions from those that arise from the stomach, first, based on whether the hallucinations appear in just one eye or similarly in both, for hallucinations that come from humoral imbalance in the stomach affect both eyes in the same way, while those that come from cataracts do not start in both eyes, nor appear identical in each. Second, one must distinguish these conditions based on continuity across time, for if the *sumptōmata*[48] of cataracts have already been present for three or four months, or even longer, but when you inspect the pupils, no cloudiness is apparent, then you will find that these people suffer because of the mouth of the cavity. In situations where not much time has passed, ask first whether the hallucinations have continued unceasingly every day since the day they began, with no intervening day being totally symptom-free, or if several healthy and symptom-free days occurred, such that the person seemed to be fully well. For continuous *sumptōmata* indicate cataract, while intermittent *sumptōmata* suggest a condition of the stomach, especially in cases when they say they experience no hallucinations whenever their digestion is excellent, even more so when at the same time as the onset of the hallucinations they feel a sharp pain at the mouth of the cavity, and further still when the *sumptōmata* cease after they vomit up acrid substances.

It is possible for you to learn these things immediately from examination on the first day that you see the person, if the eyes are, as I have said, in an entirely natural condition. But if one pupil appears hazier or muddier than the other, or is not, in short, completely clear, then this signifies the beginning of a cataract. Given that some people naturally have pupils that are not completely pure, one must examine whether both pupils appear to be similarly disposed, and, additionally, whether sufficient time has passed to allow the *sumptōmata* of cataract to develop. If this is indeed the case, then instruct the person to be satisfied with less food than usual—and with nothing unhealthy. Then, on the next day that the person has excellent digestion, ask about the visual hallucinations. If, indeed, they did not appear at all, or only faintly, then the *sumptōma* is from the stomach. If the hallucinations have persisted just the same, then one must understand that they occurred not through sympathy, but because of the particular condition of the eyes, especially if the person has taken a **drug** that includes aloe (I mean that which some call "holy bitter aloe," and others simply "bitter aloe"). For if the *sumptōma* is from the stomach, then it will be most easily treated by a dose of this drug, which also ensures good digestion, such that both goals are achieved together: the diagnosis of the affected part and its treatment.

I have, as you know, cured this condition in people who live in foreign regions through letters and without any in-person observation. Some have written to me from Iberia, some from Gaul, some from Asia, some from Thrace,[49] and some from other regions, asking if I had a reliable drug[50] for the beginning of a cataract, since no injury at all had yet appeared

---

48. We have left the Greek word *sumptōma* (plural: *sumptōmata*) untranslated because it lacks an exact equivalent in English. A *sumptōma* is something that happens, sometimes, but not always, with the implication that what has happened is bad or undesirable. See the word's glossary entry for more details.

49. "Iberia" refers to modern-day Spain and Portugal, "Gaul" to modern-day France, "Asia" to modern-day Türkiye, and "Thrace" to northern Greece.

50. The Greek word used here (*pharmakon*) makes it ambiguous whether Galen sent the people a recipe for a drug, the drug prepared from the recipe, or both.

in the pupil. I asked them first to clarify whether they had been suffering for a long time and about the other things that I described above. For those who said that six months or a full year had passed since the onset of the condition and that both eyes were in a better condition during periods of good digestion, but suffered acutely during indigestion and pain in the stomach, and were soothed when they vomited bile, I did not consider it worth investigating the pupil, since I knew for sure that the condition did not originate from the eyes, but was from the sympathy of the eyes with the stomach. When I sent them bitter aloe, I treated those people first of all, and then, through their influence, many other people in the same regions also. For all of those to whom I sent it were well-educated, and learned the diagnosis of the affected parts from the letters I sent to them, so they could easily thereafter recognize the diagnostic signs and treat the condition with the bitter drug.

Sumptōmata similar to those of cataracts often occur when the brain is suffering from certain varieties of phrenitis,[51] either different kinds or different species of it, if you wish to use these names. For there are two simple varieties of phrenitis, and a third that is a compound of both. Some people suffering from phrenitis make absolutely no errors in distinguishing visual perceptions but make judgments through unnatural reasoning. Others, on the contrary, are not at all mistaken in their thinking, but are disturbed in their perceptions, being misled by illusions. Yet others are injured in both regards.

The manner of each kind of damage is as follows. A man, left behind in his house in Rome with a wool-worker slave, stood up from the bed and went to the window, through which he could be seen and could also see the passers-by. Then he showed them each of his glass vessels and asked if they would order him to throw them down. They were entertained, clapped their hands, and agreed that he should throw them down. He did so, grabbing one after another, and they shrieked and laughed. Next, he asked them if they would order him to throw down the wool-worker, and they did. So he threw the wool-worker down. When the crowd saw him fall from high up, they stopped laughing, ran to him as he landed, and picked up his shattered body.

I am familiar with the opposite kind of damage as something that has happened not only to others, but also to myself, when I was a young man. For, when I was burning up with a high fever in summer, I believed there to be pieces of straw, dark in color, sticking out of the bed, and, similarly, threads from my clothes. I therefore tried to pluck these out. When I had caught hold of nothing with my fingers, I tried to do this again and again, and with more force. When I heard two friends who were present saying to one another, "He is picking at threads and plucking at straws," I recognized that I suffered the very thing they were describing, but was acutely aware that I was not delirious in my rational faculty. "You're speaking correctly," I said. "Now help me, so that I might not suffer from phrenitis." After they applied wet dressings appropriate to the head, troubling dreams attacked me throughout the whole

51. Ancient physicians used the word "phrenitis" to describe a type of inflammation of the brain typically accompanied with delirium.

day and night, to the point that I screamed and sprang up because of them; but on the following day all the manifestations of the condition subsided.

It is therefore clear that for those suffering in the aforementioned way because of sympathy between the brain and stomach, the *sumptōmata* have their origin from one and the same cause, in accordance with the type of phrenitis that they suffer, and not from the part of the body that is primarily affected. When some **bilious** humor gathers in the brain together with burning fever, the brain suffers in much the same way as those that are roasted by fire, and produces a smoky flame just like that from oil lamps. This smoke, descending through the channels that lead to the eye, becomes the cause of the hallucinations. For you have seen in dissections that both the arteries and the veins descend together with the nerves to the eye from the choroid plexus of the choroid membrane. But let this discussion end here, since it has made sufficient distinctions.

TEXT 15. PAUL OF AEGINA, *MEDICAL COMPENDIUM* SELECTION (3.22)

Paul of Aegina (c. 625–690 CE) was a Greek physician about whom little is known. From Aegina, an island to the north of Athens, Paul was the author of a book on pediatrics that no longer survives and the Medical Compendium, *a treatise in seven books that was meant to serve as a reference work covering many practical subjects. Paul drew heavily on the writings of earlier medical authors, including **Galen**, **Oribasius**, and **Soranus**. The* Medical Compendium *had an enormous impact on later Greek physicians, as well as Arabic physicians in the medieval period. The selection below comes from the third book, which discussed illnesses and ailments organized by the parts of the body they affected. Paul's treatments for the eye afflictions discussed here focus especially on pharmaceutical remedies, with some emphasis on regimen as a preventative measure.*

SOURCE: Translation by Brent Arehart based on the Greek text from J. L. Heiberg, *Paulus Aegineta*, vol. 1, Corpus Medicorum Graecorum 9.1 (Leipzig: Teubner, 1921).

Book 3, Chapter 22. 1. Eye problems, and firstly pain, from the works of Galen
Whenever pain in the eyes becomes very intense, consider the condition in which the eye pain occurs with inflammation. Intense eye pain occurs from an intense biting sensation caused by the sharpness of fluxes, or because the tunics are stretched when they are full, or because of an obstruction of thick **humors** or flatulence [*pneumata*]. Treat the biting sensations by draining them with purgatives and pouring liquid from an egg on them. When the inflammation has already reached a **crisis** and the body is slender, it is most appropriate to take baths. It is suitable to treat inflammation that follows a state of fullness by emptying blood, evacuating the belly, and rubbing the lower parts. Treat obstructions by emptying the entire body first, and furthermore, draw down the weight of the humors and then by using topical remedies that dispel. Warm the eyes up and pour a decoction of fenugreek on them. In cases where there is an obstruction of thick blood in the veins of the eyes without the rest of the body having a condition of fullness, use a dose of wine which has properties that create considerable heat, drain, and remove obstacles.

2. On irritation, particularly of the eye

Irritation of the eye is a state of moistness and heat accompanied by noticeable redness that occurs naturally, not because of the body, but due to some external cause such as the sun, smoke, dust, or oil. Hence, it is resolved most quickly by identifying the cause. Eye affliction is not just a form of external irritation, but it also occurs without any evident cause and lasts up to three, four, or even five days. It is most easily treated by watching out for external irritants, moderation in food, drinking water, taking a walk, and a healthy bowel movement.

3. On inflammation

If inflammation lingers in the eyes after emptying the entire body, use ointments made with things whose properties drive back the ailment and soothe the redness, such as the Nile eye-drop compound, or the Persian compound, and the compound made from nard. If there is inflammation in the conjunctiva, use the so-called single day eye salves along with pouring egg white on them. During the next day, if the inflammation does not increase in intensity, anoint with a compound of nard and use a vapor bath made from a decoction of melilot and fenugreek. If thick moisture is causing the eye affliction, we will use **drugs** that do not adhere to the liquids or thicken them but drugs with properties that scatter, moisten, and excrete, such as the Chian compound.[52] If the liquids are wedged in around the head, apply a **cupping** vessel to the occipital bone, or cut it open, or apply leeches to the brow of the aching eye, and **plaster** on clean bread in water with rose or barley boiled with a decoction of poppy capsules likewise with rose. Use a more drastic plaster made from saffron, melilots, date flesh, coriander leaves, soft-boiled eggs and boiled yolk, breadcrumbs broken into mash, a little bit of rose, and poppy capsules made smooth in a decoction. Sometimes we also mix it with poppy seed to relieve pain. If there is great necessity for this due to the pain, also mix in the smallest amount of poppy-juice, but narcotics must be avoided when the pain is not great. If the inflammation is moderate, leave aloe by itself in water or pour on an egg white. So that the remedy is ready to go, take six **drachmas** of saffron, sixteen drachmas of gum, and nine drachmas of rainwater and make them up into salves. Also appropriate are so-called saffron salves applied to the corner of the eyes. In cases where there is a swollen white mass around the eyelids and conjunctiva without pain in the tunics, so-called wet salves prepared from saffron, copper sulfate, and honey are also useful.

FEVERS

Today fevers are often considered a symptom of another illness, but in antiquity many considered fever to be an illness in and of itself. In general, fever was thought to be caused by some kind of excess in the body, such as an excess of heat. For example, Hippocratic case studies noted that fever could arise from too much exposure to the sun. So certain seasons when the weather was very hot and dry—such as the hottest days in the summer—gave rise

52. "Chian" refers to the Greek island of Chios.

to more fevers (see Text 8, *On Epidemics* 5.73). Medical writers also thought that fevers were caused by an excess of yellow bile, the hot and dry **humor**, often due to an improper regimen, especially diet and exercise. Hippocratic case studies note particular foods that, when eaten in excess, lead to fever, including meat, wine, and onions. The case studies also suggest the kinds of activities that brought on fever: excessive exercise, ill-timed exercise, and the extreme exertions of childbirth (see Text 8, *On Epidemics* 1.2 and 1.4).

Another explanation was that fever resulted not only from the excess of humors, but from humors that had putrefied or fermented before they could be expelled from the body. Medical writers reasoned that fever was the body's attempt to burn off these problematic humors, whether because they were overly abundant or had putrefied. In this respect, fever was understood as the body's natural, cleansing response. And physicians' medical treatments (as we will see below) aimed to assist the body in its work.

Galen agreed with many of these theories, and added a number of other possible causes, including blocked passages in the body, and breathing in foul-smelling air in the vicinity of stagnant water. Galen also attributed some fevers to excessive emotion, such as anger or erotic passion that violently moved about the body, creating friction and thus also heat. This would in turn affect processes in the body, such as the production of excessive bile or blood. This linkage between emotions and heat is also found in nonmedical sources, such as ancient erotic or binding spells that sought to evoke emotions of love in their intended targets by conjuring fever. For instance, in one binding spell found in a ritual handbook from Egypt, the formula for creating desire in the beloved states, "Make a flame in her body, flame in her intestines. Put madness after her heart, fever after her **flesh**" (*PDM* xiv, 660–65).

As medical writers discussed the various causes of fevers, they also classified types of fevers based on their cycles and duration, noting that some fevers were continuous, whereas other fevers were intermittent with periods when the fever symptoms were most pronounced (called a "**paroxysm**" or "attack"), followed by a remission. As we see in the Hippocratic case studies, physicians paid close attention to when crises occurred in their feverish patients. For example, in the case of Silenus, the physician notes that the patient experienced acute fever on the second, seventh, and eighth days of his illness (Text 8, *On Epidemics* 1.2). Physicians also categorized fevers based on their accompanying symptoms, such as sweating, shivering fits, weakness, delirium, and uncharacteristic pulse rate. For example, in the case study of the wife of Philinus, who became gravely ill fourteen days after giving birth, the physician documents fever accompanied by cold shivers on the first and eighth days (Text 8, *On Epidemics* 1.4).

The Hippocratic text *On the Nature of Humans* further divides intermittent fevers into quotidian fever (the patient experienced the full cycle of paroxysm and remission in a single day), **tertian fever** (the patient experienced the cycle of paroxysm and remission within a forty-eight-hour period), and **quartan fever** (the patient experienced the cycle of paroxysm and remission within a seventy-two-hour period). When we read the selection on fevers from **Celsus's** *On Medicine* (Text 16) we find a similar system of distinguishing fevers in terms of

GALEN'S CLASSIFICATION OF SEPTIC FEVERS

Humor	Type of Fever	Time for a Cycle of Paroxysm and Remission
Phlegm	Quotidian (daily)	24 hours
Yellow Bile	Tertian (every third day, counting inclusively)	48 hours
Black Bile	Quartan (every fourth day, counting inclusively)	72 hours

FIGURE 34 Galen's classification of septic fevers. Created by Jared Secord.

their periodicity (daily, on the third day, on the fourth day), and in terms of the kinds of symptoms that are most pronounced during the attack (heat, coldness, shivering).

Theories about the causes of fevers and their varying periodicity came together in the writings of Galen. In his view, some intermittent fevers were caused by humors that were clogged in the body's arteries, then fermenting there. He called these types of fevers "septic." He connected the periodicity of these fevers—that is, the different times for a cycle of paroxysm and remission—to the kind of humor that was clogged and fermenting (see fig. 34).

Fevers were treated in a number of different ways, but the main aims of treatment were to cool the body or to assist it in expelling excess or putrefied humors. Remedies could be as simple as cooling sponge baths, or they could involve the ingestion of food or drugs whose main property was to cool or purge. Both Celsus and Galen recommended that food be given to fevered patients only at times when their symptoms had abated because digestion was a process akin to cooking, requiring heat in order to distill food into more refined substances (see above on digestive and intestinal ailments). Hence, eating—and the digestive process of cooking—further exacerbated the heat of an already hot body. Physicians also attempted to eliminate the excess and putrefying humors through evacuating remedies, such as **emetics**, bloodletting, and enemas. For example, in the selection that follows, Celsus mentions that the physician **Asclepiades of Bithynia** recommended that his patients purge, especially their bowels, in the early days of a fever. Celsus criticized this practice for the way it weakened the already vulnerable patient—a criticism he likely felt was necessary because physicians were following Asclepiades's example.

TEXT 16. CELSUS, *ON MEDICINE* SELECTION (3.3–4)

On Medicine, *written by Aulus Cornelius **Celsus** (first centuries BCE and CE), was originally part of an encyclopedia that covered a range of topics, including agriculture, medicine, rhetoric, philosophy, and military science. The section on medicine, the only one to survive, is organized* *around the three major divisions of ancient medicine: regimen, pharmacology, and surgery. Scholars debate whether Celsus was himself a practicing physician, but his text offers hints of real experience, especially in the sections on surgery. In the selection below, taken from his discussion of illnesses that affect the entire body, Celsus focuses on fevers, explaining the characteristics of different types of fevers and how they should be treated.*

SOURCE: Translation by Jared Secord based on the Latin text from W. G. Spencer, *Celsus, On Medicine, Books I–IV*, Loeb Classical Library 292 (Cambridge, Mass.: Harvard University Press, 1935).

Book 3, Chapter 3. 1. Now follows the treatment of fevers, a type of illness that impacts the entire body and that is especially common. Of these, one variety is daily, another is on the third day, and another variety is on the fourth day.[53] Sometimes some fevers return in an even longer cycle, but this is rare. In the above varieties, both the illnesses and the procedures of treatment are different.

The fourth-day fevers are simpler. They generally begin with shivering. Then heat breaks out. Once the fever has stopped, there are two days free of it. Thus it returns on the fourth day.

2. There are two varieties of the third-day fever. One begins and ends in the same way as the fourth-day fever, with the only difference being that one day elapses free from fever before it returns on the third day. The other variety is the most dangerous by far because it returns on the third day, but it occupies around thirty-six out of forty-eight hours— sometimes more or less—accompanied by an attack, nor does it completely stop in its remission, but it only becomes milder. This type most physicians call "half every three days."[54]

3. The daily fevers vary and are complex. For some of them begin immediately with heat, others with coldness, and others with shivering. I call it "coldness" when the extremities of limbs become cold, and "shivering" when the entire body trembles. In turn, some fevers end so that full normality follows, but others so that the fever is somewhat diminished but some traces of it remain nonetheless until another attack comes. And others often come together so that they diminish hardly at all or not at all but continue. 4. Some have massive heat, others tolerable. Some are the same every day, others are different, and the attack by turn gentler on one day, and more severe on another. Some return at the same time on the following day, some later, and some earlier. Some fill a day and a night with an attack and a retreat, some less, and others more. Some cause sweating when they subside, and others do not. And in some normality comes through sweating, but in others the body is only rendered weaker. 5. But the attacks also sometimes occur once in a single day and sometimes twice or more. From this it often happens that there are multiple attacks and remissions daily, but in such a way that each corresponds to the previous. Sometimes the attacks are also blurred

53. These types of fevers are often identified as quotidian fevers (the kind that spikes on a daily basis), tertian fevers (the kind that spikes every third day), and quartan (the kind that spikes every fourth day).
54. In Greek, *hēmitritaion*.

together, so that neither their length nor the intervals between them can be recorded. Neither is it true, what is said by some, that no fever is irregular, unless it comes from an abscess, inflammation, or an ulceration. For, if this were true, the treatment would always be easier. But what evident causes do, hidden causes can also do.[55] 6. And when in the same illness fevers come on in different ways, people say that these are not the same fevers returning irregularly, but different fevers arising one after another, they create a controversy not about the matter itself, but about terminology. Even if what they said was true, it has no bearing on the method of treatment. The length of remissions is also sometimes considerable, but sometimes hardly any time at all.

Book 3, Chapter 4. 1. And such is, for the most part, an account of fevers. There are, however, different types of treatments, just as several authorities think. **Asclepiades** says that it is the duty of a physician to offer safe, fast, and pleasant treatment. That is the aspiration, but there is often danger in excessive speed and enjoyment. But the type of moderation to be employed to achieve these results as much as possible, with good health always held in first place, will have to be considered in the actual parts of treatment.

2. And before all things is the question of how a sick person should be sustained in the first days. The ancients sought to produce digestion by giving certain **drugs**, because they very much dreaded indigestion. Then they extracted the bodily matter that seemed to harm by frequently inducing bowel movements.[56] Asclepiades eliminated the use of drugs. He purged the bowel less frequently, but still did this for almost every illness. He professed to use the fever as a remedy against itself, for he judged that the sick person's strength should be shaken during the day with lack of sleep and immense thirst so that he would not even permit the sick person's mouth to be rinsed out in the first days. 3. Therefore the people who imagine that his habit was pleasant in all ways are quite mistaken. For, in his last days, he even approved luxuries for the bed-ridden sick person, but in the first days he played the role of a torturer. I, however, grant that doses of drugs should be given and the bowel purged only rarely. I nevertheless think that this should not be done so that a sick person's strength may be shaken, because the greatest danger comes from weakness. 4. It is therefore fitting for excessive bodily matter to be diminished, but only that which is naturally dissipated with nothing new being added. Thus, in the first days, there must be abstention from food. During the day, the sick person should be kept in the light, unless weak, because this also clears the body, and so the sick person should lie down in a room as lofty, bright, and spacious as

55. See Text 4, Celsus, *On Medicine*, Preface 14 and 18 for a discussion of evident causes and hidden causes. "Evident causes" refers to the cause of an illness, whereas "hidden causes" refers to the humoral makeup of the body. So an illness could be the result of the evident cause, for instance, of eating too much or too little, too much heat or too much cold; that in turn prompted the hidden cause of the illness, such as too much or too little blood, black bile, yellow bile, or phlegm.

56. "Bodily matter" translates the Latin word *materia* (sometimes *materies*). It refers generally to the substances that make up the body, and especially to the excess humors believed to cause imbalance and illness in the body.

possible.[57] As relates to thirst and sleep, the sick person should be guided to remain awake during the day. At night, if this is possible, the sick person should sleep. And the sick person should not drink, nor be tormented too much by thirst. 5. The sick person's mouth can be rinsed out when it is dry and if it has a bad smell, although this time is not suitable for taking a drink. And **Erasistratus** helpfully said that often when the interior part of the body does not need fluid, the mouth and throat do, and it is not suitable for a sick person to be poorly cared for in this way. And for the first day the sick person should be kept in this way.

6. Erasistratus' best drug is food given appropriately. It should be asked when food should first be given. Most of the ancients used to give it late, often on the fifth or sixth day. And perhaps the climate in Asia or Egypt allows this.[58] Asclepiades used to mark out the fourth day for food, after having worn out the sick person for three days in every respect. But recently **Themison** considered not when the fever had begun, but when it ended, or at least when it got better. And, waiting for the third day from that time, if the fever had not attacked by this time, he gave food immediately. If the fever had attacked, he gave food when it had ended, or, if it was constantly persisting, he at least gave food if the fever got better. 7. But nothing about these matters is a universal rule. For it is possible that food should first be given on the first day, or the second, or the third, or not until the fourth or fifth, or after one attack, or after two, or after many. For it depends on what type of illness, what type of body, what type of climate, what type of age, what time of the year. When there are so many differences, there absolutely cannot be a universal rule for time.[59] 8. From an illness that takes away more strength, food should be given earlier, and likewise in a climate in which a sick person uses up more. For this reason it seems right that a sick person in Africa should fast for no more than a day. Food should likewise be given earlier to a child than to a youth, and earlier in summer than winter. There is one thing that should be protected always and everywhere: the attending physician should keep constant watch on the sick person's strength. And as long as there is excess, the physician should combat it with fasting. If the physician begins to fear weakness, the physician should assist the sick person with food. For this is the physician's duty: that the sick person is not burdened with excess bodily matter, nor made weak by hunger. 9. And I also find this in the work of Erasistratus. Although he taught little about when the stomach, and the body itself, should be emptied, by nevertheless saying that these things should be seen to, and food given when it was needed by the body, he showed sufficiently that it is inappropriate for food to be given as long as one has excessive strength, but that care should be taken so that one's strength not diminish. From these things, however, it can be understood that many people cannot be treated by a single physician, and that the physician, if skilled, is suitable if he

57. The characteristics of the ideal room are missing in the Latin text here, but they can likely be restored from the description of a similar room at Celsus 1.2.7.

58. Celsus's point here is that the climate in Asia (modern-day Türkiye) and Egypt is different from the climate in Rome, meaning that physicians in different regions needed to adjust their treatments accordingly.

59. The rule for time refers to when a sick person should be given food: after one day, two days, etc.

does not stay away from the sick person much. 10. But people who are slaves to profit, because there is more profit from a crowd, gladly embrace precepts that do not demand constant attendance, as in this very instance. For it is easy even for someone who rarely sees a sick person to count days or attacks. That person must always be nearby who is going to see the only necessary thing: when the sick person is about to be too weak unless the sick person receives food. In general, nevertheless, the fourth day is the most suitable for beginning to give food.

MENTAL AND EMOTIONAL AFFLICTIONS

Most ancient depictions of mental and emotional turmoil come from nonmedical sources, such as mythological, oracular, theatrical, ethical, and legal texts, as well as images on pottery and *stelai*. These sources represent such turmoil in both positive and negative ways, as influences of benign and malign spirits and as disturbances of the body and soul. For example, the ancient Greeks regarded "madness" (*paraphrosune* in Greek, *mania* in Greek and Latin) as a mode of divine inspiration (*enthousiasmos*), and as a punishment for moral or religious failings. The celebrants of the god Dionysus, the Maenads, exemplify this concept (see fig. 35). In Euripides's play *The Bacchae*, Dionysus aroused the Maenads to an excited state and then used their divinely inspired madness to punish the "madness" of disbelief and impiety of King Pentheus and his mother, Agave, by tearing the king to shreds. Divine madness was also a feature of ancient divinatory practices. The oracles at temples to **Apollo** were reportedly inhabited by the god—falling into an ecstatic trance—as they became the mouthpieces by which the god dispensed wisdom or predictions of the future. In later periods, we have Jewish, Christian, and "pagan" stories that depicted mental and emotional turmoil when people were possessed by malevolent daemons. In the Gospel of Mark, the holy man Jesus was confronted by a man who was possessed by an "unclean spirit."

Mental and emotional distress was also medicalized. The Hippocratic corpus discussed altered mental states not as illnesses in and of themselves, but rather as symptoms of other illnesses. For instance, see the Hippocratic case study of Nicostratus's wife in which she is described as having "groped about with her fingers" and raving (Text 8, *On Epidemics* 4.14). Additionally, in early gynecology, mental distress was thought to be a symptom of women's ailments, whether because backed-up menstrual blood or a roaming womb impaired the organ responsible for mental faculties (see above on women's illnesses).

One of the earliest sustained discussions of mental and emotional afflictions is the Hippocratic text dedicated to the "sacred illness," a condition that involved chronic seizures and that historians now commonly associate with epilepsy. The Hippocratic author rejects mythological or ethical explanations of the illness in favor of an explanation based in somatic or materialist causes. More specifically, the author attempts to decipher the relationship between mind, soul, and body. Ancient thinkers understood mental activity to be carried out by the soul (*psychē*, from which we get the English word "psychological") or spirit (*pneuma*), which were thought to be made up of the finest kinds of matter, such as air, fire, or ether. Because these kinds of matter were physical, mental faculties were associated with the loca-

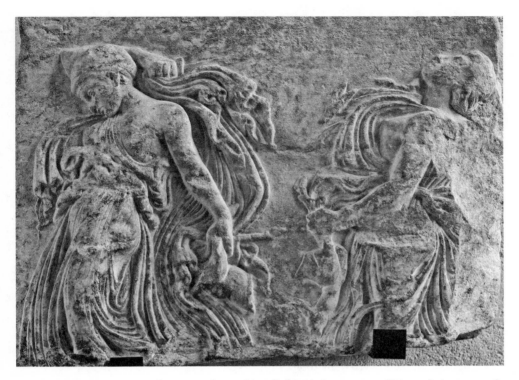

FIGURE 35 First-century CE fragment of a marble relief depicting a scene of Maenads in a state of ecstatic trance, frenzy, and madness inspired by the Greek god Dionysus. Department of Greek, Etruscan, and Roman Antiquities of the Louvre (inv. no. Ma3626). Wikimedia Commons.

tions in which they were concentrated, and debates arose about whether the mental faculties were located in the brain, heart, internal organs such as the liver, or blood (as the conduit for **pneuma**). Likewise, they discussed how disorders related to these substances could not only result in physical symptoms but also affect cognition and emotions.

Because physicians and medical writers understood the body, mind, and soul to be interconnected, we do not find a subspecialty within ancient medicine devoted solely to mental and emotional afflictions. And there were no institutions or personnel devoted exclusively to the mentally and emotionally ill. Rather, physicians applied the same pathological explanations as for any other illness (i.e., humoral imbalance, looseness and stricture). For example, there was widespread consensus that an abundance of one **humor** altered not only the state of one's physical body, but also one's disposition according to the characteristic temperaments associated with each humor: **bilious/choleric, melancholic, phlegmatic,** and **sanguine** (see fig. 16).

Over time, medical writers showed more interest in classifying different kinds of mental and emotional afflictions. In Book 3 of *On Medicine,* **Celsus** provides a systematic taxonomy distinguishing acute and chronic mental illnesses. So, a mental derangement induced by fever, for instance, would be classified as an acute condition, but if one was deranged for a longer period of time, it was classified as a chronic condition. Celsus identified a third kind of mental illness called *maestitudo*, which lasted the longest and resembled what had become known as a "melancholic" temperament. **Rufus of Ephesus** wrote an entire text on *melancholia*, a kind of mental distress caused by an excess of black bile (*melaine cholē*). Some people, Rufus thought, were prone to *melancholia* if they naturally had more black bile, but *melancholia* could also develop through improper diet and lifestyle, which produced an excess of black bile. Ancient definitions of the illness emphasized a melancholic person's tendency to despair along with a propensity for violent behavior, delusions, desire for solitude, sudden changes in mood, unreasonable desires, and excessive rage.

We do not see a single protocol specific to the detection and diagnosis of mental and emotional afflictions. **Caelius Aurelianus** recommended merely speaking with patients. **Galen** gathered an array of information from their symptoms and their home environment. For example, when encountering a woman who was experiencing disturbed sleep, Galen first hypothesized that she was experiencing some kind of melancholic despondency, with sleeplessness being the physical manifestation of the mental and emotional illness. Yet, when he noticed that her pulse quickened when a slave shared a report about a famous dancer, Galen concluded that the woman's mental distress derived from another emotional illness: lovesickness for the dancer. **Erasistratus** reports a similar episode in the diagnosis of the ruler Antiochus, who displayed other signs of mental distress, particularly when the object of his affections entered the room.

Turning to the treatments, it is important to note that care of the soul and remedies for emotional distress and excessive emotions—especially anger, grief, and sexual passion—fell under the purview of philosophical schools. There, elite men (and in rare cases elite women) devoted themselves to strengthening their rational faculty and decision-making processes, as well as to inculcating moral habits and practices, all of which enabled them to control and subdue disturbing thoughts and emotions. Within the medical realm, philosophically inclined physicians like Galen approached treatment from a similar perspective, insisting that good physicians should serve as philosophical or spiritual guides to improve the minds and emotions of their patients, just as they sought the well-being of their bodies.

Physicians who assumed that mental, emotional, and physical symptoms were connected might prescribe any of a variety of treatments to eliminate excessive or corrupt humors to restore balance to both the body and the mind. Others recommended treating mental afflictions with light therapy (either limiting exposure to light or increasing it), talk therapy (trying to cheer the patient up by assuaging fears or distracting the patient from them), or entertainment (such as listening to music or attending the theater, which would distract the patient or lead to the catharsis of troubling emotions). For seizures (*epilēpsia*), **Alexander of Tralles** describes a complicated treatment protocol that involved massaging and straightening the patient's limbs (to help relax the body), and then regulating the patient's regimen through diet and sexual activity in order to restore balance of the humors.

Some tried so-called magical and religious treatments. For example, **Archigenes of Apamea** recommends the use of a nail from a cross as an amulet for patients experiencing seizures. Other "magical" remedies—including purifications and incantations—are alluded to (albeit criticized) in *On the Sacred Illness*. And many Jewish and Christian communities who explained mental and emotional afflictions in terms of possession by evil daemons, healed community members through exorcistic rites and practices.

Finally, sometimes treatment of severe and persistent mental distress involved nothing more than physical restraint. For instance, in a vivid case history, Galen describes a Roman man suffering from *phrenitis* who was confined to an upper-story room with his slave (Text 14). In another source (potentially from the late first century CE) the **Anonymus Parisinus** suggests that when all other treatments for phrenitis failed, "nothing forbids the use of smacks and blows" (1.11). Such responses strike us as cruel, but in a time when institutional care for those experiencing mental and emotional afflictions did not exist, these cases illustrate the desperation of caregivers and how they might justify confinement and violence as a form of care.

TEXT 17. HIPPOCRATIC CORPUS, *ON THE SACRED ILLNESS*[60]

*On the Sacred Illness was attributed to **Hippocrates**, but as with all the texts in the Hippocratic corpus, the authorship is uncertain. Scholars have identified some similarities between it and other texts in the Hippocratic corpus, especially* Airs, Waters, Places *(Text 2), and believe the text was likely written in the mid- or later fifth century BCE. The author was clearly a physician writing for other physicians about the "sacred illness"—which has often been identified as epilepsy—as well as other conditions involving various types of seizures. The text is famous for suggesting that the condition known as the sacred illness was not sent by the gods, but rather caused by an excessive amount of phlegm. The author makes the case with a detailed discussion of anatomy and physiology, especially an emphasis on respiration and the impact of heredity. By arguing that the nature of divinity was all good and all beneficial to human beings, and by discrediting the view that the gods might cause illness, the author discredits practitioners who use rituals as part of their healing process, distinguishing these "shamanistic" healers from physicians such as himself.*

SOURCE: Translation by Robert Nau based on the Greek text from Jacques Jouanna, *Hippocrate, Morb. 2* (Paris: Les Belles Lettres, 1983).

Chapter 1. 1. The nature of the illness called "sacred" is as follows. It seems to me in no way more divine or sacred than other illnesses, but it has its own nature and, just as the other illnesses have a condition from which they arise, this illness also has a natural cause. 2. But people believed, on account of their inexperience and astonishment, that it was some divine act, because it is nothing like other illnesses. Because of their difficulty in understanding the illness, they insist on its divinity. But, in light of the simple manner of treatment that they apply, since they treat it with purifications and incantations, its divinity is undercut.

60. This text has traditionally been translated with the title *On the Sacred Disease*. See chapter 1 for our rationale for preferring the English translation "illness" over "disease."

3. But, if it is believed to be divine because it is wondrous, on this count there will be many sacred illnesses and not one. As I will explain, there are others no less wondrous or foreboding, and no one believes that they are sacred. As to this, I think that daily, **tertian**, and **quartan fevers**, which do not awe others, are no less sacred and come no less from a god than this illness. As to this, I see people who rage, who are out of their senses from no obvious cause, who do many strange things, and I know many people who in their sleep wail and shout, choke, jump up, and flee outside, and are out of their senses until they wake and then, just as earlier, are healthy and are of sound mind though they are pale and weak. I witnessed these things not just once, but many times. There are many other examples of every kind, but it would take too long to speak of them individually.

4. It seems to me that those who first gave a sacred character to this illness were people of the sort who are now magicians, purifiers, charlatans, and quacks, who pretend to be deeply god-fearing and to have superior knowledge. Accordingly, these people, cloaking and defending themselves with "divinity" against their powerlessness to provide something to help so that their ignorance is not revealed, deemed this suffering "sacred." Adding plausible stories, they established a treatment for their own security by proposing purifications and incantations, and having the sick abstain from baths and from many foods that are unsuitable for the sick to eat: of the fish of the seas, the red-mullet, the black-tail, the hammer, and the eel, for these are very dangerous. Of meat, goat, deer, pig, and dog, for these of all meats most disturb the **cavity**. Of birds, the rooster, turtle-dove, and bustard, meats that are believed to be very strong. Of garden greens, mint, garlic, and onion, for their pungency is not beneficial to the sick. They advise not to wear black clothes, for black is associated with death, not to wear or lie down on goatskin, and not to place foot on foot or hand on hand, for these are all obstacles. 5. They impose all these things because of the illness' sacredness and, as though they have superior knowledge, they claim various causes so that they would have a reputation for cleverness if the person becomes healthy. But, if someone dies, they would be made safe, with the defense as an excuse that they are not at fault, but the gods. For they gave no drug to eat, nor to drink, nor did they boil the deceased in baths, things that could lead them to appear at fault. 6. I guess that a Libyan,[61] one of those who lives inland, could not be healthy, if they rely upon goat skins and goat meats to any degree, since they have neither bedding, nor clothing, nor sandal that is not made from a goat. For other than goats and cattle they keep no other herds. But if things that are eaten and employed produce and increase the illness, and that heal when they are not eaten, then divinity is no longer the cause, and purifications do not help, rather the foods are what cure and harm. The power of divinity vanishes.

7. So it seems to me that those who attempt to heal in this manner believe that these illnesses are neither sacred nor divine. For when they disappear under such purifications and such treatment, what prevents these illnesses from being produced again and assailing people by techniques similar to their purifications and treatments, so that the cause is not divine but in some way human? For the person who can remove such a condition by purify-

61. The term "Libyan" refers to a person from any part of Africa other than Egypt (see fig. 17).

ing and practicing magic could also introduce them by practicing their arts, and, in this argument, divine agency perishes. 8. By saying and contriving things of this sort they pretend to have superior knowledge, and they deceive people in proposing purifications and cleansings. Much of their discourse relies upon divine and spiritual matters. And so it seems to me that they do not produce discourses based on piety, as they think, but rather on impiety and the non-existence of gods, and that their "piety" is impiety and their "divinity" is unholy, as I will explain.

9. For if they promise they can draw down the moon and conceal the sun, and make stormy and fair weather, rains and droughts, the sea and land barren, and all other such kinds of things (whether they say such things can happen from their rites or some other scheme or practice), it seems to me that those involved in these practices are impious and believe that the gods neither exist nor have any power, nor do they restrain themselves from any extreme actions, because the gods are not an object of fear for them. For if a person will draw down the moon and conceal the sun and make stormy and fair weather by practicing magic and sacrificing, I would not believe that any of these acts are divine, but human, if indeed the power of a god is mastered and has been enslaved by human intelligence. 10. But perhaps this is not so, and it is rather that people in need of a livelihood contrive and fabricate strategies of all sorts for this illness and other things, attributing to a god the cause of each type of condition. 11. For, in truth, sick people do not mimic one thing at one time and another thing at another time, but instead mimic the same things frequently.[62] If someone imitates a goat, shouts, and suffers spasms on their right side, they claim that the Mother of the Gods[63] is the cause. But if someone makes rather shrill and violent noises, they liken him to a horse, and claim that Poseidon is the cause. If someone passes some excrement, something that frequently happens to those hard pressed by the illness, the god Enodia's name is applied. If their noises are thinner and lighter, like birds, **Apollo** Nomios is the cause. If someone sprays foam from the mouth and kicks with the feet, Ares is the cause. They claim that nighttime visitation of terror, leaping from the bed and flight outside are the assaults of Hecate and onslaughts of heroes.[64] 12. They employ purifications and incantations and they perform a most unholy and most impious act, as it seems to me, for they purify those with the illness by blood and similar things as if they suffered under some **miasma** or vengeful spirits, or had been cursed by people, or had done some unholy deed. They should have done the opposite, bringing them to the shrines to sacrifice, pray, and supplicate the gods. But at present they do none of these, but they perform purifications and they conceal some of the objects of purification in the earth, throwing some into the sea and carrying some away to the hills, where no one will touch or step on them. If a god is really the cause, they should have brought them to the shrines to offer them to the god. 13. I do not,

62. This sentence may have been added as an explanatory gloss by a later scribe who copied the text.
63. "Mother of the Gods" refers to the Phrygian goddess Cybele.
64. That is, the visitations of deified humans.

though, hold the opinion that a person's body is defiled by a god, the one that is most corruptible defiled by the one that is most pure. But if it happens to become defiled with miasma through some other force or injured in some way, a god is more likely to purify and sanctify the body than pollute it with miasma. At any rate, divinity purifies, sanctifies, and cleanses us for our greatest and most impious sins. We ourselves make the boundaries of the shrines and precincts for the gods, so that no one may tread across them unless they are pure, and as we enter we sprinkle ourselves not to suffer miasma, but to cleanse any defilement we have from earlier. That is how I think it is with purifications.

Chapter 2. 1. But this illness seems to me no more divine than the rest. Like other illnesses, it has a nature and an origin from where each illness arises and a natural cause. It is divine for the same reason as all other illnesses. And it is no less treatable than the others, unless through the passage of time it has become so powerful that it is stronger than the **drugs** that are applied. 2. As with other illnesses it takes its beginnings from heredity. For if someone with excess phlegm is born from a parent with excess phlegm, and someone with excess bile is born from a parent with excess bile, and someone with consumption is born from a parent with consumption, and someone with a bad temper is born from someone with a bad temper, what is there to prevent a child from suffering the disorder when their mother or father suffers from it? For the seed comes from everywhere in the body, healthy from healthy parts and sickly from sickly parts. 3. There is another great proof that this illness is not at all more divine than other illnesses in that it naturally occurs in people with excess phlegm, but does not strike people with excess bile. But, if it is more divine than the others, this illness ought to have happened equally to all, and not to have distinguished between people with excess bile and people with excess phlegm.

Chapter 3. 1. But the brain is the cause of this condition, just as it is for the other serious illnesses. I will clearly declare by what manner and from what cause it arises. 2. The human brain is in two parts, just as it is with all other animals. A thin membrane divides it in the middle. This is why pain does not always happen in the same place in the head, but sometimes on one side or the other, and occasionally in the entire head. 3. Vessels lead into it from the entire body. Two of these are thin but there are two thick ones, one from the liver, the other from the spleen. 4. The one from the liver is like this: one part of the vessel extends downwards alongside the kidney and loins towards the inside of the thigh and comes down to the foot. It is called the "hollow vessel." The other part of the vessel extends upwards through the diaphragm and the lungs on the right and departs to the heart and the right arm while the remainder bears upwards through the collarbone to the right side of the neck to the skin itself, such that it can be seen. It hides itself beside the ear and there splits with the thickest, biggest, and most hollow branch ending in the brain, another in the right ear, another in the right eye, and another in the nostril. 5. That is how it is with the vessels from the liver. A vessel also extends from the spleen downwards and upwards to the left side, just as the vessel from the liver, but it is thinner and weaker.

Chapter 4. 1. We take in the greater part of our breath [*pneuma*] through these vessels, for these are the body's vents and draw air into themselves and conduct it via smaller vessels to the rest of the body, and they cool it off and release it back. 2. For breath [*pneuma*] cannot stand still but goes up and down. For, if it stands still and is cut off, the part of the body where it stands still becomes powerless. The proof of this is that when, while sitting or lying, one's vessels are pressed tightly enough that the air [*pneuma*] does not pass along through the vessel, and immediately numbness takes hold. This is how it is with the vessels.

Chapter 5. 1. This illness occurs in people with excess phlegm, but not people with excess bile. It begins to grow in the embryo while still in the womb. For the brain, like the other body parts, is cleansed and has growths before birth.[65] 2. In this cleansing, if the brain is cleansed properly and in due measure and if there is neither more or less shedding than required, the embryo's head is very healthy. But if too much is shed from the whole brain and there is a significant discharge, as the child grows its head will be sickly and its ears will ring intensely and the child will not be able to endure sun or cold. If the excessive shedding happens from an eye or ear, or if a vessel is reduced, that part is harmed to the degree it suffers from discharge. 3. If instead the cleansing does not happen, but there is coalescence in the brain, the infants must necessarily have excess phlegm. If, while still children, they suffer outbreaks of sores on the head, ears, and the skin in general, and from an abundance of saliva and a running nose, they will live a carefree life as they grow older, for at that time they discharge and cleanse themselves of the phlegm that ought to have been cleansed away in the womb. For the most part, those children cleansed in this way are not attacked by this illness. 4. Children whose bodies have been cleansed and who suffer neither sores, nor mucus, nor saliva, and whose brains have not been cleansed in the womb, risk being struck by this illness.

Chapter 6. 1. If the discharge makes the journey to the heart, palpitation and trouble breathing take hold and the chest is weakened, and some people also become hunchbacked. 2. For, whenever phlegm, which is cold, comes down to the lungs and heart, the blood is cooled off. The vessels, because they have been chilled forcibly, beat against the lungs and the heart, and the heart palpitates, so that necessarily difficulty in breathing and orthopnea strike (for the desired amount of breath [*pneuma*] is not received), until the influx of phlegm has been overcome, thoroughly warmed and dispersed into the vessels. 3. Then one ceases to have palpitation and difficulty breathing. This cessation is in relation to the amount of phlegm one has, for when more descends the cessation is slower, and quicker when less descends. If phlegm descends more frequently, the attack becomes more frequent. 4. One suffers these if the flux goes to the lungs and heart. If the flux reaches the cavity, bouts of diarrhea strike.

Chapter 7. 1. But if the phlegm is closed off from these passages, and flows down into the vessels mentioned before, one becomes speechless, froth flows from the mouth, there is grinding of teeth, clenching of hands, rolling of eyes, and the loss of wits; some also defecate. These attacks sometimes afflict the left side, sometimes the right, sometimes both.

65. This is a reference to the shedding of excess phlegm from the brain.

2. I will explain how each of these happen. One is speechless when phlegm suddenly comes down into the vessels and closes off the air that is not received into the brain or the hollow vessels or the cavities, but checks respiration. 3. For when a person takes a breath [*pneuma*] by the mouth and nostrils, first it comes into the brain, then the greater share into the cavity, but some of it into the lungs and some into the vessels. From there it disperses into the remaining parts via the vessels. 4. What comes into the cavity thoroughly cools it and contributes nothing otherwise, and this is the same for the lungs. But the air entering into the lungs and vessels contributes to [. . .][66] the cavities and brain and in this way furnishes thought and movement to the limbs. 5. This happens in such a way that when the vessels are shut off from air by phlegm and receive none, they cause a person to be voiceless and senseless. 6. The hands become powerless and clench when the blood does not move and is not dispersed as normal. 7. The eyes roll when the smaller vessels are cut off from air and throb. 8. Foam at the mouth comes from the lungs, for when the breath [*pneuma*] does not enter it, it foams and spouts up as if the patient were dying. 9. Defecation happens when the patient is forcefully suffocated. One is suffocated when the liver and cavity advance from above against the diaphragm and the opening of the stomach is closed off. They do this when the breath [*pneuma*] does not enter the mouth as normal. 10. One kicks with the feet when air is shut off in the limbs and cannot slip out because of the phlegm. When it shoots up and down it causes a spasm and pain, hence the kicks. 11. One suffers all these things when phlegm flows cold upon blood while it is warm, for this chills off and checks the blood. If there is a copious and thick flow, then one immediately dies, for it overpowers the blood with cold and thickens it. But, if there is less flow, it first overpowers the blood by blocking up respiration. Then, with time, when it is dispersed through the vessels and is mixed with copious and warm blood, if the phlegm is in this way overpowered, the vessels receive air and the people come to their senses.

Chapter 8. 1. Little children attacked by this illness generally die if a copious flow accompanies a south wind, for the small vessels, since they are thin, are not able to receive the phlegm because of its thickness and quantity, but the blood is chilled off and thickened, and thus one dies. 2. If the flow is slight and its downward flow makes its descent into both vessels, or one of the two, they survive, though there are marks from the disorder, for either the mouth, eye, neck, or hand becomes malformed where the smaller vessel was overcome and shrunk by being filled with phlegm. Because of the damage to the minor vessel, the part of the body that has been harmed is necessarily weaker and more deficient. 3. For the rest of their life they are generally better off, for they are no longer attacked, if they have once been so marked, for this reason: under this constraint, the remaining vessels are harmed and in some measure shriveled up, so that while they receive air, the downflow of phlegm no longer overpowers the blood to the same degree. It is still natural though, as before, for the limbs to be weaker since the vessels have been harmed. 4. Those whose flux is slight and to the right side accompanied by a north wind survive without any mark. But there is a risk, as the

66. Some words from the Greek text appear to be missing here.

infant is nourished and increases in size, of the disorder being nourished and increased as well, if they are not treated by appropriate measures. In the case of children these things, or something very close, happen.

Chapter 9. 1. Older people are not killed or deformed when the illness strikes, for their vessels are hollow and filled with warm blood. Accordingly phlegm cannot overpower or chill off the blood, so as to thicken it, but it is itself overpowered by the blood and mixed with it. Thus the vessels receive air and reason returns. The aforementioned marks are less prevalent because of the person's strength. 2. When this illness does happen to the very old, it kills or causes paralysis, since the vessels are emptied and there is a small amount of thin and watery blood. When there is much flux during the winter, the illness kills, for it chokes respiration and thickens the blood, if there is flux to both sides. But, if the flux is on one side only, it causes paralysis, for the small amount of thin and cold blood cannot overpower the phlegm, but is overpowered and thickened, so that the parts are powerless where the blood has been corrupted.

Chapter 10. 1. Flux is to the right side rather than the left, because the vessels have more room and are more numerous than on the left side, for they extend from the liver and spleen. 2. Flux and discharge happen especially to children if their heads are heated by the sun or fire, and if the brain is chilled suddenly, for then phlegm is separated off. Discharge results from the heat and the dissipation of the brain. It separates off because of the effect of the cooling and consolidation, which thus produces flux. 3. This is the cause in some cases. In other cases, a south wind that suddenly prevails after north winds [*pneumata*] relaxes the brain, which has been braced and is weak, resulting in a surge of phlegm, and thus produces flux. 4. A flux also happens when one is struck by fear during events not fully understood, and if one is frightened when someone shouts, or when one is weeping aloud and cannot quickly regain their breath [*pneuma*], the sort of things that often happen to children. Whichever of these happens to the person, their body chills immediately, and they cannot speak or take a breath [*pneuma*] and their breathing [*pneuma*] stops, the brain contracts, the blood is stopped and so phlegm is separated off and flows downward. 5. These are the causes of the seizure in children at the outset. Winter is most hostile to the old. For when someone old is warmed at a strong fire and their head and brain are heated, and then they are exposed to the cold and cool down, or come into the heat from a cold place and to a strong fire, they suffer the same things and thus an attack happens in the manner just described. There is a great risk too of suffering the same thing in the spring, if the head is warmed by the sun, but there is least risk in the summer, for there are not sudden changes. 6. When one has passed twenty years, this illness no longer strikes anyone, or only a few at most, unless it develops in infancy. For the vessels are filled with a great quantity of blood and the brain has consolidated and is solid, so that flux does not flow down to the vessels, but if flux does descend, it does not overpower the blood since it is warm and in great quantity.

Chapter 11. 1. But when the illness has grown and been nourished along with the person from childhood, this person habitually suffers from it and regularly has an attack with changing winds [*pneumata*], especially when they are south winds. Recovery becomes difficult too. 2. For the brain has become wetter than what is natural and surges with phlegm, which results in fluxes making their descent more frequently, with phlegm no longer being able to be separated and the brain being soaked and moist, rather than dried out. 3. One may clearly see that this is so from what follows with herds and flocks, which suffer attacks of this illness, especially goats, for they are most frequently afflicted. If you cut open the head, you will find that the brain is moist, overflowing with a watery discharge, and smells bad. You will clearly know from this that the god does not maltreat the body, but the illness does. 4. The same holds true for a mortal. For when the illness persists, it is no longer curable. The brain is eaten away by phlegm and it melts, and what is melted becomes water which settles around the exterior of the brain and floods it. On account of this an attack comes on more easily and frequently. For this reason the illness is long-lasting because this fluid is thin and abundant. The fluid is immediately overpowered and warmed by blood.

Chapter 12. 1. People who are already accustomed to the illness know when they are about to be attacked and they flee from people. If someone is close to home, he flees homeward, but if not, to a very remote spot, where others are least likely to see him fall and immediately he covers his head. He does this out of shame over his condition and not, as many think, from fear of divine power. 2. At first little children, from their inexperience, fall wherever they happen to be. But after they have been attacked often, when they perceive it coming, they flee to their mothers or someone whom they know well out of fear and dread of their condition. For they have not yet developed a sense of shame.

Chapter 13. 1. With the changes of the winds [*pneumata*],[67] the attacks happen for the reasons I say, in particular the south winds, next the north winds, and then the rest of the winds [*pneumata*]. For the south and north winds [*pneumata*] are the strongest, in comparison to the rest of the winds, and most opposite in their direction and power in relation to each other. 2. For the north wind condenses the air and separates from it what is muddy and damp and makes it clear and transparent. The north wind has the same effect on all other things that arise from the sea and other waters, for it separates from them what is damp and murky, and this holds true for people. Accordingly, it is the healthiest of winds. 3. The south wind acts in the opposite way to this. First it melts down and disperses the air that has been condensed in the following way. It does not immediately blow strongly, but is calm at first, since it is not able to overpower the air that earlier was thick and had been condensed, but dissolves it with the passing of time. The south wind has the same effect on the earth, sea, rivers, springs, wells, and everything that grows in the places where any moisture is present; moisture is in everything to a greater or lesser degree. All these things feel the effect of this wind [*pneuma*]: things change from clear to murky, from cold to warm and from dry to wet. Vessels filled with wine or some other liquid which are in storerooms or below ground all feel the effect of the south wind and through changes take on a different sort of appearance. The south wind makes the sun, moon, and other celestial objects dimmer than their nature. Since then it overpowers things that are so large and powerful to such an extent, it also causes the body to

67. On the characteristics of the four winds, see Text 2, Hippocratic Corpus, *Airs, Waters, Places,* and figure 17.

feel the effect and to change. 4. In relation to the changes of the winds [*pneumata*], with the south winds the brain is necessarily relaxed and filled with moisture, and the vessels become slacker. With the north winds, the healthiest part of the brain is necessarily condensed while the most injured and moistest component is separated off and washes all around the outside of the brain, and thus the descent of fluxes happens with the changes of these winds. 5. Thus this illness arises and flourishes from what comes and goes, and is not more difficult than other illnesses to treat or understand, nor is it more divine than others.

Chapter 14. 1. People must know that our pleasures, joys, laughter, and jokes arise only from inside the brain, and that the brain is also the source of griefs, sorrows, anxieties, and weeping. 2. Most of all, the brain lets us think, perceive, see, hear, and distinguish what is disgraceful from the noble, bad from good, and pleasant from unpleasant, making the decision sometimes based on custom and other times getting a sense of them through useful-ness and also distinguishing the pleasurable from the unpleasurable depending on the occa-sion. The same things do not please us all. 3. The brain likewise causes us to go mad and to lose our senses and causes terrors and fears to afflict us during the night or the day and also dreams and inopportune mental lapses, improper thoughts, ignorance of one's state of life, and strange habits. 4. We suffer all these things from the brain, not when it is healthy, but when it is warmer, moister, or dryer than what is natural, or has suffered some other condi-tion that is beyond the natural condition to which it is accustomed. 5. We are driven mad by its moistness, for whenever the brain is more moist than what is natural, it is set in motion, and when it moves neither sight nor hearing remain undisturbed, but our hearing and sight jump from one thing to another, and the tongue utters what it sees or hears moment to moment. But, as long as the brain remains at rest, a person retains their senses.

Chapter 15. 1. The brain's corruption happens from phlegm and from bile. You will know which is which in this way. People driven mad through phlegm are peaceful and do not shout or make an uproar. People driven mad through bile are noisy, hurtful, and restless, but always act inappropriately. So, if they are in a continuous state of madness, those are the reasons. 2. But, if terrors and fears afflict us, it is because of a change in the brain. The brain changes when it is heated and it is heated by bile that rushes to the brain from the body through blood vessels. Fear is present until the bile departs to the vessels and the body. Then the fear stops. 3. When the brain is chilled and compacted beyond what is its natural state, and it suffers this from phlegm, one feels grief and nausea unseasonably. Because of phlegm and the condition of the brain one becomes forgetful. 4. Shouts and shrieks happen at night when the brain is suddenly warmed. People with excess bile suffer this, but not people with excess phlegm. The brain is also warmed when much blood floods and boils it. When a person chances to see a frightful dream and is in distress, much blood comes via the vessels previously mentioned 5. Just as when awake the face is flushed and inflamed and the eyes redden out of fear and the mind intends to accomplish some evil, so too does one suffer in the same way while asleep. This ceases when one wakes up and can focus their thoughts and their blood is scattered again into their vessels.

Chapter 16. 1. Accordingly, I believe that the brain is the most powerful part in a human. For, when the brain is healthy, it is our interpreter of what happens in the air, and air provides it with understanding. 2. The eyes, ears, tongue, hands, and feet comply with what the brain perceives. For there is some element of understanding everywhere in the body, while it takes in air.[68] 3. The brain is what carries messages for the consciousness. For when one draws a breath [*pneuma*] into oneself, it arrives first into the brain, and so the air is spread out to the rest of the body, though it does leave behind in the brain what is best, which is to say what has consciousness and thought. 4. For if it reached the body first and the brain after it had left behind discernment in **flesh** and vessels, it would go into the brain while warm, impure, and mixed with the moisture from flesh and blood so that it would no longer have its true nature.

Chapter 17. 1. Therefore I claim that the brain interprets what is comprehended. 2. The diaphragm has a name unconnected to this by chance and custom, not by reality or nature, and I myself do not know any power that the diaphragm (*phrenes*) has to understand and perceive (*phronein*)[69] except that if a person is overcome with joy or grief unexpectedly, the diaphragm throbs and causes a spasm because of its thinness and because it is stretched to the utmost in the body. Further, it does not have a cavity into which it can receive what suddenly happens, good or bad, but it is disturbed by both of these because of the weakness of its nature. Since it perceives nothing before any other part of the body, it but falsely has this name and attribution, just like the parts near the heart are called "ears,"[70] but contribute nothing to the hearing. 3. Some people say that we also think with the heart and that this is what is grieved and what thinks. But this is not so. Rather, the heart is convulsed just as the diaphragm is, but more so for the following reasons. Vessels from the whole body extend to the heart which encloses them in such a way that it perceives if any disturbance or tension happens to a person. The body is forced to shudder and to tense up when pained and to shiver and to suffer the same thing when overjoyed, since the heart and the diaphragm are most affected by perceptions. Neither, however, shares in intelligence, but the brain is the source of all these things. 4. So, just as the brain is the first of the parts of the body to feel the effect of the intelligence of air, so too, if any strong change happens in the air because of the seasons and the air differs from itself, the brain first feels its effect.[71] Accordingly, I say that illnesses that attack it are most acute, gravest, deadliest, and hardest for the inexperienced to interpret.

Chapter 18. 1. This so-called sacred illness arises from the same causes as the others, namely from what goes in and goes out of the body, from the cold and the sun, and from the changing of the winds [*pneumata*] and their never being at rest. These things are divine, so that there is no need when classifying the illness to consider it more divine than the rest.

68. The Greek text in this sentence is suspect, so the translation is uncertain.

69. The author is claiming that there is no connection between the Greek word for "diaphragm" (*phrenes*) and the word for "perceive" (*phronein*), despite their similarity. This claim is responding to a debate in Greek antiquity about whether the brain or the heart was the seat of perception.

70. These parts are called "auricles" because they resemble ears.

71. The Greek text of this sentence is uncertain.

Rather, all illnesses are divine and all are human. Each has its own nature and peculiar power and not one baffles our understanding or lacks the potential for treatment. 2. Most can be cured by the same things from which they arise. One thing is nourishment for one illness and another thing for another illness, and for another a detriment. And so this is what the physician must know, so that he may, in consideration of the advantage of each thing, provide to one patient food or increase it, but remove another patient's food or diminish it. 3. For, in the case of this illness and all others, one must not strengthen the illnesses, but wear them out by administrating what is most hostile and unaccustomed to each illness. For an illness flourishes and is augmented by what it is accustomed to, but it withers away and is diminished by what is hostile. 4. Whoever knows how to cause in people a dry, moist, cold, or warm condition through regimen could also heal this illness, if this person could distinguish the right time for beneficial treatment, without purifications, spells, and all such quackery.

EPIDEMICS

As we saw in chapter 3, the epidemiological conditions of ancient Mediterranean cities were ideal for pathogens to flourish and for communicable illnesses to spread. When a high percentage of residents experienced an illness, the city was said to have an "epidemic"—from the Greek word describing an illness that fell "upon" (*epi*) everyone within a "city" (*dēmos*).[72] Sometimes, even when contagious diseases exploded in a city, they remained relatively contained. Other times illnesses spread more widely: these were called "pandemics" from the Greek word describing an illness that fell upon "all" (*pan*) of the "cities" (*dēmoi*) of the known world.

Local outbreaks of illness could explode into full-blown pandemics because communities across the Mediterranean were connected by basic infrastructure (such as the 250,000 miles of roads constructed by the Romans) that made travel and trade between regions more accessible, and also became a vector by which illness spread. As people moved between regions, they carried local strains of pathogens that were novel to faraway communities who did not have immunity to them. It is not surprising, therefore, that we hear about several waves of pandemics sweeping across the ancient Mediterranean.

And it is not surprising that the most devastating epidemics were centered in densely populated cities. The plague of Athens (430–427 BCE), for instance, exploded within the city while it was under siege during the Peloponnesian War. As Athenian citizens who lived in the countryside clamored for protection within the city's fortified walls, the highly concentrated living conditions exacerbated the spread of the communicable illness. Likewise, we hear of the rampant transmission of the illness in the close quarters of army encampments and naval ships. One eyewitness reports that the epidemic devoured his unit, killing 1,050

72. See the introduction to Text 8, the Hippocratic *On Epidemics,* for alternative meanings of this word.

out of 4,000 hoplites in just forty days, and another remarked that, when naval ships were struck by the plague, the fleet became floating tombs. Scholars estimate that in three years this deadly plague killed 75,000–100,000 people in Athens, wiping out 25–35 percent of the city's population.

Several centuries later (541–543 CE), we hear about an even more catastrophic epidemic that ravaged the city of Constantinople during the reign of emperor Justinian (hence this epidemic is called "the Justinianic plague"). Accounts from the time report that the city's death toll climbed until 10,000–16,000 people were dying each day. Scholars believe these numbers to be inflated, but even conservative estimates conclude that the Justinianic plague killed one-third to one-half of the population of Constantinople.

We are fortunate to have firsthand accounts for both of these epidemics: a report on the plague of Athens from the Athenian general **Thucydides** (Text 18) and reports on the Justinianic plague from the ancient historian **Procopius** (Text 19). Historians learn a myriad of things from these accounts. First, we glean a complex understanding of the experience of living through mass disease events. The description of symptoms helps us imagine the physical agony of being stricken with the illness. For example, Procopius describes the fever, extreme fatigue, violent delirium, bloody vomiting, and "bubos" (swollen, blackened lymph nodes that sometimes discharged pus; see fig. 36) that characterized the Justinianic epidemic. Our sources also give us a window into people's emotions: from the hardship, disgust, and repulsion that caregivers and family members felt upon seeing their loved ones ravaged by the illness, to the fear of coming into contact with even beloved friends, to the overwhelming emotional distress caused by so much death and grief. Our sources paint a vivid picture of the effect mass disease events had on cities: because the digging of mass graves could not keep pace with the number of dead, our sources report that corpses were strewn about the city, piled up on seashores, or were thrown into the sea; and a putrefying stench permeated the city. But worse than that was the inability to perform burial rites that Greeks and Romans believed necessary for the dead to find peace and rest in the afterlife. Thus the jeopardy of loved ones' eternal well-being further exacerbated the grief over their death. Taken together, our sources give us a nuanced sense of what it was like to live through devastating pandemics.

Firsthand accounts also provide information about how the sick were cared for. On the one hand, we hear that fear of contagion prevented some from offering aid to friends and family, resulting in the sick being abandoned and perishing uncared-for. On the other hand, we hear about people who, at the expense of their own health, provided nursing care to the sick and dying. Procopius gives us a picture of the weary caregivers who were "driven to exhaustion" because of the need to keep an ever-watchful eye on the sick, who "kept falling out of bed and rolling around on the floor" and who, because of their delirium needed to be "pushed and pulled" to stay still. Because this care was so difficult, people pitied caregivers as much as those suffering from the illness itself (Text 19, Procopius, *History of the Wars* 2.22.23).

Our sources also teach us about the impact epidemics and pandemics had on societal structures and norms. Some of our accounts report that people set aside their enmity

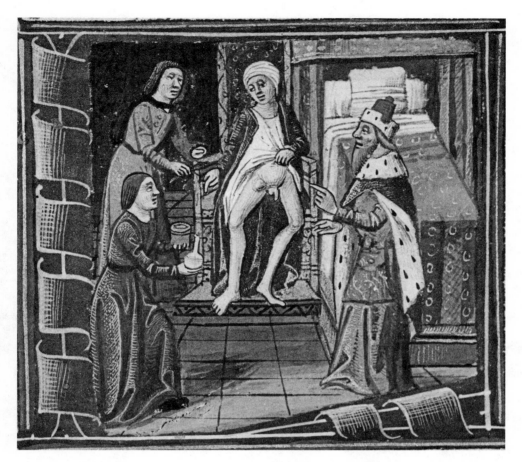

FIGURE 36 Illustration in a medieval manuscript of the Hippocratic text *On Epidemics* depicting Hippocrates treating a victim of the plague of Athens (430–427 BCE). The plague victim is portrayed with a bubo (swollen, blackened lymph nodes that sometimes discharged pus) in his groin. Reports from the plague of Athens do not in fact describe bubos among the symptoms; rather it was a symptom belonging to the sixth-century Justinianic plague and in the fourteenth-century Black Death (also known as the "bubonic" plague), which was likely projected anachronistically in time by the medieval illustrator. Likewise, stories that Hippocrates visited Athens during the plague were invented by later biographers and perpetuated by illustrations like this. Photo credit: Sächsische Landesbibliothek, Staats- und Universitätsbibliothek, Dresden; http://digital.slub-dresden.de/id337794197/281; Mscr.Dresd.Db 93, fol. 458r.

for former rivals and united in acts of mutual care, yet more often our accounts paint a picture of social unrest, confusion, and disorder. Out of weariness or fear, people abandoned their work. Grain and fruit rotted in the field, as there was no one to harvest it. Cattle, sheep, goats, and pigs roamed wild. As production and trade came to a grinding halt, supplies and food at the markets became scarce. When faced with such shortages, desperate people resorted to riots and looting. As a result, people gave up all hope—thinking they would soon die or that the end of the world had come—abandoning social norms and engaging in lawlessness.

Finally, our sources reveal the ways people made sense of what was happening to them. Some appealed to religious explanations, believing catastrophic illnesses to be divine punishment. Thus, people of different religious affiliations flocked to the sanctuaries of their gods to atone for anything they might have done to draw the gods' ire, and also to petition the gods for help. Others made sense of epidemics with medical explanations. To their mind, the cause of the illness must be something everyone in the community shared, such as a water source, climate, or—the most popular theory of this kind—the air they all breathed. This latter explanation came to be known as **miasma** theory, derived from the Greek and Latin term that described the "stained" quality of air that was adverse to human health.[73] The Hippocratic authors who advanced miasma theory advised people who found themselves in the throes of an epidemic to flee from the region with contaminated air and, if they could not relocate, to reduce what they ate and drank so that they would become thinner and weaker and in turn take in fewer and shallower breaths of this bad air (see Text 5, *On the Nature of Humans* 9).

Despite such attempts to make sense of catastrophic illness and death, our sources report that pandemics often remained inexplicable to many who lived through them. Procopius, for example, discussed the frustration of physicians who could not understand the illness even after they dissected the bubonic swellings from corpses. Thucydides and Procopius both noted that there was no pattern as to whom the illness would strike down and whom it would spare. And both writers bemoaned the fact that a remedy that worked for some sick people proved useless—or even harmful—to others. Overall, our sources report that the seemingly arbitrary and incomprehensible nature of epidemics was in part what made them so frightful.

Historians and scientists too have attempted to identify the cause of ancient epidemics, with guesses including bubonic plague, influenza, typhoid fever, typhus, smallpox, and measles. Until recently, these scholars conducted retrospective diagnosis using symptomatology: attempting to match the symptoms described in historical sources with symptoms of known illnesses today. This problematic approach, however, assumes that eyewitnesses described symptoms accurately, even though we know their intent in writing their accounts was to depict the horror of what they were seeing, not to take meticulous medical case notes. Moreover, diagnoses based on symptoms are complicated by the fact that pathogens mutate over time; thus we cannot be sure that the symptoms related to various strains of an illness remain stable over time and therefore usable for diagnostic purposes.

73. Writers such as Diodorus of Sicily and **Galen** attempted to identify what caused pathogenic air. They concluded that it must derive from putrefying matter, whether the putrefaction of stagnant, marshy waters or putrefying human corpses, especially when they piled up in mass graves or on the battlefield.

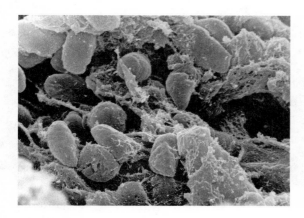

FIGURE 37 Scanning electron microphotograph depicting a mass of *Yersinia pestis* bacteria, the pathogen responsible for the sixth-century Justinianic plague and the fourteenth-century bubonic plague (i.e., Black Death). This bacterium was found in the foregutte (the first part of the digestive tract) of a flea who was a vector for the disease. Photo credit: Rocky Mountain Laboratories, NIAID, NIH. Wikimedia Commons.

Fortunately, in the past two decades scientists have developed a more exact approach to diagnosing historical illnesses: paleogenetics. The value of this approach becomes immediately clear when we look at the case study of *Yersinia pestis*. Scientists interested in the pathogen responsible for the fourteenth-century bubonic plague (i.e., Black Death) worked with archaeologists to unearth human remains from a cemetery in which victims were buried. Then, geneticists extracted pathogen DNA from the human remains, and sequenced the genome to identify the culprit behind the Black Death: the bacterium *Yersinia pestis* (see fig. 37). Finally, scholars compared their results against genetic material harvested from human remains from other gravesites across Europe, including bodies of people who died in the Justinianic plague. By this method, scientists confirmed that the same pathogen, *Yersinia pestis*, was the source of three separate pandemics: the Justinianic plague in the sixth century, the Black Death in the fourteenth century, and another pandemic in the nineteenth century.

TEXT 18. THUCYDIDES, *HISTORY OF THE PELOPONNESIAN WAR* SELECTION (2.47–54)

Thucydides *(c. 460–395 BCE) was an Athenian general and historian. He lived through the Peloponnesian War (431–404 BCE) fought between Athens and Sparta, serving on the Athenian side until he was exiled from Athens, and then observing the remainder of the war as a noncombatant. Thucydides's History of the Peloponnesian War draws from his own observations and conjectures, as well as from his interviews with eyewitnesses. The selection below provides a detailed account of what happened to Athens in the summer of 430 BCE. The Athenians withdrew from the countryside and took refuge inside the city's defensive walls (they were still kept well-supplied by ships via the connecting port of Peiraeus). Meanwhile, the attacking Spartan forces controlled the land outside the walls. This led to overcrowding in Athens, and created conditions where infectious diseases could spread easily. Thucydides's account describes an epidemic that broke out in Athens, killing many people and leading to a deterioration of the city's social* *norms and institutions. Thucydides, who was himself infected, describes the characteristics of the illness, demonstrating familiarity with the language and concepts of the Hippocratic physicians active in Athens during his lifetime.*

SOURCE: Translation by Martin Hammond based on the Greek text from H. Stuart Jones and J. E. Powell, *Thucydidis Historiae*, 2nd ed., Oxford Classical Texts (Oxford: Clarendon Press, 1963). First published in *Thucydides: The Peloponnesian War* (Oxford: Oxford University Press, 2009). Reprinted with permission of Oxford University Press.

Book 2. 47. Such was the funeral held in this winter: and with the passing of winter there ended the first year of this war.

At the very beginning of the next summer the Peloponnesians and their allies invaded Attica, with two-thirds of their forces as on the first occasion, under the command of Archidamus the son of Zeuxidamus, king of Sparta. They settled in and began to ravage the land.

They had not been in Attica for more than a few days when the plague first broke out in Athens. It is said that the plague had already struck widely elsewhere, especially in Lemnos and other places, but nowhere else was there recorded such virulence or so great a loss of life. The doctors could offer little help at first: they were attempting to treat the disease without knowing what it was, and in fact there was particularly high mortality among doctors because of their particular exposure. No other human skill could help either, and all supplications at temples and consultations of oracles and the like were of no avail. In the end the people were overcome by the disaster and abandoned all efforts to escape it.

48. The original outbreak, it is said, was in Ethiopia, the far side of Egypt: the plague then spread to Egypt and Libya,[74] and over much of the King's territory. It fell on the city of Athens suddenly. The first affected were the inhabitants of the Peiraeus, who went so far as to allege that the Peloponnesians had poisoned the wells (at that time there were no fountains in the Peiraeus). Afterwards the plague reached the upper city too, and now the number of deaths greatly increased. Others, doctors or laymen, can give their individual opinions of the likely origin of the plague, and of the factors which they think significant enough to have had the capacity to cause such a profound change. But I shall simply tell it as it happened, and describe the features of the disease which will give anyone who studies them some prior knowledge to enable recognition should it ever strike again. I myself caught the plague, and witnessed others suffering from it.

49. It so happened that this year was commonly agreed to have been particularly free from other forms of illness, though anyone with a previous condition invariably developed the plague. The other victims were in good health until, for no apparent cause, they were suddenly afflicted. The first symptoms were a high fever in the head and reddening and inflammation of the eyes; then internally the throat and tongue began to bleed and the breath [*pneuma*] had an unnaturally foul smell. There followed sneezing and hoarseness of voice,

74. "Libya" refers to any part of Africa other than Egypt (see fig. 17).

and shortly the affliction moved down to the chest accompanied by a violent cough. When it settled in the stomach the turmoil caused there led to the voiding of bile in every form for which the doctors have a name, all this with great pain. Most then suffered from an empty retching which brought violent spasms: in some this followed as soon as the vomiting had abated, in others much later.

The surface of the body was not particularly hot to the touch or pallid, but reddish and livid, breaking out in small pustules and ulcers. But the sensation of burning heat inside the body was so strong that sufferers could not bear the pressure of even the lightest clothing or sheets, or anything other than going naked, and their greatest wish was to plunge into cold water. Many who had no one to look after them did in fact throw themselves into cisterns, overcome by an insatiable thirst: but as a rule the quantity of water drunk made no difference. A constant infliction was desperate restlessness and the inability to sleep. Throughout the height of the disease there was no wasting of the body, but a surprising physical resilience to all the suffering, so that there was still some strength in them when the majority died from the internal fever after six to eight days. If they survived this period most others died from the consequent weakness when the disease spread down to the bowels causing heavy ulceration and the onset of completely liquid diarrhea.

The disease first settled in the head then progressed throughout the whole body from the top downwards. If any survived the worst effects, symptoms appeared when the disease took hold in their extremities. It attacked genitals, fingers, and toes, and many lived on with these parts lost: some too lost their sight. There were those who on recovery suffered immediate and total loss of memory, not knowing who they were and unable to recognize their friends.

50. Indeed the pathology of the disease defied explanation. Not only did it visit individuals with a violence beyond human endurance, but there was also this particular feature which put it in a different category from all other diseases with which we are familiar: although many bodies lay unburied, the birds and animals which prey on human flesh kept away from them, or, if they did eat, died of it. Evidence of this was the notable disappearance of carrion birds, nowhere to be seen in their usual or any other activity: the dogs, being domestic animals, allowed more immediate observation of this consequence.

51. This then, leaving aside the many variants in the way different individuals were affected, was the general character of the disease. Throughout this time there were no attacks of the usual illnesses: any that did occur ended in the plague.

Some died in neglect and others died despite constant care. Virtually no remedy was established as a single specific relief applicable in all cases: what was good for one was harmful to another. No particular constitution, strong or weak, proved sufficient in itself to resist, but the plague carried off all indiscriminately, and whatever their regime of care. The most dreadful aspects of the whole affliction were the despair into which people fell when they realized they had contracted the disease (they were immediately convinced that they had no hope, and so were much more inclined to surrender themselves without a fight), and the cross-infection of those who cared for others: they died like sheep, and this was the greatest cause of mortality. When people were afraid to visit one another, the victims died in isolation, and many households were wiped out through the lack of anyone to care for them. If they did visit the sick, they died, especially those who could claim some courage: these were people who out of a sense of duty disregarded their own safety and kept visiting their friends, even when ultimately the family members themselves were overwhelmed by the scale of the disaster and abandoned the succession of dirges for the dead. But the greatest pity for the dying and the distressed was shown by those who had had the disease and recovered. They had experience of what it was like and were now confident for themselves, as the plague did not attack the same person twice, or at least not fatally. These survivors were congratulated by all, and in the immediate elation of recovery they entertained the fond hope that from now on they would not die of any other disease.

52. The suffering was made yet more acute by the influx from the country into the city, and the incomers suffered most of all. With no houses of their own, and forced to live in huts which at that time of year were stifling, they perished in chaotic conditions: the dead and the dying were piled on top of each other, and half-dead creatures staggered about the streets and round every fountain, craving for water. The sanctuaries in which they had encamped were full of corpses—people dying there were not moved: all sacred and secular constraints came to be ignored under the overwhelming impact of the disaster, which left men no recourse. All previously observed funeral customs were confounded, and burial was haphazard, any way that people could manage. Many were driven to shameful means of disposal for lack of friends to help them, so many of their friends already dead: they made use of other people's funeral pyres, either putting their own dead on a pyre constructed by others and quickly setting light to it, or bringing a corpse to a pyre already lit, throwing it on top of the other body in the flames, and then running away.

53. In other respects too, the plague was the beginning of increased lawlessness in the city. People were less inhibited in the indulgence of pleasures previously concealed when they saw the rapid changes of fortune—the prosperous suddenly dead, and the once indigent now possessing their fortune. As a result they decided to look for satisfactions that were quick and pleasurable, reckoning that neither life nor wealth would last long. No one was prepared to persevere in what had once been thought the path of honor, as they could well be dead before that destination was reached. Immediate pleasure, and any means profitable to that end, became the new honor and the new value. No fear of god or human law was any constraint. Pious or impious made no difference in their view, when they could see all dying without distinction. As for offenses against the law, no one expected to live long enough to be brought to justice and pay the penalty: they thought that a much heavier sentence had already been passed and was hanging over them, so they might as well have some enjoyment of life before it fell.

54. Such was the affliction which had come on the Athenians and was pressing them hard—people dying inside the city, and the devastation of their land outside.

TEXT 19. PROCOPIUS, *HISTORY OF THE WARS* SELECTION (2.22–23)

Procopius *(c. 507–after 555 CE) was a Greek historian and eyewitness to the wars fought by the emperor Justinian (who reigned from 527 to 565 CE). From 540 to the end of his life, Procopius lived in Constantinople, the capital of the Eastern Roman Empire (also called the "Byzantine Empire"). In 542, most of the Mediterranean world was struck by an epidemic. Procopius's account focuses on the impact of this epidemic on the city of Constantinople. The manner in which he describes the plague in his time seems inspired by the historian* **Thucydides***'s account of the plague that struck Athens nearly 1,000 years before (compare Text 18).*

SOURCE: Translation by H. B. Dewing, revised by Anthony Kaldellis based on the Greek text from Jakob Haury, *Procopii Caesariensis Opera omnia*, vol. 1, revised by Gerhard Wirth (Leipzig: Teubner, 1962). First published as *The Wars of Justinian* (Indianapolis: Hackett, 2014), with minor edits. Reprinted with permission of Hackett Publishing Company, Inc. All rights reserved.

Book 2, Chapter 22. 1. During those times there was a plague that came close to wiping out the whole of humankind. Now for all the calamities that fall upon us from the heavens it might be possible for some bold man to venture a theory regarding their causes, like the many marvelous theories about causes that the experts in these fields tend to dream up which are, in reality, utterly incomprehensible to humankind. Still, they make up outlandish theories of natural science, knowing well that they are saying nothing sound and they are content with themselves if only they manage to deceive a few people whom they meet into accepting their argument. 2. But about this calamity there is no way to find any justification, to give a rational account, or even to cope with it mentally, except by referring it to God. 3. For it did not afflict a specific part of the earth only or one group of people, nor did it strike during one season of the year, based on which facts it might have been possible to contrive some subtle explanation regarding its cause; instead, it embraced the entire earth and wrecked the lives of all people, even when those lives were as different from each other in quality as can be imagined, nor did it respect either gender or age. 4. For people differ from each other in the places that they live, the customs that govern their lifestyle, the manner of their personality, their professions, and many other ways, but none of these factors made the slightest difference when it came to this disease—and to this disease alone. 5. It struck some during the summer, others during the winter, and the rest during the other seasons. So each person should state his own opinion about how he understands all this, and so too should our subtle theorists and astrologers, but I, for my part, will now state where this disease originated and how it destroyed people.

6. It originated among the Egyptians who live in Pelusium.[75] From there it branched out in two directions, the first moving against Alexandria and then to the rest of Egypt, the

75. Pelusium was located in Egypt at the eastern edge of the Nile Delta on the Mediterranean Sea.

second coming to the Palestinians who live by the border of Egypt. From here it spread to the entirety of the world, always moving along and advancing at set intervals. 7. For it seemed to move as if by prearranged plan: it would linger for a set time in each place, just enough to make sure that no person could brush it off as a slight matter, and from there it would disperse in different directions as far as the ends of the inhabited world, almost as if it feared that any hidden corner of the earth might escape it. 8. It overlooked no island or cave or mountain peak where people happened to live, and if it passed through a region upon whose inhabitants it did not lay its hands or whom it did not affect in some way, it would return to that place at a later time: those whom it had previously ravaged it now left alone, but it did not let up from that place before it had exacted the proper and just toll in dead people, the very death toll that the inhabitants of the surrounding areas had paid earlier. 9. This disease always spread out from the coasts and worked its way up into the interior. It arrived at Byzantium[76] in the middle of the spring of its second year, where I happened to be at the time. And it struck as follows.

10. Visions of demons taking every imaginable human form were seen by many people, and those who encountered them believed that they were being struck on some part of their body by that man whom they met; the disease set in at the very moment when they saw this vision. 11. At first, those who met these creatures would try to turn them away by invoking the most holy names and otherwise exorcizing them in whatever way each knew how, but it was all perfectly futile, for even in the churches where most people sought refuge they were perishing constantly. 12. Later they would not bother to notice even when their friends were calling out to them, but instead they shut themselves up in their rooms and pretended not to hear, even while the others were pounding on their doors; this was, of course, because they feared that the caller was one of those demons. 13. But others were not affected in this way by the plague; instead, they saw a *dream* vision in which they suffered the same thing at the hands of the entity standing over them, or else they heard a voice predicting to them that their names would be placed on the lists of those who were about to die. 14. Most people, however, were taken ill without the advance warning of a waking vision or a dream. 15. They fell ill in the following way. Suddenly they became feverish, some of them when they rose from sleep, others while they were walking about, and still others while they were doing any odd thing. 16. The body did not change its color or become warm as during a regular fever, nor did it burn up; rather, the fever was so feeble from its beginning all the way to the evening that it gave no cause for worry either to the victims themselves or to their doctors who touched them. 17. In fact, no one who fell ill in this way believed that he would die from it. But then on the same day for some people, or on the next for others, at any rate no more than a few days later, a bubonic swelling appeared. This happened not only in that part of

76. Byzantium was the original name of the city of Constantinople, modern-day Istanbul in Türkiye.

the body, below the abdomen, which is called the *boubon*,[77] but also inside the armpit, in some cases by the ears, while in others at various points on the thigh.

18. Up to this point the symptoms of the disease were more or less the same for everyone who contracted it. But as for what followed, I am not able to say whether the variation in its progression was due to the differences in bodies or because it followed the will of him who introduced the disease into the world. 19. While some fell into a deep coma, others developed acute dementia, but both felt the fundamental effects of the disease. Those who became comatose forgot all about their loved ones and seemed to be always asleep. 20. If someone cared for them, they ate in the meantime, but those who were abandoned died of starvation. 21. Those gripped by the madness of dementia, on the other hand, could not sleep and became delusional. Imagining that people were attacking them in order to kill them, they became hysterical and fled at a run, shouting loudly. 22. So those who were caring for their needs were driven to exhaustion and constantly faced unheard-of difficulties. 23. For this reason everyone pitied the latter no less than their patients, not because they were at all affected by the disease through proximity—for no doctor or layman contracted this misfortune by touching any of the sick or the dead, given that many who were constantly burying the dead or caring for the sick, even those unrelated to them, continued to perform this service against all expectation, whereas many who contracted the disease from an unknown source died directly—rather, they pitied them because they had to endure a great hardship. 24. For their patients kept falling out of bed and rolling around on the floor, and they would have to put them back; and then they would long to rush out of their houses, and they would have to force them back by pushing and pulling them. 25. If any came near to water, they wanted to throw themselves in, but not because they needed to drink (for most rushed into the sea); rather, the cause was mostly the mental illness. 26. Food also caused them much pain, as it was not easy for them to eat. Many died because they had no one to look after them, were done in by hunger, or threw themselves from a height. 27. Those who did not became delirious or comatose died unable to endure the pain brought on by the mortification of the bubos. 28. Now one might deduce that the same thing happened to the others too but, as they were utterly beside themselves, they were unable to sense the pain; the illness of their minds took all sensation away. 29. Some doctors were at a loss because the symptoms were unfamiliar to them and, believing that the focus of the disease was to be found in the bubos, decided to investigate the bodies of the dead. Cutting into some of the bubos, they found that a kind of malignant carbuncle had developed inside.

30. Some died immediately, others after many days. In some cases, the body blossomed with dark pustules about the size of a lentil. These people did not survive a single day; they all died immediately. 31. Many others suddenly began to vomit blood and perished immediately. 32. I have this to state too, that the most eminent doctors predicted that many would die who shortly afterward were unexpectedly freed of all their maladies, and they also

77. In Greek, *boubon* means both "groin" and "swelling." It was a characteristic feature of the illness, which sometimes is called the "bubonic" plague.

claimed that many would survive who were destined to perish almost immediately. 33. Thus there was no cause behind this disease that any human reason could grasp, for in all cases the outcome made little sense. Some were saved by taking baths, others were no less harmed by it. 34. Many who were neglected died but many others paradoxically survived. Likewise, the same treatment produced different results in different patients. In sum, no method of survival could be found by man, whether to guard himself that he not be exposed to the disease at all or to survive that misfortune once he had contracted it; for its onset was inexplicable while survival from it was not under anyone's control. 35. As for women who were pregnant, death could be foreseen if they were taken ill with the disease. Some had miscarriages and died while others perished in labor along with the infants they bore. 36. It is said, however, that three new mothers survived while their infants did not, and that one died in childbirth though her child was born and survived. 37. In cases where the bubos grew very large and discharged pus, the patients overcame the disease and survived, as it was clear that for them the eruption of the carbuncle found relief in this way; for the most part, this was a sign of health. But in cases where the bubos remained in the same condition, these patients had to endure all the misfortunes that I just described. 38. It happened for some that the thigh would become withered and because of this the bubo would grow large but not discharge pus. 39. In the case of others who happened to survive, their speech was not unaffected, and they lived afterward with a lisp or barely able to articulate some indistinct words.

Book 2, Chapter 23. 1. The disease lasted four months while it ran its course in Byzantium but it was at its peak for three. 2. At first only a few people died above the usual death rate but then the mortality rose higher until the toll in deaths reached five thousand a day, and after that it reached ten thousand, and then even more. 3. In the beginning each would arrange in person for the burial of the dead from his own household, whom they would even throw into the graves of others either by stealth or using violence. But then confusion began to reign everywhere and in all ways. 4. Slaves were deprived of their masters; men who were previously prosperous now suffered the loss of their servants who were either sick or dead; and many households were emptied of people altogether. 5. Thus it happened that some notables were left unburied for many days because there was no help to be had.

So the responsibility of handling this situation fell, as was natural, upon the emperor. 6. He posted soldiers from the palace and made funds available, appointing Theodorus to supervise this task; this was the man in charge of imperial responses, that is, his job was to convey to the emperor all the petitions of suppliants and then inform them of his decisions. In the Latin tongue the Romans call this office a *referendarius*. 7. So those whose households had not fallen so low as to be entirely deserted provided in person for the burial of their own relatives. 8. Meanwhile, Theodorus was burying the dead that had been abandoned by giving the emperor's money and spending his own as well. 9. And when the existing graves were full of dead bodies, at first they dug up all the open sites in the city, one after another, placed the dead in there, each person as he could, and departed. But later those who were digging these ditches could no longer keep up with the number of those dying, so they climbed up the towers of the fortified enclosure, the one in Sycae,[78] 10. tore off the roofs, and tossed the bodies there in a tangled heap. Piling them up in this way, just as each happened to fall, they filled up virtually all the towers; and then they covered them again with their roofs. 11. A foul stench [*pneuma*] would waft from there to the city and bring even more grief to its people, especially if the wind was blowing from that direction.

12. All the customs of burial were overlooked at that time. For the dead were neither escorted by a procession in the customary way nor were they accompanied by chanting, as was usual; rather, it was enough if a person carried one of the dead on his shoulders to a place where the city met the sea and threw him down; and there they were thrown into barges in a pile and taken to who knows where. 13. At that time also those elements of the populace who had formerly been militants in the circus fan-clubs set aside their mutual hatred and together attended to the funeral rites of the dead, carrying in person and burying the bodies of those who did not belong to their color. 14. Even more, those who previously used to delight in the shameful and wicked practices in which they indulged, well, these people gave up the immorality of their lifestyles and became religious to an extreme degree. However, this was not because they really understood what it means to be wise nor because they had suddenly become lovers of virtue. 15. For it is impossible for a person to so quickly change what nature has implanted in him or the habits he has acquired over a long period of time—unless, of course, some divine goodness touches him. For the time being, however, almost everyone was so astounded by what was happening, and believed that they were likely to die immediately, that they temporarily came to their senses out of pure necessity, as could only be expected. 16. In fact, as soon as they overcame the disease and were saved, thinking that they were now in the clear given that the evil had moved on to some other people, they completely reversed course again in their character and became even worse than they had been before, making a spectacle of the inconsistency in their behavior; their malice and immorality now quite overpowered their better selves. One would not, therefore, utter a falsehood if he were to assert that this disease, whether by some chance or providence, carefully picked out the worst people and let them live. But these things were understood only afterward.

17. It was not easy in those times to see anyone out and about in Byzantium, for all were holed up in their homes. Those who happened to be healthy of body were either tending to the sick or mourning for the dead. 18. If you happened to chance upon someone going out, he was carrying one of the dead. All work came to a standstill and the craftsmen set aside all their trades as did anyone who had some project at hand. 19. And a true famine was careering about in a city that nevertheless abounded in all goods. It seemed difficult to find enough bread or an adequate supply of anything else; such a thing was, in fact, worthy of mention. Therefore it seemed that some of the sick too lost their lives before their time because they lacked the necessary sustenance. 20. The whole experience may be summed up by saying

78. This area was located just to the north of the walled city of Constantinople, across a small channel of water called the Golden Horn.

that it was altogether impossible to see anyone in Byzantium wearing the chlamys,[79] especially when the emperor himself fell sick (he too developed a bubo).[80] In a city holding dominion over the entire Roman empire, everyone was wearing civilian clothes and privately minding his own business. 21. That was how the plague affected Byzantium and the other Roman lands. It spread also to the Persian lands as well as to all the other barbarians.

79. Public officials in the later Roman Empire wore colorful garments embroidered with the insignia and standards of their office.
80. The emperor referred to here is Justinian, who reigned from 527 to 565 CE.

TEN

Common Treatments and Therapeutics

Once ancient physicians diagnosed a patient, they would prescribe a course of medical treatment (called "therapeutics"). From the fourth century BCE, therapeutics fell into three main categories: regimen (sometimes called "dietetics"), pharmacology (the use of **drugs**), and surgery (on this division, see Text 4, *On Medicine,* Preface 9). As we study each of these categories of treatment, however, it is important to be attentive to the wider range of practices included across them: prescriptions for diet, exercise, sleep, sexual activity, mental activity, massage, pharmacological remedies (ingested or topical), bloodletting (also called "venesection" or "phlebotomy"), **cautery, cupping,** scarification, and various kinds of surgery (from treatment of shallow wounds to amputation). Other treatments outside of the three categories included the use of incantations and spells (written or spoken), music therapy, incubation at healing shrines, and dream therapy. It is also important to remember that most physicians created treatment plans that involved multiple practices spanning these categories and that physicians were as interested in the preservation of physical and mental health (i.e., routine care of the patient), as they were in returning a sick person to a healthy state (i.e., cure of the patient).

As we study therapeutics, we quickly run into some challenges. First, although medical writers discussed treatments in almost every extant text, only a few texts talk about treatments in a systematic and comprehensive way. Second, even texts devoted to the subject do not always stay on task. For instance, much of **Galen**'s two texts *On the Therapeutic Method* and *Therapeutics to Glaucon* were devoted more to diagnosis than to treatment. So, to gather information about physicians' approaches to treatment, we have to read and synthesize a wide range of writings.

For Rationalists, therapeutics were primarily based on the principle of opposites: treatments that countered imbalances. For example, an illness that was characterized by excessive heat would be treated with cooling remedies, such as cooling foods or cold baths. This approach meant that physicians needed an extensive knowledge of the properties of various ailments, as well as knowledge of the effects various treatments had on the body.

Empiricists did not base their therapeutics on an assessment of the nature of the illness, nor did they use a set of principles to guide their therapeutic reasoning. Rather, they followed a process of trial and error for determining the course of treatment. They relied on knowledge of which treatments had worked in similar cases in the past. For instance, if an eye salve worked for an ingrown eyelash in the past, then physicians would use the same salve the next time they encountered the same ailment, and if they encountered a new eye ailment that was similar to an ingrown eyelash, they might try the same drug.

Methodist physicians based much of their therapeutic system around something they called the *diatritus*, which literally meant "the third day." They believed that a patient would experience a **paroxysm** forty-eight hours after the first appearance of symptoms.[1] During these first forty-eight hours, Methodist physicians would have their patients abstain from eating. The *diatritus* also regulated later stages of treatment, with the Methodists checking on patients' condition every forty-eight hours and then determining whether they were strong enough for bloodletting or other more drastic forms of treatment. More generally, Methodists tended to follow the model of the physician **Asclepiades of Bithynia** (c. 124–40 BCE?), who claimed to provide "safe, fast, and pleasant treatment" (Text 16, Celsus, *On Medicine* 3.4.1), preferring gentle forms of therapy, including walking, singing, and rocking or swinging on a swing.

Ancient physicians prescribed activities—or restrictions on activities—that today would more clearly fall under the purview of other health and lifestyle professionals, such as nutritionists, dietitians, herbalists, pharmacists, fitness trainers, massage therapists, spa attendants, counselors, parenting experts, life coaches, sex therapists, sleep experts, personal chefs, gardeners, and sommeliers. Most of these recommendations were understood to be part of regimen (see below). From the outset, we wish to emphasize that these areas of life were considered a component of medical practice.

Finally, we must also keep in mind that, in addition to medical treatments, many people suffering from illness would have sought help from others, such as visiting healing shrines or ritual experts. Some may have also taken matters into their own hands, following the treatment advice of knowledgeable family members and friends and devising treatments for themselves (see chapter 12 on patients). For example, **Cato the Elder** relied heavily on cabbage as a panacea for almost anything that ailed him (Text 25).

---

1. The "third day" was counted inclusively, meaning that a patient who became ill on Monday would be expected to have a paroxysm on Wednesday, with Monday counting as the first day, Tuesday as the second day, and Wednesday as the third day. To use modern language, this meant that a paroxysm would be expected to occur every other day for the duration of the illness.

REGIMEN

A significant portion of ancient physicians' work was to devise regimens for their patients. By regimen, we mean a systematic plan—taking into account various aspects of the patient's lifestyle—that would either preserve or restore health. While the most significant features of a regimen plan included diet, exercise, and bathing, physicians also advised their patients on how to occupy their minds and spend their leisure time. And physicians might also prescribe a regimen of bloodletting, **emetics**, or purgatives. Because Greco-Roman medicine was as intent on preventing illnesses as it was on curing them, physicians could prescribe a healthy regimen for anyone—even those not currently enduring an illness—and thus everyone could be regarded as a potential patient.

Physicians based their prescriptions for regimen on one of a few guiding principles. Most often, they devised a regimen that would balance the **humors** or qualities (hot, cold, wet, dry; see fig. 16). Given that every individual patient's body was slightly different and because their lifestyles and living conditions varied, physicians needed to formulate a regimen tailored precisely to the uniqueness of each patient. The physician might start with general considerations, such as season or the particular climate of the region. For instance, in the winter (or in wet and cold climates) they might advise eating roasted meats and drinking undiluted wine in order to heat and dry the body, whereas in the summer (or in hot and dry climates) they might recommend eating boiled meats and diluted wine to cool and moisten the body. They also took into consideration the age of their patients (young people tended to be hot and wet, whereas older people tended to be cold and dry; see chapter 14 on life stages) or gender (women were thought by most to be wet and cold; see chapter 9 on women's illnesses). Additionally, physicians took into account their patients' activity levels (including, for instance, their occupation), and the nature of their physique (for example, soft bodies were presumed to absorb moisture more readily, whereas hard bodies were thought to be drier). And, finally, physicians asked patients about the events of the past few days: What had they eaten or what activities had they been engaged in? With all of these variables in mind, the physician could better understand the current state of their patient's body and fine-tune a regimen best able to encourage balance. We can see many of these principles at work in selections below from the Hippocratic *Regimen in Health* (Text 20) and **Paul of Aegina**'s *Medical Compendium* (Text 22).

Another approach was to devise a regimen that would deal with problematic humors. **Galen**, for instance, thought that some illnesses were caused by a humor becoming overly thick and stagnant, and then putrefying. In these cases, the solution was to create a regimen that would dilute thick humors so they could be more easily purged and evacuated. His text entitled *On the Thinning Diet* was not a weight-loss manual, but rather a guidebook outlining how to make thin and evacuate thick humors. In other circumstances, Galen was concerned about conditions that arose from food not being properly digested (i.e., **concocted**) into humors, which in turn either blocked up or flowed too loosely through the digestive system. In these cases, Galen prescribed a diet that would stabilize digestion.

Just as regimen was central to the work of physicians, so too we find regimen at play in the medico-religious contexts of temples of **Asclepius.** For example, the famous orator **Aelius Aristides** (117–after 181 CE) suffered from a slew of digestive complaints, as well as a very large tumor in his groin. For his digestive complaints, Asclepius purportedly instructed Aristides to take a compound **drug;** and for his tumor, the god told him to run barefoot in winter, go horseback riding (a particularly painful endeavor), and sail across the harbor and eat acorns with honey and then vomit before sailing back. Although these instructions might appear strange to our modern logic, ancient medical theorists understood riding and sailing to be forms of passive exercise akin to rocking a child. As we peruse the many accounts of healing at Asclepian temples, we see that it was quite common for the god (and his temple attendants) to orchestrate comprehensive treatment plans that included alterations in diet, exercise, and bathing, as well as drugs.

When it came to dietetics (food-based therapies), we must keep in mind that all food was regarded as medicinal. Since all food was understood to be made up of elements (earth, water, air, and fire), it had heating or cooling, moistening or drying effects. The properties of the foods were likewise thought to alter a body's humoral makeup. Physicians thus paid attention to the properties of various foods and prescribed food that would rebalance their patients' bodies: drying foods for people who were overly wet, cooling foods for people who were hot, and so forth. For this reason, the prescribed use of food is similar to pharmacology. That is, foods could be thought of as drugs if food was taken in a different manner than usual (for example, breast milk applied to the eyes of an adult as a remedy for an ophthalmological ailment) with the purpose of enhancing one's health. Finally, physicians might also prescribe fasting, whether abstaining from specific foods or from all food for a certain period of time. To help alleviate the discomfort associated with fasting, **Erasistratus** (who was reported to have regularly prescribed fasting) recommended the Scythian practice of binding the belly.

In their recommendations regarding exercise, physicians again employed the principle of opposites: certain kinds of exercise would warm a person suffering from a cold condition, other kinds of exercise would dry someone suffering from a damp condition, and so forth. Physicians also prescribed exercise to maintain a steady bodily balance, customized to the conditions of the season or weather, or to gender, age, or occupation. For instance, ancient medical writers discussed the need to exercise more vigorously in winter than in summer, calibrating one's body temperature with the temperature of one's surroundings. And gentler exercises were prescribed for women and older people (who were thought to be naturally colder), given that more vigorous exercises might burn off too much of their precious innate heat, leaving them in a weakened state.

The wealthy could afford even more guidance with respect to their exercise regimen. Wealthy men would exercise in *gymnasia* or the *palaestra* often under the direction of either a professional trainer or a physician (see fig. 38). Galen, ever disdainful of competition from other professionals, argued that physicians were better at overseeing their patients' exercise regimens. And in his texts we find him giving instructions on exercises such as wrestling,

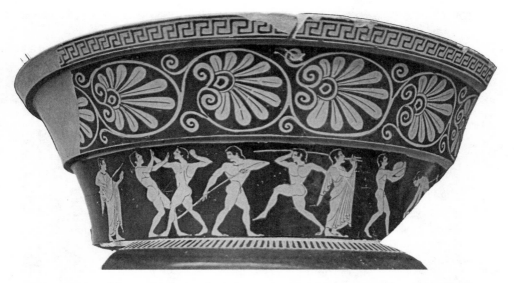

FIGURE 38 Attic red-figure Greek vase depicting men engaged in a variety of sports, including wrestling, javelin, and discus. From the Glyptothek museum, Munich. Photo Credit: Matthias Kabel. Wikimedia Commons, Creative Commons Attribution 3.0.

boxing, the *pancratium* (a mix of wrestling and boxing), running, shadow fighting, punching a *corycus* (an earth- or flour-filled ball), ball play (to which he devotes an entire treatise entitled *Exercises with the Small Ball*), and pulling ropes. Women too found ways to exercise, as illustrated in depictions of women lifting weights, throwing the discus, running, and tossing a ball (see fig. 39). And, according to Galen, lower-class people got exercise in the manual labor they engaged in daily—digging, rowing, plowing, pruning, carrying, reaping, riding, fighting, walking, hunting, and fishing—obviating their need to exercise in the *gymnasium*.

Although bathing had been part of prescribed regimens from the earlier periods of Greek medicine, the Romans developed bathing into a central feature of Roman life, building monumental public bathing establishments that used elaborate systems of channels and pipes under the floors to heat the bathhouse rooms and pools of water. Some of the most elaborate bathhouses included multiple rooms of varying temperatures. Some of these rooms housed tubs of water for soaking and plunges, while others were devoted to sweating (see fig. 40). People would start in the *caldarium* (the hot room), which was closest to the furnaces. After sweating, they would be coated in oil and cleaned off with a *strigil* (a metal scraper), leaving the skin free of dirt and sweat as well as softened. Then they would move to the *tepidarium* (the warm room), and finally to the *frigidarium* (the cold room), which often contained a pool for a cold plunge. After working their way through the rooms, people would often be massaged with unguents and oils (on massage, see below).

Although diet, exercise, and bathing were the three primary components of regimen, physicians also directed patients in matters of sex and sleep. Depending largely on one's

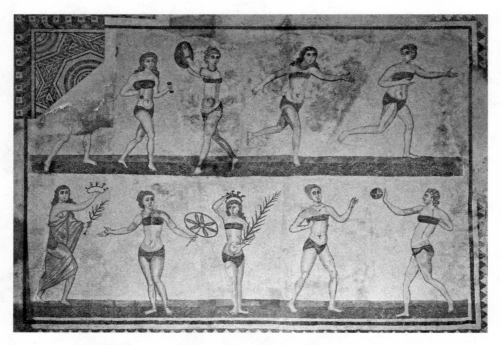

FIGURE 39 Fourth-century CE floor mosaic depicting women engaged in a variety of exercises and sports, including weightlifting, discus throwing, running, and tossing a ball (perhaps a weighted ball). They wear clothing—a breastband and undergarment—that would have allowed for free and easy movement while engaged in these activities. The woman in the lower left holds out a crown and palm frond, and another girl dons the crown and holds the frond, apparently as the victor of an athletic competition. This mosaic was found in a small room, perhaps a bedroom, in an expansive estate with over 3,500 square meters of mosaic floors. From the Villa Romana del Casale (Piazza Armerina, Sicily). Wikimedia Commons.

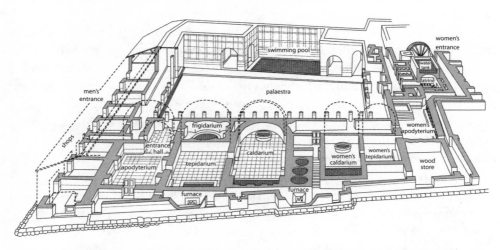

FIGURE 40 Illustrator's rendering of the Stabian bath complex in Pompeii. This illustration depicts the multiple rooms of the bathhouse, including rooms with pools of water (of varying temperatures) for soaking and plunges, and steam rooms for sweating. Adjacent to these rooms is the palaestra, where people exercised, sometimes with professional trainers or as part of athletic clubs. After *Cambridge Latin Course Book I*. Reproduced with permission of Cambridge University Press through PLSclear. Redrawn and amended by Gina Tibbott.

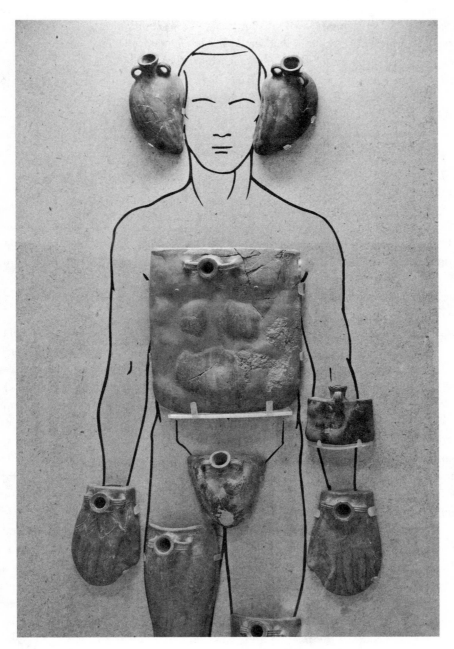

FIGURE 41 First-century BCE to first-century CE clay hot-water bottles (Pafos, Cyprus). In addition to going to bath complexes, ancient people used water therapies tailored to particular parts of their bodies. The clay vessels pictured here were shaped to fit onto different parts of the human body, and had very thin walls, so we assume they were filled with warm liquid (probably hot water or maybe hot olive oil) and then applied to the sick, injured, or painful part of the body. Limassol Archaeological Museum, Cyprus. Photo credit: Carole Raddato (CC BY-SA 2.0).

gender, physicians regarded sexual intercourse as either a debilitating activity or a cure. On the one hand, physicians thought that semen was blood that had been concocted to a frothy state; thus when it was ejaculated from a man's body, it resulted in a detrimental reduction to his vital heat. On the other hand, sexual intercourse was considered a remedy for a variety of women's illnesses, such as backed-up menstrual blood and a roaming womb (see chapter 9). As we see in Text 22 (*Medical Compendium* 1.53), Paul of Aegina recommended that sexual activity be adjusted according to the seasons. For example, one should be more restrained in one's sexual activities in autumn because of the need to retain innate heat when transitioning to a cooler season.

Unlike in our time, sleep does not figure prominently in ancient discussions of healthy lifestyles. That said, some commented on the ideal conditions for good sleep. For example, Clement of Alexandria (second and third centuries CE), a Christian philosopher and moralist steeped in medical thought, went into detail about the kind of mattress one should use, noting that a harder bed was better than a softer one because it afforded the ability to move around in one's sleep, which was a kind of salutary night-time exercise. He even went so far as to call it a natural *gymnasium* for sleep. Additionally, as we discuss further below, dreams were often used diagnostically by physicians to determine regimen for patients.

As we see in the selections from **Celsus** included below, when physicians suspected that one of the humors in their patient's body was in excess, was too thick, or had become corrupt, they prescribed one of several treatments to evacuate the problematic substance. Bloodletting (which could take the form of venesection [see fig. 42] or the application of leeches) was regarded as one of the most effective methods, and it became so common in antiquity that we find the practice mentioned across many medical texts. There was, however, disagreement about how best to do it, how often, and under what conditions. **Agnellus of Ravenna** outlined basic principles for bleeding patients based on season, region, age, temperament, habit, strength, and weather (see also Celsus's discussion of various opinions in Text 21). And several authors remarked on the dangers of bloodletting if performed improperly or by unskilled practitioners. Celsus sounds a cautionary note about bleeding patients who are weak or feverish, since the bleeding will further sap their strength, as well as bleeding patients who have undigested food (likely because the process of digesting food was thought to require heat, and blood was associated with heat as a humor). He also warned against excessive bleeding in a single session. We understand, therefore, why some patients were reluctant to undergo the procedure. And this might explain why Erasistratus refused altogether to perform the treatment, instead recommending binding and bandaging body parts to encourage the pooling and redistribution of blood into different parts of the body.

The selections below from Celsus also discuss **cupping** as a way to deal with putrefying blood and swelling in the body (see fig. 48). Physicians would light a flame inside a cupping vessel to create a vacuum and then suction the cupping vessel to the body part being treated. Before applying the cupping vessel they sometimes made a small incision on the spot first

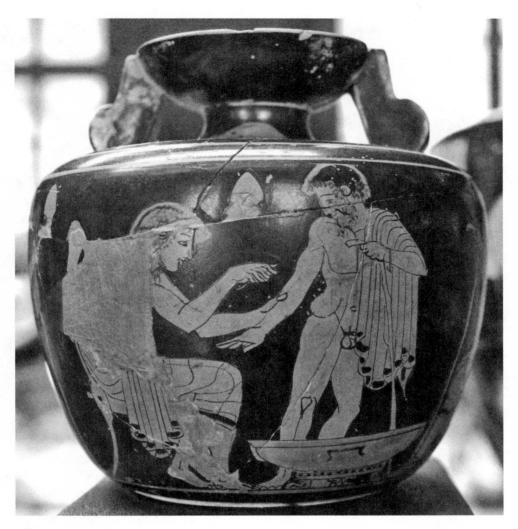

FIGURE 42 Circa 480–470 BCE red-figure Greek vase depicting a seated man holding the arm of another man and reaching toward him with a scalpel, presumably poised to start the practice of bloodletting. A shallow bowl sits on the ground, likely to catch the blood that is drained from his body. Department of Greek, Etruscan, and Roman Antiquities of the Louvre (CA 1989; CA 2183). Photo credit: Bibi Saint-Pol. Wikimedia Commons.

(wet cupping), and sometimes not (dry cupping). This was thought to draw out the bad matter, whether blood or air.

Finally, physicians also prescribed emetics (substances that induced vomiting), laxatives (substances that induced movement of the bowels), and other purgatives in the event other more gentle means failed to return patients to health (for a more detailed discussion, see below on pharmacology).

In general, we see that regimen in antiquity was comprehensive in its approach to dealing with or preventing illness, involving physicians' considerations of diet, exercise, bathing, sleep, sexual activity, and many other things when devising treatment plans for patients.

TEXT 20. HIPPOCRATIC CORPUS, *REGIMEN IN HEALTH* SELECTION (1–9)

Regimen in Health *was attributed to* **Hippocrates***, but as with all the texts in the Hippocratic corpus, the authorship is uncertain. The text offers advice about how people of different ages, genders, and physical conditions should manage their bodily intake and outtake at different times of the year in order to be healthy. Like all ancient discussions of regimen, this text focuses on eating, drinking, exercise, bathing, and the prevention or promotion of vomiting and other evacuations from the body. With content that appears elsewhere in the Hippocratic corpus,* Regimen in Health *might be largely a compilation of insights drawn from other texts. In the manuscript tradition* Regimen in Health *was transmitted along with the Hippocratic text* On the Nature of Humans *(Text 5), so scholars debate whether they were two separate texts or merely two parts of the same text. If the latter is the case, then* Regimen in Health *could be attributed to Polybus, Hippocrates's son-in-law, and dated to the late fifth century BCE.*

SOURCE: Translation by Robert Nau based on the Greek text from Jacques Jouanna, *Hippocratis De natura hominis*, 2nd ed., Corpus Medicorum Graecorum 1.1.3 (Berlin: Akademie Verlag, 2002).

Chapter 1. Regular people[2] ought to follow a regimen in this way. During the winter, eat as much as possible and drink as little as possible. Drink must be wine as undiluted as possible. Food should be wheat bread and all meats should be roasted. In this season, eat as few vegetables as possible. For in this way the body will be especially warm and dry. When spring sets in, drink more and make it more diluted, a little at a time. Take softer foods in smaller amounts. Choose barley bread in preference to wheat bread. Meat, according to the same principle, must be boiled instead of roasted. Already during the spring one must eat few vegetables, so that a person settles into summer by taking all their grains soft, meats boiled, vegetables raw and boiled, and the greatest quantity of drinks that are as diluted as possible. For someone who takes their barley-bread soft, their drink watery in a great amount, and all their meats boiled, the change will not be great and sudden during the summer. Take food and water in this way when it is summer, so that the body may become cold and soft. For the season is warm and dry and it naturally makes bodies feverish and parched. And so people must counteract these conditions through their habits. According to the same principle, the transition from spring to summer should be prepared in the same way as that

2. "Regular people" refers to those who do not follow a specialized diet and exercise plan, in contrast to the specialized diets of athletes or soldiers discussed later in the text.

from winter to spring. Less food should be eaten and more should be drunk. Start doing the opposite when moving from summer to winter. In the autumn make more food and make it drier, and the same principle for meats. Drinks should be smaller and not as diluted, so that the winter will be good and a person may drink a small quantity mixed as little as possible, and eat a great quantity of the driest possible food. For in this way a person will be especially healthy and not at all cold. For the season is both cold and wet.

Chapter 2. People with physiques that are fleshy, soft, and reddish benefit from following drier regimens for most of the year, for the nature of these physiques is moist. People who have physiques that are compact and taut, with reddish or dark complexion, benefit from following a moister regimen more often, for their bodies tend to be dry. Young people also benefit from following softer and moister regimens, for that time of life is dry and their bodies are still firm. But older people must more often employ a drier habit for more time, for at this time of life bodies are moist, soft, and cold. Regimens should be followed accounting for time of life, the season, and physiques, counteracting the prevailing heat and cold. This is how one would best attain health.

Chapter 3. During the winter, one should walk quickly, but during the summer one should walk leisurely, unless under the hot sun. People who are fleshy must walk faster, but those who are lean [must walk] more leisurely. People should bathe much during the summer, but less during the winter. People who are lean should bathe more than those who are fleshy. In the summer, people should dress in clothes soaked with oil, but pure in the winter.

Chapter 4. Fat people who want to become thin should exert themselves strenuously while they are hungry, and eat their foods while still gasping, not yet having caught their breath, and drink wine beforehand, not diluted nor too cold. They should prepare their meats with sesame seasoning and other similar things. Also let their foods be rich, for in this way they would become filled with the least amount of food. They should eat one main meal a day, not bathe, sleep on a hard bed, and walk about wearing as little clothing as possible. Thin people who wish to become fat should act differently and opposite to this, including not strenuously exerting themselves while hungry.

Chapter 5. Use **emetics** and purges of the **cavity** as follows. Induce vomit during the six winter months, for this time is more productive of phlegm than the summer and illnesses of the head and the region above the diaphragm arise then. But, when it is warm, use enemas, for the season induces fever and the body contains more bile, there is heaviness of the loins and the knees, fevers occur, and there is colic of the belly. And so the body must be cooled and what has come up from these regions must be drawn downwards. For people who are somewhat fat and moist, let their enemas be saltier and thinner. But for people who are rather dry, compact, and weak, let their enemas be fattier and thicker. Fatty and thick enemas are made from milk, or broth from boiling chickpeas and other similar things. Thin and salty enemas are made from things like brine and seawater.

Use emetics in this way. Fat people should use emetics while running or walking quickly at midday. The emetic should be half a cup of hyssop ground into twelve cups of water, and after pouring vinegar in and adding salt, so that it turns out to be as agreeable as possible, a person should drink this. The person should drink this rather leisurely at first but then more quickly. Thinner and weaker people, after eating, should use emetics in this manner. After bathing in warm water, they should drink a cup of undiluted wine. Then they should eat all kinds of food and not drink during or after eating. Instead, they should pause for as long as it takes to travel about a mile, and then drink a mixture of three wines (dry, sweet, and sharp) at first rather undiluted and little by little over a long period of time, and then more diluted, more quickly, and in greater amounts.

A person who has been accustomed to take an emetic twice a month would do better to take emetics on two days in a row rather than every fifteenth day, but people do entirely the opposite. People who should vomit their food and who have problems with digestion benefit from eating many times a day and by having a variety of foods and meats that have been prepared in every way, and by drinking two or three types of wines. All people who do not vomit up their food or have moist cavities benefit by acting in an opposite manner.

Chapter 6. Infants should be bathed in warm water for a long time and provided with wine to drink that is diluted and not entirely cold, which makes the belly distend least and produce gas. These things should be done so that they may be less susceptible to convulsions and so that they may become bigger and have a healthier complexion. Women should follow a regimen drier in character, for dry foods are more beneficial for the softness of their **flesh** and less diluted drinks are better for the womb and nourishing the fetus.

Chapter 7. People who train should run and wrestle during the winter, but during the summer should wrestle little and not run, but rather walk a lot in the cold. People who ache from exhaustion after their runs should wrestle and people who ache from exhaustion while wrestling should run. For in this way the part of the body that fails during exertion would be thoroughly warmed and given rest. People who are struck by diarrhea when training and whose excrement consists partly of undigested food should reduce their exercises by no less than a third measure and should eat half as much food. For it is clear indeed that the cavity cannot warm enough to digest the amount of the foods entering. Their foods should be thoroughly baked bread crumbled into wine and what they drink should be as undiluted and as little as possible, and they should not take walks after eating. During this time, they must only eat one main meal. In this way, the cavity would be warmed and able to manage whatever enters. This type of diarrhea is found in people whose bodies are extremely solid when they are compelled to eat meat because their nature is of this sort, for the veins now contracted do not cope with the foods entering. This nature itself is quick to change and turns to extremes, and in such types of bodies good condition flourishes only for a short time. People with physiques that are less firm and hairier are receptive to forced feeding, and especially strenuous exertion, and their good condition flourishes for a longer time. People who vomit up their food the day after eating it, and whose upper abdominal regions distend because their foods are undigested, benefit from sleeping longer and should force their bodies to different strenuous exertion. They should drink a greater quantity of rather undiluted wine and eat less food at this time. For clearly the cavity, in its weak and cold state, cannot digest the amount of food. People who are seized by thirst must reduce their food and strenuous exertions and should drink wine that is diluted and as cold as possible. People who have pains in their innards after exercises or some other serious exertion benefit from taking a break without food, and from drinking what, when it enters the body in the smallest quantity, will expel the most urine, so that the veins along the innards are not strained through being filled. For it is in such a way that growths and fevers occur.

Chapter 8.[3] In the case of people whose illnesses arise from the brain, first a numbness seizes the head, urinating is frequent, and one suffers the features of strangury. A person suffers this for nine days. If water and mucous discharge from the nostrils or the ears, the illness will cease and the strangury will end. A person passes without trouble much white urine until twenty days pass. The pain also leaves from the person's head but the light is taken from the eyes.

Chapter 9.[4] An intelligent man should recognize that health is the most valuable blessing for people. He should learn from his own judgment how to benefit himself in his illnesses.

TEXT 21. CELSUS, *ON MEDICINE* SELECTION (2.10–11)

On Medicine, *written by Aulus Cornelius* **Celsus** *(c. 25 BCE–50 CE?), was originally part of an encyclopedia that covered a range of topics, including agriculture, medicine, rhetoric, philosophy, and military science. The section on medicine, the only one to survive, is organized around the three major divisions of ancient medicine: regimen, pharmacology, and surgery. Scholars debate whether Celsus was himself a practicing physician, but his text offers hints of real experience, especially in the sections on surgery. In the selection below, Celsus discusses one of the main areas of regimen—dietetics—which included not only the food physicians ought to have their patients eat, but also how physicians might expend bodily* materia *(a Latin word that here means something like "bodily matter") before it has a chance to cause harm. One method of treatment in this respect was bloodletting, which Celsus suggests might be employed for nearly every illness or condition, though he warns that physicians ought to be cautious about letting only bad blood and that only skilled physicians ought to perform the procedure. At the end of the section, Celsus offers advice on another method by which to draw blood out of the body—***cupping***—which had less severe effects and was thus more appropriate for sick persons who could not endure bloodletting.*

SOURCE: Translation by Jared Secord based on the Latin text from Guy Serbat, *Celse, De la médicine,* vol. 1 (Paris: Les Belles Lettres, 1995).

3. Chapter 8 also appears in another Hippocratic text, *On Diseases* 2.12.
4. Chapter 9 also appears in another Hippocratic text, *On Affections* 1.

Book 2, Chapter 10. 7. Nevertheless, it can happen that an illness may require bloodletting, though the body seems hardly able to endure it. But if it appears that there is no other option, and the person in distress is about to die unless there be some help, even in a reckless way, in this situation it is the job of a good physician to point out that there is no hope without letting blood, and to acknowledge how much fear this action may produce, and then eventually, if it is demanded, to let blood. 8. It is unfitting to hesitate in a matter of this sort. For it is better to try an uncertain option than none. And this should especially be done when there is paralysis of the muscles, when someone becomes suddenly speechless, when a throat infection becomes suffocating, when the attack of a prior fever was nearly fatal, and it is likely that a similar onset will follow and it seems that the strength of the sick person will not be able to endure it.

9. Blood should absolutely not be let from a sick person with undigested food,[5] but even this is not a universal rule. For the situation does not always wait for digestion. Therefore if someone falls from a height, if someone is bruised, or if someone vomits blood suddenly, even if this person has eaten food a little before, bodily matter must be taken from this person immediately so that it might not afflict the body if it settles. The same advice will also hold in other unexpected situations that lead to suffocation. 10. But if the nature of the illness permits bloodletting, it will only happen when we suspect there is no undigested food remaining. Therefore the second or third day of poor health seems most suitable for this procedure. But while it is sometimes necessary to let blood on the first day, it is never useful after the fourth day, since by that time the bodily matter itself is used up and has corrupted the body, so that bloodletting can make the body weak rather than whole. 11. If a severe fever oppresses, letting someone's blood during the attack itself is to slit this person's throat. One must wait, therefore, for remission. If the fever does not weaken, but ceases to increase, and remission is not expected, then the opportunity must not be missed, though it is remote and quite dangerous.

12. When the procedure of bloodletting is necessary, it should generally be broken up into two days. For it is better on the first day to comfort the sick person, and then purge the sick person fully, rather than potentially hastening the sick person's end at once by having let all of the sick person's strength drain away. If this approach is effective for pus or water under the skin, it should necessarily be that much more effective for blood. If the cause impacts the entire body, blood should be let from the arm. If it impacts a particular part, then blood should be let from that part itself, or at least from the closest part to it, because blood cannot be let from everywhere, but only from the temples, arms, and near the ankles. 13. I also know that some people say blood should be let from as far as possible from where

5. Celsus's reasoning here is that excess bodily matter in the sick person will clear up once the food is digested and expelled from the body, meaning that there is no need to speed the process along with bloodletting.

the sick person is injured.[6] For, they say, the course of the bodily matter is diverted, but in that way the bodily matter is summoned into the very part that burdens the sick person. But this is false, for bloodletting draws out from the nearest spot first, and blood from the furthest spots follows so long as it is being let. When it is stopped, no more blood comes because it is not being drawn. 14. Nonetheless, experience itself seems to have taught that if a head is broken, blood must rather be let from the arm. If the problem is in the upper arm, blood must be let from the other arm. I believe this is so because, if something bad results, the parts that are already doing badly are more liable to be injured.[7] Blood is also sometimes diverted when it rushes out from one part and is discharged from another part. For if blood is given another passage to flow, it stops flowing from a place where we don't want it when something placed in front of it stops it there.

15. Letting blood may be performed most easily by someone who has experience, but it is extremely difficult for someone without experience. For the artery is joined to a vein, and to these are joined tendons.[8] Thus, if a scalpel touches a tendon, a spasm of the tendons follows, and this kills a person cruelly. But an artery cut open neither closes up nor heals. It also sometimes leads to blood spurting forth violently. 16. As for the vein itself, if by chance it is cut with its severed ends pressed together, it emits no blood. But if the scalpel is brought down timidly, it cuts the top layer of the skin, but does not cut into the vein. Sometimes even the vein lies hidden and is not easily found. Thus many things make a task that is easiest for an experienced person difficult for an unskilled person.

The vein must be cut in its middle. When blood spurts forth, one ought to pay attention to its color and condition. 17. For if the blood is thick and black, it is bad and therefore useful for it to be shed. If it is red and transparent, it is good. Letting this blood is truly unhelpful, and even harmful; the blood must immediately be stopped. But this cannot happen with a physician who knows from what sort of body blood should be let.[9] 18. It is more likely that blood will flow black continually on the first day. Although this is so, if enough has already flowed, it must be stopped, and an end must always be made before consciousness fades. The arm must be bandaged up with a pad that has been wrung out with cold water. On the next day, the vein should be struck with the back of the middle finger, so that its recent

6. Celsus is referring to the idea expressed in other medical texts (such as Hippocratic Corpus, *On the Nature of Humans* 11) that blood vessels extended for long distances across the body, allowing a physician to let blood from an area far away from where the injury or problem was located, and yet still have an effect on the injury or problem.

7. Here we see Celsus's general belief that bloodletting can be dangerous, with the potential to cause injury especially to the part that is already injured.

8. The Latin word Celsus uses here is *nervus,* which can be translated variously as "nerve," "sinew," or "tendon." These three terms, which modern anatomical knowledge recognizes as distinct, were regarded by Celsus as being basically the same.

9. Celsus is suggesting that physicians with knowledge of the different qualities of blood will not make the mistake of letting blood that show signs of being good.

coagulation may be loosened and it may shed blood again. 19. If the blood on the first or second day begins to be red and transparent, after initially having flowed thick and black, enough bodily matter has been drawn off, and what remains of the blood is pure. The arm must therefore be bandaged immediately and kept this way until the little scar is strong. This is formed most quickly on a vein.

Book 2, Chapter 11. 1. There are two types of cups, one bronze and the other horn. The bronze type of cup is open on one side, and closed on the other. The horn type of cup is also open on one side, but has a small hole on the other. Into the bronze cup is piled burning linen, and in this way its mouth is applied and pressed upon the body until it adheres. 2. The horn cup is put upon the body as it is, then, when air is drawn away by its mouth from the side where the small hole is, and the hole has been closed with wax, it also begins to adhere. Either type of cup can be made not only from these kinds of materials, but also from whatever else is appropriate. And if other types are unavailable, a small cup or a cooking pot with a narrow mouth may be suitably adapted for the task. 3. If the skin has been cut before with a scalpel, when the cup has adhered, it extracts blood. If the skin is whole, it extracts air. Therefore when there is harmful bodily matter inside, the first method should be employed, but when there is swelling, the second. The use of a cup, however, is particular to situations when the problem is not in the whole body but in a certain part, the draining of which is enough to establish good health. 4. This very fact is evidence that— when a limb is being relieved—blood must be let with a scalpel from the part that has already been injured. Unless someone is diverting a discharge of blood in that direction, no one puts a cup on a different part rather than the part itself which is in pain and must be relieved. There can also be a need for cupping in chronic illnesses, even if they have already lasted for some time, whether there is corrupt bodily matter or bad air. 5. There can also be a need in certain acute cases, if the body must be unburdened and the sick person's bodily strength does not allow for blood to be let from a vein. And this option is less violent, so it is safer, and not ever dangerous, even if it is during an attack of a fever, and even if it is applied with undigested food. 6. Therefore, when there is a need for blood to be let, if a cut vein is a great danger, or if the problem even now is in one part of the body, one must rather take recourse in cupping, although we know that there is no danger in it, it is nevertheless less help, and one cannot relieve something severely harmful except with an equally severe option.

TEXT 22. PAUL OF AEGINA, *MEDICAL COMPENDIUM* SELECTION (1.53–56)

In the first book of his Medical Compendium, ***Paul of Aegina*** *(c. 625–690 CE) offered advice about diet, health, and what we now might call "preventative medicine." The selection below provides guidance to readers about how to manage the balance of their **humors** at different times of the year and under different circumstances. Paul's suggestions relate primarily to eating and drinking, but he also suggests other means of balancing the humors, including exercise and bathing, as well as the use of **emetics**, laxatives, and bloodletting to rid the body of excessive humors.*

Paul's advice illustrates the range of components involved in regimen, as well as the centrality of regimen as one of the primary branches of ancient medicine (alongside pharmacology and surgery).

SOURCE: Translation by Brent Arehart based on the Greek text from J. L. Heiberg, *Paulus Aegineta*, vol. 1, Corpus Medicorum Graecorum 9.1 (Leipzig: Teubner, 1921).

Book 1, Chapter 53. On the Appropriate Regimen by Season
It is good to conduct our regimen relative to the seasons. During winter, engage in more physical activities and eat more, especially when the weather conditions are dominated by northern winds. When there is wet weather, engage in a similar amount of physical activity but partake of less food and drink. In general, make the body dry when the season is mostly wet, just as we make the body warmer when it is cold. Eat warm meat and vegetables and drink more wine. When spring begins, some people should empty themselves through emetics, others through their belly, and others should take out blood by cutting a vein— whatever method happens to be the habit and desire of each individual. During the summer, it is beneficial to take a rest from physical activities and to reduce food intake. The types of food consumed should be more cooling. Take plenty of drinks. Everything should contribute to chilling and moistening the body. During the autumn, when conditions are irregular, erratic, and contribute to all kinds of sicknesses, one should conduct a very cautious regimen, making sure not to make mistakes involving the cold. Use a great deal of restraint when it comes to sexual activity and cold beverages.[10] Stay away from cold air in the early morning and burning air in the afternoon. Do not overfill on fruits, for it causes harm not only in abundance, but also by making bad humors and flatulence. Furthermore, the best kinds of fruit, namely figs and grapes, produce air [*pneuma*] if one does not take them before other foods, and they ruin meals. If taken in advance, they neither create flatulence nor completely ruin meals. When the air gets colder, heat the body proportionally and do everything as though winter is coming. After the equinox, it would also be good to employ one of the methods of emptying mentioned earlier so that nothing excessive gets retained during the winter and becomes harmful.

Book 1, Chapter 54. Regimen for People that Become Engaged in a Busy Lifestyle
A person that becomes engaged in a busy lifestyle must consider whether he was in the habit of exercising previously, or if he does not exercise in due measure, whether he tolerates this habit without becoming constantly sick when he has a good sweat. A bodily constitution of this sort should not change habits, nor in general should people change their habits who are sick for a long time. If someone appears to be constantly sick, when it is caused by abundance, your goal should be a regimen that is healthy overall, so that the humors will always be balanced. But if the illness is due to a state of bad humors, your goal should be for the best humors. Now, as for people that accumulate an abundance, those that go

10. Some ancient authors believed that sexual activity had a cooling effect on the body.

straightaway to bathe should engage in massage afterwards and some light exercise before-hand. As for people who were already doing these things, we will recommend that they do the same things and increase the frequency a little bit, but also that they reduce some of their food and take in less nourishing food. When it comes to people that accumulate bad humors, there is not just one thing to consider because there is no single form of this. Some people accumulate a colder and more **phlegmatic** state of bad humors, while some accumu-late a warmer state with more bile, just as others accumulate a state with more black bile. Thus, they need to abstain from every kind of food and drink that naturally and readily gen-erates the accumulating humor. In all these cases, a common remedy is a downward purge of the belly.

Book 1, Chapter 55. Regimen for Travelers
It is easiest to depart for journeys if one does so with empty bowels and does not walk intensely. Furthermore, during the summer, wrap the loins up to the flanks with a soft band six or seven fingers in width and no more than five cubits in length. A cane is also useful for journeys. Throwing a cane forward while going downhill holds back the body as it bends forward like a pole, while leaning on a cane when going uphill makes moving the body upslope easier. Now, when there is a pause during the journey, oil, a small amount of some summer food, and a good amount of a drink is fitting for this season, along with a break after lunch before proceeding. For someone that is forced to travel continuously and gets thirsty, it is fitting to drink threshed barley in water with a moderate amount of salt. It is necessary to beware of the heat and the sun, making sure that the body is not exposed to the sun naked but covered up, so that it does not harden and dry out along the journey. This way, the fatigue should be minimized and none of the aforementioned condi-tions should occur to the same extent. When it is winter, it is fitting to empty the bowels and anoint oneself before the journey, and to take a good bit of winter food and a small drink. With a longer band, wrap not only the loins but also the spine and the chest properly well. When resting in comfort, if it is very cold, then it is better neither to anoint oneself nor to have food and drink nor any other comfort unless one is going to stay in the same spot. Even if someone is not fatigued after long journeys and other kinds of intense activity, one must treat him just like fatigued people. This way, something unpleasant should be less likely to happen.

Book 1, Chapter 56. Regimen for Sailing
As for the vomiting that happens to people while sailing, it is not easy or useful for first tim-ers to resist, as it tends to help with everything for the most part. After vomiting, one should not take in a lot of food or just any kind of it. Eat lentils dry and cooked with a little bit of pen-nyroyal, or bread broken into watery and fragrant wine. Take a small amount of drink, either weak wine that is entirely watery or vinegar made from honey. It will be necessary to boil the lentils and then, when they become soft, to crush them so that they are smooth. Then dry them and put them together this way in a clay container. Later on, if more vomit-

ing occurs, reduce the intake of food even further and take a small drink: vinegar made from honey with water in which thyme has been steeped, or pennyroyal and water with fine barley meal, or weak fragrant wine with meal that is likewise watery. For the disagreeable odors on the ship, one should go smell quinces or thyme or pennyroyal. One should also look out at sea as little as possible until one gets in the habit of spending time on the ship. And pay attention to the drinking water, making sure that it is not muddy, malodorous, or salty.

PHARMACOLOGY AND DRUG THERAPIES

As we learned in the previous section, all food was thought of as medicine in terms of the ways it could affect the balance of the body by changing its properties (hot, cold, wet, and dry) and its **humors**. Thus we find many of the same plant, animal, and mineral substances showing up in cookbooks, discussions of regimen, and pharmacological literature. For instance, the passage from **Oribasius** discusses the medicinal properties of the humble legume, the chickpea (Text 27). The line between food therapy (dietetics) and drug therapy (pharmacology) was often blurry in the ancient world.

However, from very early on in the ancient Greek world (and even earlier in Mesopotamia and Egypt), certain substances were recognized as **drugs** on account of their ability to act on the body in a wider variety of ways; these abilities were called a drug's "power" (*dunamis*). In addition to heating/cooling and moistening/drying, drugs could have analgesic, anesthetic, anodyne, aphrodisiac, anti-inflammatory, **astringent**, cathartic, condensing, contraceptive, diuretic, drying, **emetic**, emollient, **expectorant**, hallucinatory, laxative, narcotic, purgative, sedative, stimulating, and thickening powers. Pharmacologists, physicians, healers, and laypeople in the ancient world classified drugs according to the specific kinds of effects they had on the body.

The Greek words *pharmakon* (singular) and *pharmaka* (plural) had many meanings, some of them strictly medical, while some had supernatural or ritual connotations, both sinister and sacred. For instance, *pharmakon* could mean simply "remedy" or "drug," but it could also mean "poison," "charm," "spell," and even "scapegoat." (There is a similar ambiguity of meaning in the Latin words *medicamentum* and *venenum*, which meant both "drug" and "poison.") We see this complex of associations with drug-based remedies reflected in a number of the entries from **Pliny the Elder's** *Natural History* (see Text 28). And such opposing sets of meanings for the word *pharmakon* are understandable given that some medicinal substances could both heal and cause harm depending on dosing or how they were administered. For example, hellebore could increase menstrual flow, but it could also act as an abortifacient. Given the negative connotations associated with the word *pharmakon*, it is no wonder **Scribonius Largus** spends so much time insisting on the usefulness of drugs in medical treatment. In the selection below (Text 24), he is responding to opponents who argued that physicians should not use drugs to treat their patients.

The ritual or "magical" meanings of the word *pharmakon* remind us that most remedies were associated with the divine prior to the emphasis of early Greek natural philosophy and Hippocratic medicine on scientific explanations. Yet we should not think about these ritual and medical meanings as alternative or competing understandings. Rather, we find both sacred and medicinal dimensions overlaid in pharmacological literature. For example, the famous Alexandrian physician **Herophilus** (c. 330–c. 260 BCE) reportedly said that "drugs are the hands of the gods" (Text 24, Scribonius Largus, *Recipes*, Preface 1). This saying is important in a number of respects for understanding Greek and Roman pharmacology. First, even scientific thinkers assumed, for the most part, that plants, animals, and minerals had healing properties because the gods created them to have such properties. They were sacred gifts for humans to use to make life better: to cure human illness and reduce suffering. Second, some people regarded discoveries of new drugs to be revelations from the gods, and thought it necessary to show gratitude to the gods for disclosing scientific knowledge to humans (see, for example, Text 41, *Oath of Asaph and Yoḥanan*). Some thought that the gods even implanted clues in the physical characteristics of the plants themselves to signal how they were to be used (an idea that later came to be known as the doctrine of signatures or similitudes). For instance, the plant lungwort, with flowers that resemble lungs, was thought to be a remedy for illnesses affecting respiration. Third, we hear about elaborate ritual processes involved in the collection of drugs. For instance, in one of our earliest Greek botanical texts, *Inquiry into Plants*, **Theophrastus** noted that some of the root cutters (*rhitozomoi*) whose remedies he cited observed sacred and apotropaic rituals when collecting plant materials, practices that were thought to involve danger (see examples in Text 23). For instance, if one gathered a plant sacred to a certain deity without acknowledging it as a divine gift, one might incur divine displeasure. Fourth, drug sellers were not only purveyors of medicinal remedies, but they often also sold protective amulets and even poisons. Finally, many plants had long-standing associations in popular thought with particular divinities and astral phenomena (the sun, moon, stars, and constellations). And it was commonly thought that body parts and internal organs were likewise connected to constellations and their attendant divinities. Hence we find an extensive web of connections between drugs, the sacred, and so-called magic in ancient pharmacological texts.

Although all genres of ancient medical texts discuss pharmacology intermittently and although we find pharmacological remedies discussed in many nonmedical sources (such as Text 25, **Cato the Elder's** *On Agriculture*), we are fortunate to have a number of pharmacological collections and handbooks that are devoted solely to the topic (such as the collections of Scribonius and **Dioscorides**; see Text 26 for the latter). And these sources represent— more than in most other areas of ancient medicine—the influence and influx of knowledge from laypeople, popular healers, and other kinds of professionals who mixed sacred and scientific thinking. For instance, Pliny the Elder, who compiled a book of remedies in his encyclopedia, *Natural History*, mentions assembling his collection of drugs as he traveled, sourced from local customs across the provinces. And Theophrastus notes that some of his

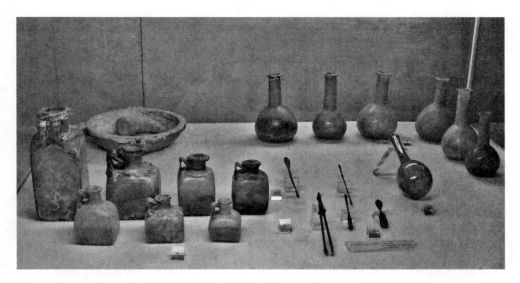

FIGURE 43 Glass cruets, mortar, and pestle from Pompeii. Medicinal mixtures were stored in glass cruets like those pictured here (*front left, back right*), and also in pottery vessels that sometimes had a label describing their contents impressed into the clay. A mortar and pestle (*back left*) were used to crush and mix ingredients for cooking and also for medicinal remedies. Naples Archaeological Museum. Photo credit: © Carlo Raso.

knowledge about plants derives from conversations with root cutters, drug sellers, and potion makers.

These pharmacological collections were organized systematically. In each entry, they recorded the powers of the plant and the ailments it could be used to treat. They also provided information to help people identify and harvest the plants, such as the plant's morphology (i.e., its form and structures, especially distinguishing features like a colored stem or a scalloped leaf), the geographic areas in which it grew, and its growing and harvesting seasons. And, finally, they provided instructions on how to store, prepare, and administer or apply the remedy (e.g., ingested, as a salve, as a **pessary**, etc.), and the precise measurements and doses to use.

Ancient pharmacological texts often divided drugs into simple and compound medicines. A simple medicine was a drug that was made based on the main power(s) of a single substance—for instance, opium poppy, cabbage, verdigris (copper patina), or goat dung. Sometimes, as we see in the texts below, pharmacological writers combined these single substances with other ingredients with the aim of either making the simple substance usable for different applications (such as combining with wine so the remedy might be ingested, or combining with wax so the remedy could be made into a suppository), or enhancing the powers of the drug (see, for example, Text 26, where Dioscorides explains that opium poppy becomes more effective when mixed with the juices of hypocist and shittah tree). Compound drugs, on the other hand, were a combination of multiple substances, each of which was necessary to produce the drug's powers. Some of these remedies had their roots in toxicology more so than in ancient botany and pharmacology; in other words, some of the earliest compound remedies were created to counteract poisoning or bites and stings of venomous animals. Reliance on and enthusiasm for compound medicines then developed over time. Compound drugs could include up to sixty ingredients and require elaborate processes and multiple steps to produce; hence the need for specialists: pharmacologists. And some individuals or regions came to be known for specialty compounds (such as the eye salves from Persia and Chios discussed in Text 15, **Paul of Aegina's** *Medical Compendium*).

One of the most famous compounds from antiquity was known as theriac. Theriac had its earliest roots in the legendary efforts of the Hellenistic ruler Mithridates IV of Pontus to create a universal antidote for all possible poisons, especially those found in the bites and stings of venomous creatures (see chapter 9 on bites and stings). Eventually theriacs were regarded as a panacea, a remedy for all illnesses. For instance, **Galen** was in charge of creating the theriac that the Roman emperor Marcus Aurelius took every day as a kind of ancient multivitamin. *Collyria* (eye medicines) were another popular class of compound drug, mixed as semisolid sticks that would be dissolved as needed. Physicians specializing in ophthalmological problems (a common complaint in antiquity; see chapter 9) would often carry different kinds of these compound remedies to treat a wide variety of ophthalmological conditions, such as eye inflammation, blurred vision, or skin lesions around the eye.

Although most drugs in ancient pharmacological texts are plant-based, writers such as Pliny and Dioscorides also record many remedies that derive from human or animal parts, as well as from minerals (metals or stones). For example, Pliny explains that people experiencing epilepsy should drink human blood—especially from gladiators, those thought to possess exceptional strength—to restore their vitality. Turning to animals, Pliny records several remedies that seem to assume a transfer of the animal's special powers or potency through the body part most associated with those powers. For example, the tooth of a mole or a dog—animals known for the intensity of their bites—could be used to cure toothaches or to soothe children who were teething. In terms of drugs derived from minerals, it appears that knowledge of these remedies developed from the experiences of miners and metalworkers. Copper miners, for instance, observed that their wounds tended to heal more quickly than those of people working in other occupations, prompting innovations in the medicinal use of copper.

Readers of ancient pharmacological sources are often surprised at the preponderance of drugs composed of substances that today we would consider unhealthy, dangerous, or disgusting, such as human or animal feces, blood, ear wax, milk, urine, sweat, and spit (see Text 28, Pliny, *Natural History* 28.35–38). In antiquity, physicians and other healers assumed that all substances, even off-putting or sometimes harmful ones, could have powers that might be used to treat certain illnesses under certain conditions. For example, menstrual

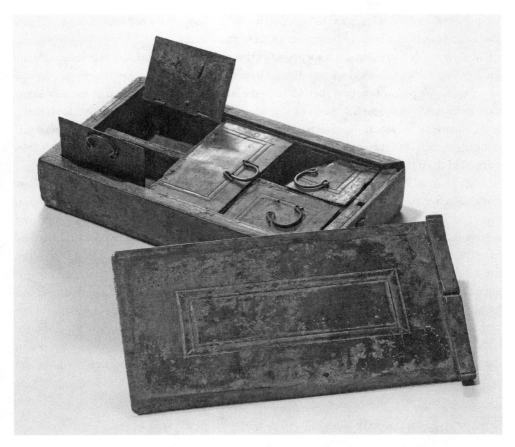

FIGURE 44 First- to second-century CE bronze medicine box, Roman, from Yortan (modern-day Türkiye). Medical boxes like the one pictured here contained a sliding lid and several internal compartments in which physicians could keep different kinds of drugs. These boxes were small and lightweight enough to be easily portable as physicians traveled from patient to patient. Some medical boxes had a long compartment for medical instruments, though instruments were often kept in their own cylindrical containers. British Museum (1921,1220.122). © The Trustees of the British Museum. All rights reserved.

blood was thought to be able to spoil crops, rust metal, and corrode mirrors, but there were times when its powers could have healing applications as well (possibly related to the view that menstrual blood was partially digested food, and thus possessed nourishing properties). Additionally, Dioscorides recommended using grime from the walls and floors of bathing complexes. This grime—a kind of compound drug containing everything from dirt, human sweat, oils used to rub down bathers, condensation, and residues from perfumes and cosmetics—was thought to be good for healing injuries of the perineum and for joint pain because of its heating and softening properties. Although such remedies might seem strange to modern readers, we must attempt to discern how ancient pharmacologists understood the powers and healing properties of these substances.

Modern readers are also often surprised by the effectiveness of ancient remedies. Despite the fact that ancient medical writers did not have a sophisticated notion of germ theory nor had they developed antibiotics, they identified a number of substances that we now know have antimicrobial properties, such as copper and frankincense, when applied to wounds. Additionally, as we see in the selection from Dioscorides below (Text 26), ancient pharmacologists recognized the soporific and analgesic effects of the poppy plant even while they warned of the dangers of overdose, which could result in coma and death.

Finally, in addition to the wealth of information that scholars of ancient pharmacology can obtain from textual sources, we can also learn about drug therapies from archaeological evidence. We have many well-preserved bowls in which drugs were mixed, jars and vessels in which drugs were stored, and small portable boxes in which physicians would have transported drugs to their patients' homes (see figs. 43, 44). Scholars can test residues from these artifacts to determine the drugs they contained, and some jars were labeled with the names of the drugs they contained, enabling us to gather information about drugs commonly in use. We also have *collyrium* stamps that were impressed on the solid sticks of eye ointment before they hardened, providing information about the ingredients or kind of medication (see fig. 30). Finally, archaeologists have also unearthed many instruments used in the preparation and administration of drugs, such as mortars and pestles, weights and scales, and spoons.

TEXT 23. THEOPHRASTUS, *INQUIRY ON PLANTS* SELECTION (9.8)

Theophrastus (c. 372/1–287/6 BCE) was a philosopher and student of **Aristotle**, whom he succeeded as head of the Lyceum in Athens. A prolific author of more than 200 texts, Theophrastus had wide-ranging interests, including natural science, and especially botany, earning him the title "Father of Botany." His text, Inquiry into Plants, categorizes and organizes the plants known to Theophrastus, carefully detailing the features that distinguished them one from another. The selection below is taken from the ninth book of Inquiry into Plants, which contains material from another of Theophrastus's texts called On the Properties of Medicinal Plants. As the title suggests, this text explains how various parts of plants might be used for medicinal purposes. In this selection, Theophrastus also discloses root cutters' beliefs about how to harvest plants safely.

The translation includes some passages in square brackets. These were added to the Greek text by an unknown editor who combined several of Theophrastus's botanical texts. This editor also added headings, transitions, and commentary designed to make the text more readable and comprehensible.

SOURCE: Translated by Jared Secord based on the Greek text from Suzanne Amigues, *Théophraste, Recherches sur les plantes*, vol. 5 (Paris: Les Belles Lettres, 2006).

Book 9, Chapter 8. 1. [Concerning the juices that have not previously been discussed—I mean, those that are medicinal or that have other properties—we must attempt to discuss in a similar way. At the same time, we must discuss roots, for some of the juices come from them and, apart from this, have many properties of all kinds on their own. Speaking generally, we must discuss all medicinal things: fruit, juice extracted from plants, leaves, roots, and herbs. For the root-cutters also call some medicinal things an herb.]

[Concerning the roots that are medicinal and have whatsoever kinds of properties whether in themselves, or in the juices, or in some other of their parts, or, in general, of the shrubby or herbaceous plants with such properties, and the differences of flavors and odors and of all those that produce no odors, which are certainly no less natural.]

There are many properties of "roots"[11] and they are used for many purposes. But those that are medicinal are especially sought after because they are the most useful, and they are different in that they do not have the same uses and property in the same parts, [just as he said a little earlier.] In general, most "roots" have the property in themselves, and also in the fruits and juices; some also have it in their leaves. The root-cutters call the properties belonging to the leaves in almost all cases "herbs."

2. The extraction of juice from the plants that are extracted happens for the most part in the summer, sometimes when it is beginning, and other times at the end of the season. The cutting of roots happens in some instances when wheat is being harvested, but more of it is done in late autumn after the rising of Arcturus,[12] when the leaves have fallen, and when plants that have useful fruit have shed it. The extraction happens either from the stems (such as spurge, wild lettuce, and most plants), or from the roots, or, thirdly, from the head (such as with the poppy). This is the only plant for which this applies; this extraction is peculiar to it. In some plants the juice gathers on its own like tears, such as the tragacanth, for it is not possible to cut it. But in most cases the juice comes from an incision. In some cases the juice collects right away into receptacles, such as the spurge or the poppy (for they call it both names), and generally with all the plants that happen to be full of juice. For those plants that are not full of juice, they take it with a piece of wool, such as the wild lettuce. 3. In some instances there is no juice but still an extraction of sorts happens: they cut down and crush the plants and pour water over them, then strain off the water and collect the residue. But it is clear that the juice of these plants is dry and inferior. The juice extracted from other "roots" is less powerful than the juice of the fruit, but that of hemlock[13] is stronger, and a quite small pill of it given to someone results in an easier and quicker death. It is also more effective for other uses. The extracted juice of the deadly carrot is also stronger, but that of

11. The Greek word used here (*rhiza*) can refer both to the root of a plant, but also to a medicinal plant. When the word "root" appears in quotation marks, it refers to a medicinal plant, rather than the root of a plant.

12. Arcturus is the brightest star in the constellation Boötes.

13. Hemlock was the substance used for the death of the Athenian philosopher **Socrates.**

all the other plants is less powerful. And thus the extractions of juices generally happen in these ways.

4. There is no such difference for the cutting and gathering of roots, except for the seasons—for example, whether it is summer or autumn—and for the parts of the roots—for example, the lower and delicate parts of hellebore. For they say that the upper and thick part that is like a head is useless and that it is given to dogs when one wants to purge them. And they say there are differences of this sort for certain other plants.

5. In addition, pharmacists and root-cutters say other things, some of these probably true, but others that are exaggerations. For they advise that people should stand into the wind when cutting roots, such as the deadly carrot and some others, and anoint themselves with fat. They say that the body will swell up if one stands in the opposite direction. They also advise that those gathering the fruit of the white rose should stand into the wind. If not, they say there is danger to the eyes. And they advise that some roots should be cut at night, and others during the day. They say some should be cut before the sun falls upon them, such as the honeysuckle.

6. These suggestions and those similar to them may perhaps seem not out of place, for the properties of these plants are harmful. They say that these plants cause inflammation, like fire, and actual burns. For instance, hellebore quickly causes a headache, and those digging it up cannot do this for a long time. For this reason they eat garlic before digging and drink unmixed wine right after. But ideas of this sort, so to speak, are implausible and far off the mark, such as their advice to dig up the peony (some call it the sweet pomegranate) at night. For, they say, if someone does this in the daytime and is seen gathering the fruit by a black woodpecker, there is danger for his eyes. And if someone is seen cutting the root, his anus prolapses.

TEXT 24. SCRIBONIUS LARGUS, *RECIPES*[14] SELECTION (PREFACE 1–14)

Recipes, written by **Scribonius Largus** *(first centuries BCE and CE), is a major text of pharmacology that includes 271 medicinal recipes. Scribonius was a medical professional in Rome. The selection below is the letter of dedication for* Recipes. *It emphasizes the importance of pharmacology in the practice of medicine (opposing physicians who refuse to prescribe* **drugs***), and also sets out the ethical standards required for physicians. The remainder of the text was organized according to the parts of the body, providing recipes from head to toe, and beginning with the simplest remedies.*

SOURCE: Translated by Jessica Wright based on the Latin text from Joëlle Jouanna-Bouchet, *Scribonius Largus, Compositions médicales* (Paris: Les Belles Lettres, 2016).

14. This text is often referred to by its Latin title, *Compositiones*, which we have translated here as "Recipes."

Scribonius Largus Sends Greetings to His Friend Callistus

1. It is reported, Caius Julius Callistus,[15] that **Herophilus**—once considered among the greatest physicians—said, and not without reason, in my opinion, that drugs are the hands of the gods. For drugs, tested through use and experience, offer precisely what divine touch has the power to accomplish. Thus we have often noticed, during the consultations and disputes among physicians who are distinguished in authority, when it is being investigated what is to be done or by what method a sick person is to be cured, that certain people who are humble and even unknown, but who have more practical experience, or—shameful as it is to admit—are far removed from the discipline of medicine and not even adjacent to the profession, immediately free the patient from all pain and danger by giving them an effective drug, as if through the presence of divine power.

2. On this account, we must reject those who attempt to deprive medicine of the use of drugs—even though "medicine" itself is so called not from "healing" but from the potency and efficacy of drugs.[16] It is necessary, however, to commend those who study every method for helping those who are in danger. Certainly, I myself have several times obtained great distinction in knowledge based on the successful use of drugs, and I recall many who have won exceptional glory for the same reason. For this part of medicine is actually the most necessary, and is certainly the oldest, and on account of this was first celebrated and made famous, if indeed it is true that the ancients cured problems of the body with herbs and their roots, since the timid race of mortals did not easily commit itself to iron and to fire at the beginning.[17] Even now, very many people—I would not say everyone—do this, and, except when forced by great necessity and hope of deliverance itself, do not allow things that are scarcely bearable to be done to them .

3. Why, therefore, some deprive medicine of the use of drugs I cannot discover, unless it is to expose their own ignorance. For, if they have no experience of this kind of remedy, then they deserve to be accused, since they have been so negligent in such a necessary aspect of the art. If, on the other hand, they are in fact experienced in the usefulness of drugs, but deny their use, then they are more blameworthy, since they are troubled by the fault of jealousy, which is an evil that should be reviled by all living beings, and especially by physicians, who ought to be reviled by all gods and humans if their mind is not filled with pity and gentleness, in accordance with the objective of the profession itself.

4. Therefore, let no one who is legally bound by the sacred oath of medicine give a bad drug even to an enemy—although let him attack them when the situation demands it, so

---

15. Caius Julius Callistus was a freed slave who held an influential place at the Roman imperial court under the emperor Claudius (who reigned from 41 to 54 CE).

16. Scribonius's point depends on the Latin names for these words: "medicine" is *medicina*, "healing" is *medendo*, and "drugs" is *medicamentorum*. His etymological argument links the word *medicina* with *medicamentorum*, but not with *medendo*.

17. Here "iron" refers to surgery (which used metal instruments) and "fire" to cautery (which involved burning bodily tissue).

that as both soldier and citizen he may be good in every way—because medicine does not value humans based on fortune or status but promises itself equally to all who beg for its help, and never offers itself as a source of harm for anyone.

5. **Hippocrates**, the founder of our profession, transmitted the first principles of the discipline by swearing an oath, in which it is ordained that no drug may be given or shown by any physician to a pregnant woman by which an embryo is expelled, long ago instructing the minds of students in human kindness.[18] For, if they have considered it unlawful to injure the uncertain hope of a human being, how much more wicked will they judge harming someone already brought to completion? Therefore, he considered it of great value for whoever lived according to his way of life to protect the name and dignity of medicine with a pious and sacred mind, for medicine is the knowledge of healing and not harming. If medicine does not remain fully vigilant in every way with regard to help for those who are in distress, it does not provide the compassion that it promises to humankind.

6. Therefore, those who are unwilling or unable to help the afflicted and who discourage others by denying sick people help that is often delivered by the power of drugs should cease what they are doing. For, indeed, medicine comes to the aid of those who are in distress through specific steps, as it were. First, with food, given reasonably and at a suitable time, medicine attempts to benefit those who are weak. Then, if a successful treatment does not result, medicine has recourse to the power of drugs, for these are more potent and effective than food. After, when obstacles to good health do not yield even to drugs, then medicine is forced to turn to surgery or, finally, to **cautery**.

7. But **Asclepiades**, the greatest medical author, denied that drugs should be given to patients. Some people use this false claim in place of an argument. If this were true, I would nonetheless be able to say that Asclepiades saw what he discerned with the senses; perhaps he did not direct his full attention to this subject. He was human and acted with little success in this matter. I am not deterred by an authority when I see that the thing itself is clearly helpful. But for now, since they fabricate stories about him so shamelessly, what can I say but that those who say these things commit a kind of parricide and sacrilege?

8. For that man denied that drugs should be given to those who are feverish and who have been seized by serious problems, which the Greeks call "urgent conditions,"[19] because he believed that they could be cured more safely with food and wine given at suitable intervals. Elsewhere, in the book titled *Paraskeuastikōn,* that is, "Of Preparations," he asserts that the physician who does not have two or three recipes—both tested and prepared on the spot for each problem—is of the lowest rank. You see, therefore, how much the use of drugs displeases Asclepiades! For him, anyone who does not have many drugs mixed for each kind of problem does not seem worthy of the medical profession.

18. See Text 40, the Hippocratic *Oath.*
19. In Greek, *oxea pathē.*

9. But, through the negligence of some people, audacity of this sort by those who are physicians only in name has spread widely. For rarely does anyone, before entrusting themselves and their kin to a physician, make a careful judgment about this person, even though there is no one who entrusts even the painting of their own image to a craftsperson who has not been tried and approved in advance through certain tests. Furthermore, in non-necessary things, everyone has weights and exact measures to avoid error. Clearly, this is because there are some people who value all other things more than themselves. Therefore, each person should take up studying, and some people are not only ignorant of ancient authors, through whom the profession might be brought to perfection, but even dare to invent false stories about them.

10. For when someone has been chosen without consideration of character, but bad and good are considered of equal rank, reverence for the discipline and the school perishes, and everyone instead pursues what can be achieved without labor and what seems capable of offering the same authority and usefulness. Thus, everyone practices medicine just as they wish. For nobody is able to move some people from perverse practice, and the scope of the profession allows everyone free judgment. And so we observe many people who have pursued the full name of "physician" with knowledge of only one aspect of healing.

11. We, however, have followed the right path from the beginning with no prior judgements in our perception of the whole art, as much as is possible for a human being, because we believed that in this way we would attain all useful things. We were driven, I swear, not so much by desire for money or glory as by knowledge of the art itself. For, to be able to protect and restore good health, one's own and that of another person, we have considered it great and beyond the natural intuition of any human. And so, just as we did with other parts of the discipline, we studied attentively those aspects of it that display its power through drugs, all the more so because we observed its effects through daily practice, demonstrating this beyond the faith and belief of most people.

12. But what need is there to prove further that it is necessary to use drugs, especially to you, who, precisely because you have perceived their usefulness, have sought certain recipes from me? Attentive to your kindness and the brilliance of your mind, which indeed you offer fully to all people, but especially to me, I have compiled in this book not only what you desired, but also anything else I happened to have at hand from experience. For I desire, I swear, to reciprocate in whatever way I am able your enduring good will toward me, since I have been helped by you at all times, but especially in these recent days.

13. For the duty of your loyalty to me did not prevent you from giving to our divine Caesar,[20] as soon as you could, my Latin medical writings which I had entrusted to you, after you had read and shared your opinion of them with me. I place much importance on your judgment. You, again, with a mind that was most pure and benevolent toward me, approved the diligence of my work not just with words, but by the act of its publication under

20. "Caesar" refers to the Roman emperor Claudius, who reigned from 41 to 54 CE.

your distinguished name. When you dedicated the work with your divine hands by praising it, you took on as much risk through your judgment as I did through my pen.

14. And so I confess that I willingly offer you unparalleled gratitude, because even before you were asked you answered my own prayers with friendliest affection, and because with your fullest favor I plucked riper fruit and pleasure from this study of mine. May you be forgiving, however, if it seems to you that there are few recipes, and that they have not been written up for every problem, since we are, as you know, far from home, and a number of necessary books did not accompany us. Later on, however, if it should please you, we will compile many recipes for each individual problem. It is appropriate for many recipes to be selected for inclusion, since indeed some of them are more suitable for some people, and all of them are not suitable for all people, on account, obviously, of the difference among bodies.

TEXT 25. CATO, *ON AGRICULTURE* SELECTION (156–157)

On Agriculture was written by the Roman statesman and soldier Marcius Porcius **Cato** *(234–149 BCE), often referred to as Cato the Elder. In this work Cato shares his experience and expertise as an owner of a successful estate with other wealthy men who own farms or wish to acquire them. The text offers wide-ranging advice for nearly anything that the master of an estate might want to know, including advice about medical practices the master might perform himself on family members and slaves. In the selection below, Cato praises the medicinal properties of cabbage. Chapter 156 is certainly Cato's own work, but chapter 157 may have been written by someone else and subsequently added to manuscripts of Cato's* On Agriculture.

SOURCE: Translated by Andrew Dalby based on the Latin text from R. Goujard, *Caton, De l'agriculture* (Paris: Les Belles Lettres, 1975). First published in *Cato: On Farming (De agricultura)* (London: Prospect Books, 1998). Reprinted with permission of Prospect Books.

Chapter 156. On Cabbage as an Aid to Digestion
Cabbage surpasses all vegetables. Eat it either cooked or raw: if you eat it raw, dress it with vinegar. It aids digestion remarkably and does the bowels good, and the urine will be beneficial for all purposes.

If you want to drink a lot and eat copiously at a party, eat as much cabbage as you want, raw, dressed with vinegar, before dining. Then, when about to dine, eat about 5 leaves. You will feel as if you had eaten nothing, and you can drink as much as you want.

If you want to purge by vomiting, take 4 *lb.* of the tenderest cabbage, divide into three equal bunches and tie. Then put a pot of water on the fire, and when it begins to boil plunge one bunch into it briefly. It will stop boiling. Then, as it boils, plunge the bunch again while you count five, and take it out. Do the same with the second bunch, and then the third. Then put all together and pound. Remove into a linen bag, and express about 1 pint of juice into an earthenware mug. Add a salt crystal about the size of a bitter vetch seed, and roasted cumin seed enough to give a flavor. Then put the mug outdoors, in good weather, overnight.

The person who is to take the medicine should have a hot bath, drink honey water, and go to bed without dinner, then in the morning drink the juice and walk for four hours, and do any business required. When the urge comes and nausea is felt, recline and vomit. So much bile and phlegm will be thrown up that the patient will wonder where it all came from. Later, after moving the bowels, drink half a pint or a little more. If the motions are too frequent, take two spoonfuls of fine flour, crumble into water and drink a little, and they will stop.

For those who are troubled by colic, cabbage should be steeped in water. When steeped, put it into hot water. Boil until thoroughly soft. Pour off the water. Then add salt and a little cumin; also add fine barley meal and olive oil. The boil,[21] pour into a dish and allow to cool. This is to be included in the patient's next meal, or, preferably, to be eaten on its own. Unless there is fever, give also harsh red wine mixed with as little water as possible; if there is fever, give water. Do this daily, early in the morning. Do not give too much, or the patient will become sick of it instead of continuing to take it freely. Treat a man, a woman or a child in the same way.

Now as to patients for whom urination is painful or dribbling. Take cabbage, put in boiling water, boil briefly till half cooked. Then pour out some of the water, add plenty of oil and salt and a little cumin. Bring to the boil briefly. Then take the juice, cold, and eat the cabbage itself, digesting it as quickly as possible. Do this each day.

Chapter 157. On the Pythagorean Cabbage and Its Good and Health-Giving Properties
First you must know the different kinds of cabbage and their nature.

It blends all healthy influences and ever adapts itself with the application of heat, being at once dry and wet, at once sweet and sour and bitter. Cabbage, in its mixed nature, has all of the so-called Seven Good Things.

Garden Cabbage and its Uses
First, then, to explain this nature. The first kind is called *levis*, delicate. It is large, broad-leaved, long-stemmed, and has a powerful nature and great force. The second is crinkled, called *apiaca*: good in nature and appearance, it is more powerful in medicine than the first. So is the third, called mild: thin-stemmed, it is tender and the bitterest of all, with a very active thin juice, and you must know first of all that of all the kinds of cabbage none is as effective a medicine as this.

Put it, ground fine, to all wounds and swellings. It will clean up and heal all sores painlessly. It brings boils to a head and makes them burst.

It will clean up and heal septic wounds and cancers, as medicines cannot. Before you apply it, wash with plenty of hot water, then apply ground cabbage twice a day. It will remove all decay. Black cancer gives off a smell and a foul slime; the white is purulent but fistulous and suppurates under the **flesh.** Grind cabbage for illnesses of this kind. It will cure them, and is the best thing for illnesses of this kind.

21. "The boil" refers to the mixture of things that have been boiled together.

In case of dislocation, foment with hot water twice a day and apply ground cabbage: it will soon cure it. Apply twice a day: it will remove the pain. If there is any bruising, it will break it up; apply ground cabbage: it will cure it.

If any sore or cancer develops in the breasts, apply ground cabbage: it will cure it. If the sore cannot bear the bitterness of the cabbage, mix with barley flour and apply the mixture: it will cure all sores of this kind, while other medicines cannot cure them or clean them up. If a boy or girl has a sore of this kind, again, add barley flour.

If you want your cabbage chopped, washed, dried, sprinkled with salt or vinegar, there is nothing healthier. To enjoy it more, sprinkle with honey vinegar. Washed and dried, with chopped rue and coriander and sprinkled with salt you will enjoy it a little better. It does you good, permits no disease to remain in the body, and does the bowels good. If there was any disease present internally, cabbage will cure all, remove all sicknesses from the head and the eyes and cure them. Take it in the morning before eating.

If there is black bile, if the spleen swells, if the heart or liver or lungs or diaphragm are painful, in a word, it will cure whatever organ is painful.

Grate *silpium* over it: that is good.

When all the veins are blown up with food they cannot breathe through the body, and that gives rise to illness. When from overeating the bowels will not move, if you take (as I advise) an appropriate amount of cabbage, you will develop no illness from overeating.

Now nothing clears illness of the joints as well as raw cabbage, whether you eat it chopped, with rue and coriander chopped in, dry, with grated *sirpicium*, or as cabbage in honey vinegar sprinkled with salt. If you take this, you will have the use of all your joints. It costs nothing, and even if it did you should try it for the sake of health. Take it in the morning before eating.

One who suffers from insomnia or senility will find the same cure effective. Give this patient, before eating, cabbage fried in fat, hot, and a little salt. The more that is eaten, the quicker will be the recovery from this illness.

Those who are troubled by colic are to be treated as follows. Soak cabbage thoroughly, then place in a cooking pot and boil thoroughly. When well cooked, pour off the water and add plenty of oil and a little salt, cumin and fine barley meal. Then boil thoroughly. When it has boiled put in a dish. Give this to the patient to eat, without bread if possible; if not, allow bread, with this dish as relish, but nothing else. If there is no fever, give red wine to drink. The cure will be rapid.

Whenever necessary this will cure anyone who is weak: take cabbage as just described.

Cabbage Eaters' Urine

In addition, store the urine of anyone who habitually eats cabbage; warm it, bathe the patient in it. With this treatment you will soon restore health; it has been tested. If you wash feeble children in this urine they will be weak no longer. Those who cannot see clearly should bathe their eyes in this urine and they will see more. If the head or neck is painful, wash in this urine, heated: they will cease to be painful.

Also, if a woman foments her parts with this urine, they will never irritate. Foment as follows: boil in a basin and place under a commode; the woman is then to sit on the commode, covering the basin with her clothing.

Wild Cabbage and its Uses

Wild cabbage has the greatest strength. It should be heated and ground thoroughly fine.

If you intend to purge someone, the patient should not take dinner on the preceding day. In the morning, before eating, give ground cabbage and 4 **cyathi** of water. Nothing will purge so well, not even hellebore or scammony, and safely too: you must know that it is healthy for the body. Use it on those you despair of curing. When giving this purge, administer as follows: give this for seven days as a liquid food. When there is appetite, give donkey meat. If the patient will not eat that, give boiled cabbage and bread, and a mild wine mixed with water to drink. The patient should wash only occasionally, using oil instead. One thus treated will long remain healthy and suffer no sickness unless self-induced.

If there is a suppurating or fresh sore, sprinkle this ground wild cabbage with water and apply: you will cure it.

In the case of a fistula, insert it as a pack. If the pack will not stay in, dilute the ground cabbage, put in a bladder, attach a reed, squeeze into the fistula. This will soon effect a cure.

Also apply, ground, with honey, to any wounds old or recent. This will cure them.

If there is a nasal polyp, put dried ground wild cabbage in a tuft of wool; put to the patient's nose to aspire as much as possible. Within three days the polyp will fall out. When it has done so continue the treatment for an equal number of days to heal up the roots of the polyp completely.

If you are hard of hearing grind cabbage with wine, press out the juice, drop into the ear warm. You will soon be aware of hearing more.

Apply cabbage to a suppurating scab. It will cure it without causing a sore.

TEXT 26. DIOSCORIDES, *MEDICAL MATERIAL* SELECTION (4.64)

Medical Material, *written by* **Dioscorides** *(second half of first century CE), is the most influential text of pharmacology from Greco-Roman antiquity. In five books, this text discussed the pharmacological properties of roughly 700 herbs, plants, fruits and vegetables, animal products, and minerals. This collection of information was based on Dioscorides's travels throughout the Eastern provinces of the Roman Empire: Egypt, Syria, Palestine, Asia Minor (modern-day Türkiye), and Greece, among other regions. The selection below discusses the properties of the opium poppy, and provides instructions on how to process the plant for medicinal treatments (see fig. 45).*

SOURCE: Translated by Lily Y. Beck based on the Greek text from Max Wellmann, *Pedanii Dioscuridis Anazarbei De materia medica libri quinque*, vol. 2 (Berlin: Weidmann, 1906). First published in *Pedanius Dioscorides of Anazarbus: De materia medica*, third, revised edition, Altertumswissenschaftliche Texte und Studien Band 38 (Hildesheim: Olms, 2017). Reprinted with permission of Georg Olms Verlag AG.

Book 4, Chapter 64. Opium poppy

1. The opium poppy: there is one kind that is cultivated and that is grown in gardens; its seed is used roasted for a health-promoting diet; they also use it with honey instead of sesame; it is called *thylacitis*, having an oblong little head and its seed is white. And there is another kind that is wild, having a capsule that hangs down, and black seed; this one is also called *pithitis*, but some call even this one *rhoias*, because of the juice that flows from it. A third kind is wilder, smaller, and more medicinal than these, having the capsule oblong.

2. Their common property is cooling; it is for this reason that the leaves and capsules, boiled in water and fomented, are soporific; the decoction is also drunk for insomnia and the capsules, ground up and mixed with barley groats, are suitable for inflammations and erysipelas. Brayed when green, they must be molded into little troches, and after they have dried, they must be stored and so used. The capsules, boiled in water until they are half-cooked, then boiled again with honey until the liquid condenses, make anodyne lozenges for coughs, rheums of the trachea, and for conditions relating to the abdomen.

3. And it does become more effective if one mixed with it juice of hypocist and of shittah tree. The seed of the black poppy, ground up, is given to drink with wine for diarrhea and leucorrhea, and it is plastered on with water on the forehead and temples of insomniacs. And the juice, since it, too, cools a great deal, befuddles, and dries, taken in an amount as small as a bitter vetch is analgesic, soporific, helpful for digestion, and comes to the aid of coughs and abdominal conditions; but when too much of it is drunk, it plunges into a coma and it is deadly.

4. Soaked with unguent of roses, it is good also for headaches, but for earaches it is good when instilled with unguent of almonds, saffron, and myrrh; it is good for eye inflammations with a boiled egg yolk and saffron; for erysipelas and wounds with vinegar, and for gout with a woman's milk and saffron. Inserted into the anus as a suppository, it is soporific.

5. The best juice is thick and heavy, it induces sleep when smelled, it is bitter in taste, it easily dissolves in water, it is smooth, white, not rough nor lumpy, nor hardens when soaked as does wax. Additionally, it flows easily when exposed to the sun, when dripped on a lamp the flame is not dark-colored, and it preserves the intensity of its scent after it has been quenched. Some, however, adulterate it by mixing it with juice of horned poppy or with gum or with juice of wild lettuce. But the juice that is mixed with juice of horned poppy is yellow, the one made with juice of wild lettuce is faint in scent and rather rough, and the one with gum is weak and translucent.

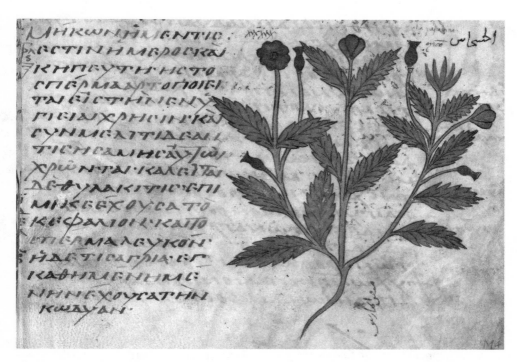

FIGURE 45 Ninth-century CE manuscript entry on the opium poppy in Dioscorides's *Medical Material*. In addition to providing information about the opium poppy's healing properties, how to prepare it, what ailments it is useful for, and how to harvest the plant's juices, the manuscript also includes an illustration of the plant so that it would be easily identifiable for those wishing to harvest it. Gallica Dioscorides, BnF Gr. 2179, folio 91r. Permission: Bibliothèque Nationale de France.

6. Some reach such madness as to mix even suet with it. It is roasted for eye medication in a new clay vessel until it becomes soft and appears to be of a more orange-tawny color. You should know, however, that **Diagoras** says that **Erasistratus** rejects its use for earaches and ophthalmia because it weakens the sight and it is soporific. **Andreas** says that if it were not adulterated, those anointed with it would be blinded, and **Mnesidamos** that the only suitable use of it is for sleep through smell, otherwise it is harmful; these assertions are decidedly false, being refuted by experience, because the efficacy of a **drug** is confirmed by its performance.

7. Nor is it inappropriate to describe also how they collect the juice: and so, some people after braying the capsules together with the leaves squeeze them through a press and after pounding them in a mortar, shape them into troches. Such a product is called *meconion;* it is less efficacious than the juice. In extracting the juice after the dew dried off, it is necessary to scratch all around the capsule with a knife in a way as not to pierce through its inner part and to make superficially straight cuts at the side of the capsule, then wipe up the tear that flows with the finger into a spoon and repeat the process shortly thereafter, for a tear is

found formed, and it is found also on the following day. This, too, must be pounded in a mortar, shaped, and stored. But, as the cuts are made, one must stand back so that the juice does not come in contact with the clothing.

TEXT 27. ORIBASIUS, *MEDICAL COMPILATIONS* SELECTION (1.20)

Medical Compilations is a large medical encyclopedia compiled by physician and author **Oribasius** *(c. 325–400 CE). This text collected, edited, and organized extracts from earlier medical writers, including the many texts written by* **Galen.** *The selection below, taken from one of the books devoted to the properties of different types of food, extols the medicinal virtues of chickpeas.*

SOURCE: Translated by Mark Grant based on the Greek text from J. Raeder, *Oribasii Collectionum Medicorum Reliquiae,* vol. 1, Corpus Medicorum Graecorum 6.1, 1 (Leipzig: Teubner, 1928). First published in *Dieting for an Emperor,* Studies in Ancient Medicine, vol. 15 (Leiden: Brill, 1997). Reprinted with permission of Brill.

Book 1, Chapter 20. 1. Chickpeas are no less flatulent than broad beans and they are no less nourishing than the same, but they arouse the urge for sexual intercourse and at the same time are productive of sperm. 2. There is also a purgative power in them to a greater degree than that in broad beans, so that some varieties of chickpeas even clearly break up the stones condensed in the kidneys; these are black and small and are called "rams"; it is better to drink their juice alone after boiling them in water. 3. Green chickpeas happen to be extremely excrementitious like all green pulse, just as chickpeas that are toasted lose their flatulent quality, but become harder to digest and more **astringent** and give less nourishment to the body.

TEXT 28. PLINY, *NATURAL HISTORY* SELECTIONS (27.14–20, 28.35–38)

The Natural History, *written by* **Pliny the Elder** *(c. 23 or 24–79 CE), is an encyclopedic text that covers a range of topics, including geography, botany, agriculture, horticulture, zoology, mineralogy, and medicine. The* Natural History *records information Pliny drew from reading widely, and from observations picked up during his administrative work and travels throughout the Roman Empire. In the selections below, Pliny discusses the medicinal properties of aloe and saliva.*

SOURCE: Translated by Molly Jones-Lewis based on the Latin text from Alfred Ernout, *Pline l'Ancien, Histoire naturelle, Livre XXVII* (Paris: Les Belles Lettres, 1959), and *Livre XXVIII* (Paris: Les Belles Lettres, 1962).

Book 27. 14. Aloe has a certain resemblance to squill, but it is larger and has more succulent leaves, with streaks running lengthwise. Its stalk is tender, reddening at the center, not unlike an asphodel stalk; its single root is embedded like a stake in the earth. The plant itself has a strong odor and is bitter to the taste. The most popular variety is imported from India, but it also grows in Asia.[22] However, the Asian variety is only used for wounds, applying fresh-cut leaves—they do an amazing job of closing them—or sap. For this reason, they grow the plant in conical pots, just as they grow house-leeks.

15. Some people also incise the stalk before it goes to seed in order to extract the sap, and some people also incise the leaves. Sap can also be found on its own sticking to the plant in a droplet; for this reason, some people advise paving the area where it has been planted so the droplet is not soaked up. There were some who reported that there is a mineral source of this sap in Judaea beyond Jerusalem, but no variety is of poorer quality, nor is any darker or moister.

16. And so it will follow that the best kind is fatty and clear, ruddy in color, crumbly and compact like liver, and easily liquified. Dark and hard aloe should be rejected, as should sandy aloe, and aloe that has been adulterated with gum and acacia resin, which can be recognized by taste. Its nature promotes condensation, thickening, and gentle warming. Its uses are many, but the primary one is to loosen the bowel since it is almost the only drug that is effective as a laxative while also strengthening the stomach, and without disturbing it with any harmful property.

17. A **drachma** of it is drunk, but for looseness of the stomach, a spoonful mixed in 2 drinking cups of lukewarm or cold water is taken two or three times over the course of a day, as the situation demands. However, for a proper purge, a dose of 3 drachmas is usual; the drink is more effective if taken with food. When mixed into sour wine and massaged into the head against the direction of growth, it slows hair loss. Aloe relieves headache when applied on the temples and forehead with vinegar and rose-oil, or a more dilute mixture of it may be poured on them.

18. It is agreed that aloe heals all problems of the eyes, especially itching and scabbing of the eyelids, and that it is also good applied with honey—especially Pontic[23] honey—as a salve for bruises and purple skin lesions. It treats the tonsils, gums, and all sores in the mouth. A drachma's weight drunk in water treats **expectorations** of blood, if these are moderate, and if not, drunk in vinegar. It also stops the flow of blood from wounds or any other cause, either by itself or in vinegar.

19. Additionally, it is also extremely useful for encouraging scar tissue to form in wounds. It is also sprinkled over male genitals that have been badly ulcerated, and it is applied to bulging growths and fissures of the anus, sometimes in wine, sometimes in raisin wine, sometimes by itself, dried, depending on whether soothing or shrinking action is needed for the treatment. Also, it gently stops bleeding from bulging hemorrhoids.

20. It is administered for dysentery and, if food is not being digested properly, it is drunk a little after dinner. For jaundice, three **obols** in water are drunk. For purging the internal

---

22. "Asia" refers to Asia Minor, which is roughly equivalent to modern-day Türkiye (see fig. 17).
23. "Pontic" refers to the ancient area of Pontus, located in modern-day north-central Türkiye, south of the Black Sea.

organs, pills made with a honey reduction or terebinth resin are swallowed. It softens nail cuticles. For **drugs** of the eyes, it is washed in order to rinse out any sandiness, or it is heated in an earthenware vessel and stirred frequently with a feather so that it can be evenly toasted. . . .

Book 28. 35. I have, however, explained that a fasting person's saliva is really one of the best ways to protect against snakes,[24] but lived experience also endorses other effective uses for it. We spit at epileptic illnesses, that is, we throw back contagion. In a similar way we also ward off magic spells and the bad luck of meeting someone who limps on their right leg.

36. We also ask the gods' pardon for wanting some particularly ambitious outcome by spitting into our lap. And by the same logic it is now customary to spit three times as an advance announcement when using any medicine and in this way help the treatment along, and to mark erupting boils three times with the saliva of a fasting person. I am saying something astonishing, but it is easy to test. If someone regrets a blow inflicted either from a distance or in hand-to-hand combat and immediately spits into the center of the hand that struck the blow, the resentment felt by the victim will be minimized immediately. This point is proved often when a beast of burden's strength has faded, and after this kind of remedy the animal's stride is fixed immediately.

37. Some people, however, add weight to the blow before they strike by spitting into their hand in a similar fashion. Therefore we should also believe that ringworm and inflammatory skin conditions can be prevented with regular application of a fasting person's saliva. Likewise, crusty eyes are treated with a daily morning application of saliva, and growths with the root called apple of the earth kneaded with saliva. Pains of the neck are treated by applying a fasting person's saliva with the right hand to the right knee, and to the left knee with the left hand. If some bug has flown into the ear and someone spits on it, the bug flies out.

38. Among the charms that avert evil, there is also the practice of spitting on urine when it is excreted, and similarly spitting into the right shoe before putting it on, and also whenever someone crosses the place in which one has encountered some danger. **Marcion of Smyrna**, who wrote about the properties of simple ingredients, tells us that sea-centipedes are ruptured when spat upon, and that the same is true of toads and other frogs as well. **Ofillius** tells us that the same is true of snakes, if someone spits into their open mouths, and **Salpe** writes that whenever a body part is numb, the numbness can be relieved if someone spits into the lap or if the upper eyelid is touched with saliva.

SURGERY

The Greek and Latin terms for "surgery" (Greek *kheirourgia* and Latin *chirurgia*) translate literally as "work done with the hands." In antiquity, this category included many treatments that involved cutting or opening the body, such as the excision of gangrenous tissue from

24. Pliny, *Natural History* 7.13–15.

wounds and eye surgeries. But the category of surgery in antiquity also included noninvasive manipulations of the body using one's hands. For example, the reduction or immobilization of a broken bone (discussed in the section on wounds and fractures in chapter 9) would have been considered a form of orthopedic surgery. That said, the majority of surgical procedures in antiquity were conducted to treat a traumatic injury of one sort or another, such as a battlefield wound or an occupational injury.

From our earliest medical sources, it is clear that surgery was controversial for a number of reasons. First, there was no way to fully anesthetize patients, and ancient analgesics (mainly narcotics such as opium, henbane, and mandrake) were not likely to have been completely effective in eliminating the pain involved in many procedures. In many of our descriptions of surgery, we hear of a team of people—physicians' assistants, as well as family and friends—tasked with restraining patients who were writhing in pain as the surgeon attempted to complete the procedure as quickly as possible. Second, many surgical treatments were vulnerable to rot and putrefaction. Although ancient physicians and surgeons used substances such as copper and frankincense (which we now know have antimicrobial properties), ancient surgical patients were at grave risk of life-threatening septicemia. Third, practitioners with varying levels of skill performed surgeries. On the one hand, some were highly trained specialists with a good deal of experience studying and practicing surgical techniques (see Text 34, **Galen**, *On Anatomical Procedures*). But some practiced the risky specialty of surgery—with its low rates of success and high rates of patient death—because they were struggling to find clients. As a result of this variation, surgery as a medical practice was often regarded with suspicion and fear.

The controversial nature of surgery provides context for part of the Hippocratic *Oath*, which vows, "I shall not cut, not even those who suffer from stones, but shall yield to the men who practice this trade" (Text 40). Scholars have long debated how to interpret this part of the oath. The oath's specific mention of a stone—likely meaning a kidney or bladder stone—refers specifically to the physician's choice either to remove stones surgically (through a procedure called "lithotomy") or to wait to let the stone pass naturally (an excruciatingly painful experience); the author of the oath prefers the latter option. But scholars wonder if this vow was meant more generally as a pledge not to undertake surgical treatments of any kind, instead leaving them to specialists, or if the vow was merely a pledge not to perform elective surgeries. Scholars also wonder if the author of the oath was trying to distinguish professional physicians who exhibited caution about undertaking unnecessary and dangerous procedures from other kinds of healers who were less scrupulous and rushed into surgery.

Our knowledge of ancient surgery is relatively detailed. We know that many surgical advances occurred in Alexandria, Egypt, under the Ptolemaic rulers, and these advances were, in part, a result of the burgeoning of anatomical and physiological research involving human dissection (see chapter 2). A similar emphasis on anatomy persisted centuries later in the Roman Empire. For example, in Galen's *On Anatomical Procedures*, he discussed the need for physicians to learn anatomy through careful practice of dissection in order to be

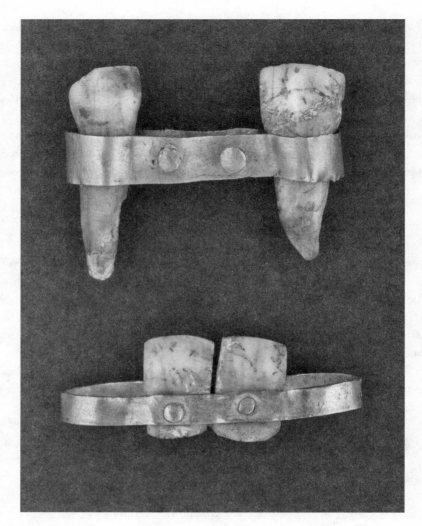

FIGURE 46 Circa seventh-century BCE Etruscan dental prostheses with human teeth mounted onto a gold band. These prostheses (for the upper and lower jaw) would have been anchored into the mouth in the place of missing teeth. Roman medical writers like Celsus also recommended gold wire to bind teeth that had been damaged or loosened by a blow or accident to adjacent teeth. Gold was the preferred material for dental appliances because it was the most malleable metal, able to be hammered and rolled into thin wires. National Museums Liverpool, World Museum (inv. nos. M10334 and M10335).

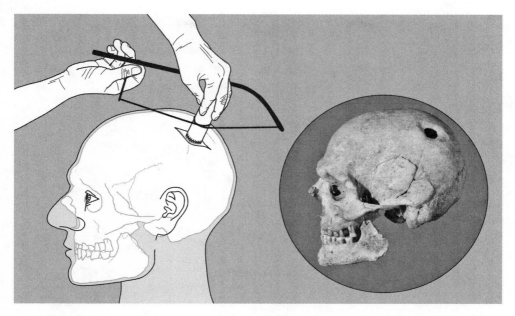

FIGURE 47 Illustrator's rendering of trepanation procedure; second-century CE trepanned skull of Chios, Greece. Trepanation was the surgical process of drilling a hole, often down to bone, using an instrument called a trephine. The illustration on the left shows how the procedure worked: a saw-toothed drill was placed on the body part to be bored into. Then the string of a bow was wrapped around the drill and, with one hand, sawed back and forth to rotate the serrated edge of the drill into the skin/bone. With the other hand, downward pressure was applied onto a metal cap placed on the top of the drill. The ancient Greek skull on the right bears a hole that was created by trepanation. Because of the healed linear fracture below the bore hole, we know that the patient survived the procedure. Illustration by Gina Tibbott. Photo credit: Copyright Hellenic Ministry of Education and Religious Affairs, Cultural Sector. Photographic archive of the Ephorate of Antiquities of Chios.

able to perform surgical operations with skill and to avoid inflicting further damage on patients (Text 34).

We have a variety of texts from the Roman Empire that discuss in detail a range of particular surgeries. These sources give us a sense of the ailments that so troubled ancient people they were willing to undergo surgery. For example, in his text *On Medicine*, **Celsus** describes procedures for treating cataracts and severe wounds, including those involving prolapsed intestines (Text 29, 7.7 and 7.16). Another intervention regularly described in our sources was anal surgeries, particularly those relating to hemorrhoids and fistulas (abnormal channels that branched off from the anal canal, and that often became infected because of fecal matter that accumulated there). These occurred frequently because of the unsanitary conditions of toilets (see chapter 3) and regular travel on horses, donkeys, or camels. They would have been quite painful, especially during defecation, given their proximity to the rectum. The Hippocratic text devoted wholly to the subject of anal fistulas recommends several

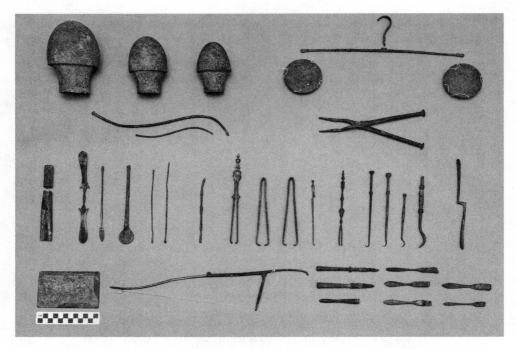

FIGURE 48 Circa first- to second-century CE surgical kit from Colophon (modern-day Türkiye). The collection includes cupping vessels of various sizes, a slab (likely for mixing compound drugs), a pair of scales (to weigh drugs or their ingredients), catheters, forceps, knives, spoons, scalpels, probes, cauteries, tweezers, hooks, and a bow and drills for trepanning. The Johns Hopkins Archaeological Museum (Buckler Collection #1–35). Image by James T. VanRensselaer.

procedures for dealing with them. The goal was to cut open the **flesh** between the anal canal and the abnormal channel in order to allow it to heal together as continuous tissue.

Dental surgery was also sometimes performed by specialized dental practitioners. For example, Celsus described tooth extraction, a procedure that involved scraping around the gum, attempting to loosen the tooth prior to pulling it using either one's fingers or forceps. Celsus cautioned against attempting to pull a tooth without loosening it first, as one could dislocate the patient's jaw, or cause damage to his or her eyes and temples. Archaeologists have uncovered dental forceps that were used to extract teeth, and also recovered human remains that show evidence of dental bridges, caps, wiring loose teeth to solid ones, and dentures (see fig. 46).

One of the most fascinating surgical procedures was cranial **trepanation**, which involved boring, drilling, sawing, or scraping the skull in order to gain access to the brain cavity or to relieve pressure on the brain (see Text 8, *On Epidemics* 5.16). This procedure was used to treat severe headaches, to remove projectiles or weapons lodged in the head, or to remove fractured cranial bone resulting from violent blows to the head. Remarkably, archaeologists have unearthed human remains with trepanned skulls that have fully healed (see fig. 47).

However, because the operations posed significant risk of brain damage or death, it is also not surprising that evidence of unhealed trepanation has been found, indicating that the individual likely died as a result of the procedure.

We are also fortunate to have many surgical instruments from the period that, when paired with descriptions of treatments in the literary sources, give us an even clearer sense of surgical procedures. Our largest collections of surgical instruments come from a house in northern Italy that was destroyed by fire and then built over, and from the towns around Mt. Vesuvius that were encased by the falling ash; both disasters preserved the surgical instruments in situ (see fig. 70). Surgical instruments have also been found buried in the graves of physicians. From such sites, scholars have cataloged about 500 kinds of instruments from antiquity: scalpels, probes, forceps, **cauteries**, **cupping** vessels, catheters, drains, specula (vaginal and rectal), hooks, suturing needles, **fibulae**, syringes, **clysters**, plungers, spoons, scissors and shears, and tools for bone and dental surgery such as chisels, saws, rasps, and files, and **trephines** (see fig. 48). Given this wide range of instruments (many of which came in different sizes and designs), and given that many of these tools are still in use today in relatively unchanged form, we should be deeply impressed by the complexity and comprehensiveness of ancient surgical instrumentation.

And although any surgery in antiquity posed significant danger to patients, we should be impressed by the wide range of procedures performed in antiquity: from the basic surgical procedures depicted in the Hippocratic corpus to the more complicated procedures that developed in later periods. The fact that surgeries as complex as strumectomy, herniotomy, arteriotomy, aneurysmectomy, rhinoplasty, transvaginal hysterectomy, mastectomy, and tracheotomy were performed should dissuade anyone from underestimating ancient surgeons' knowledge and skills.

TEXT 29. CELSUS, *ON MEDICINE* SELECTIONS (7.PROEM, 7.5, 7.7, AND 7.16)

On Medicine, written by Aulus Cornelius **Celsus** *(first centuries BCE and CE), was originally part of an encyclopedia that covered a range of topics, including agriculture, medicine, rhetoric, philosophy, and military science. The section on medicine, the only one to survive, is organized around the three major divisions of ancient medicine: regimen, pharmacology, and surgery. Scholars debate whether Celsus was himself a practicing physician, but his text offers hints of real experience. In the section on surgery, Celsus sketches a history of the field of surgery and describes the traits of an ideal surgeon. Then Celsus provides detailed instructions for a range of different types of procedures. The selections below focus on surgeries to extract weapons of war (such as arrows or lead pellets), a surgery to remove cataracts from the eye, and surgeries on intestines that have spilled out of the body.*

SOURCE: Translated by Jared Secord based on the Latin text from Innocenzo Mazzini, *A. Cornelio Celso, La chirurgia, Libri VII e VIII del De medicina* (Pisa: Istituti editoriali e poligrafici internazionali, 1999).

Book 7, proem. 1. The third part of medicine is that which treats by the hand, as is generally known and has been said by me.[25] It does not disregard **drugs** and the regulation of diet, but it does most things by hand, and its effects among all the parts of medicine are most obvious. Because fortune accomplishes much in illnesses, and the same things are sometimes beneficial and sometimes empty, it can be questioned whether favorable health results from the help of medicine, the body, or fortune. 2. Moreover, in instances when we depend especially on drugs, although progress is more obvious, it is nevertheless often clear that health is sought in vain through drugs and is restored without them. This can be understood from the eyes, which sometimes after being harassed for a long time by physicians, get better without them. But in this part of medicine which treats by the hand,[26] it is apparent that all progress derives mostly from this surgery, even if it is helped somewhat by other factors. This part of medicine, though it is extremely ancient, was developed more by **Hippocrates,** that parent of all medicine, than by earlier physicians. 3. Later, separated from the other parts of medicine, it began to have its own teachers. In Egypt it grew especially with **Philoxenus** as founder, who dealt with this part of medicine most thoroughly in many written volumes. **Gorgias,** too, and **Sostratus** and **Hero** and the two **Apolloniuses** and **Ammonius,** all of them Alexandrians, and many other famous men each made additional discoveries. And in Rome, too, distinguished teachers, especially in recent times Tryphon the father and **Euelpistus** and, as can be understood from his writings, **Meges,** the most erudite of these, have added certain changes for the better and improved the discipline.

4. A surgeon ought to be young, or at least closer to youth, with a strong and stable hand that never trembles, ready no less with the left hand than the right, with the pupil of the eyes sharp and clear. A surgeon ought to have an undaunted spirit, so merciful that he wants to heal the sick person he has admitted into care, but not disturbed by the sick person's cry of pain in such a way to hurry more than the situation demands, or to cut less than necessary, but in the same way to do everything as if he is not affected by the other person's cries.

. . .

Book 7, Chapter 5. 1A. Weapons, too, which have been stuck in the body and are fixed within it, are often removed with considerable trouble. There are certain difficulties associated with different types of weapons, and other difficulties from the places in which they have penetrated. Every weapon, however, is extracted either from the part where it entered, or from the part in which it pointed. In the first case, the weapon has made for itself a passage by which it may return. In the second, the scalpel provides a passage, for the **flesh** is incised against its point. But if the weapon has not penetrated deeply, and is in the top layer of flesh, or if it at least has not crossed the large blood vessels and areas containing tendons, there is nothing better to do than to pull it out by the way it came. 1B. If, however, the distance through which the weapon must be turned back is greater than it has pierced, and it has already crossed the blood

25. See Text 4, Celsus, *On Medicine,* Preface 9.
26. The "hand" refers to surgery, one of the three divisions of ancient medicine, along with regimen and pharmacology.

vessels and areas containing tendons, it is more appropriate to open up the path that remains, and to extract it, for the weapon is more easily reached and pulled out more safely. In a larger limb, if the weapon has crossed the middle with its point, a wound that has gone all the way through heals more easily because it can be treated with a drug on both sides. 1C. But if the weapon is to be drawn back, the gash must be enlarged with a scalpel, so that the weapon may follow more easily, and so that there may be less inflammation. Inflammation increases if the body is torn by the weapon itself while it comes out. Likewise if the wound is opened from the other side, it should be wider than would be filled by the weapon as it comes out. The greatest care, however, must be taken in both cases that there be no incision of a tendon, a larger vein, or artery. When any of these situations is detected, the weapon must be removed by a blunt hook, and drawn away from the scalpel. When the incision is large enough, the weapon must be removed, in the same manner and with the same care so that, while the extraction is taking place, there is no injury to any one of the parts that I said should be protected.

2A. These are general rules. There are some particular rules for different types of weapons, which I will now disclose. Nothing penetrates into the body as easily as an arrow, and it also sinks in very deeply. This happens both because it is propelled with great force and because it tapers to a point. Thus it is more often removed from the other side from where it entered, and especially because it is generally encircled with barbs that wound more if the arrow is withdrawn backwards than forwards. 2B. But when a passage has been opened, the flesh should be spread out with an iron tool shaped like a Greek letter.[27] Then, when the arrow is in view, if the shaft is attached to the point, it must be pushed forward until it can be grasped and removed from the other side. If the shaft has already come off and only the arrowhead is inside, the point should be grasped with the fingers or with forceps and extracted in this way. 2C. When it is preferable for it to be pulled out from the side where it entered, the method of removal is no different. For, once the wound has been enlarged, either the shaft, if it is attached, must be pulled out, or, if it is not attached, the arrowhead itself. But if the barbs appear to be short and thin, they should be broken up on the spot with forceps, and the weapon drawn out free from them. If the barbs are larger and thicker, they should be covered up with broken reed-pens of a writer, and thus pulled out so that they do not cause harm. This is what to look out for in the case of arrows.

3A. If the weapon that has penetrated is wide, it is inappropriate for it to be drawn out from the other side, so that we do not add another large wound to an existing large wound. Therefore a wide weapon must be pulled out with a particular type of iron tool that the Greeks call the "Dioclean scoop"[28] because **Diocles** was its inventor, whom I already placed among the greatest of the ancient physicians.[29] It is a sheet of iron or bronze that has two

27. Which Greek letter Celsus intended to mention has been lost in the manuscript tradition. The likeliest possibility seems to be a capital letter upsilon (Y). This would make the instrument look something like a bivalve speculum (see fig. 22).

28. Among the ancient medical instruments that are still extant, we have not identified for certain any Dioclean scoops.

29. On Diocles, see Text 4, Celsus, *On Medicine,* Preface 8.

hooks curved downwards on one end. 3B. On the other end, it is folded over on its sides, and its end is lightly inclined to that side, where it is bent, and is also perforated in that spot. This instrument is inserted at an angle next to the weapon. Then, when it has come to the top of the point, it is turned a little, so that it catches the weapon with its perforation. When the point of the weapon is in the hole, immediately fingers placed under the hooks on either side extract the tool and the missile at the same time.

4A. There is a third type of weapon, which sometimes has to be pulled out: a lead ball, stone, or something similar, which has broken through the skin and has sunk inside without breaking. In all these instances the wound must be opened wider, and what is inside must be extracted with forceps through the path by which it entered. Some difficulty, however, is added with every injury if the weapon has become stuck in a bone or sunk in the joint between two bones. 4B. In a bone, the weapon must be moved around until the point is loosened from the part it has dug into, and then the weapon must be extracted either by hand or forceps (this is also the method for teeth to be extracted), and hardly ever does the weapon not come out. But if it stays behind, it can be shaken out by the blow of an iron tool. When it is not pulled out, the last step is to bore a hole with a **trephine** and from that hole to cut away the bone against the weapon in the shape of the letter delta[30] so that the lines dividing the letter point at the weapon. After this is done, the weapon will inevitably loosen, and be removed easily. 4C. If the weapon has forced its way into the joint between two bones, the two limbs around the wound must be bound with bandages or straps and by means of these they are pulled apart so that they stretch out the tendons. When these are stretched, the space between the bones is wider, so that the weapon may be recovered without difficulty. Care must be taken, just as I have stated in other places, so that no tendon, vein, or artery is injured by the weapon while it is being extracted, with the same method stated above.[31] 5A. But if the wounded person is struck by a weapon that has been poisoned, after all the same things are done, with more speed if possible, add to this the treatment employed for someone who has drunk poison or who has been bitten by a snake. Once the weapon is extracted, the practice of medicine for the wound itself is no different from what it would be if nothing had lodged in the wounded body. On this topic enough has been said in another place.[32]

. . .

Book 7, Chapter 7. 13A. I have already mentioned cataracts elsewhere because when a new cataract occurs, it is often also broken up by drugs.[33] But when one is more chronic, it requires treatment by hand, a surgery that can be considered one of the most delicate. Before I speak

---

30. The Greek capital letter delta: Δ. Based on Celsus's description, the pointed top of the letter would be pointing at the weapon.

31. See 7.5.1C above.

32. See Text 12, Celsus, *On Medicine* 5.26.21.

33. Celsus, *On Medicine* 6.6.35. Celsus is explaining here that he has discussed cataracts that have been acquired recently elsewhere in the text (the section on drugs); his discussion of cataracts that a patient has had for a long time is included in this section on surgery because they require surgical, rather than pharmaceutical, treatment.

about this, a few things must be pointed out about the nature of the eye. Knowledge of the eye is relevant for many things, but it is especially relevant in this case. The eye, then, has two outer tunics, the higher of which is called "horn-like" by the Greeks.[34] In the part of the eye that is white, the horn-like tunic is adequately thick. In the area of the pupil, it is thinner. 13B. The lower tunic is joined to this tunic. In the middle part, where the pupil is, it is concave with a small hole. Around this the layer is thin, and in the further parts it is thicker, and is called by the Greeks "like the afterbirth."[35] These two tunics, while they enclose the inner parts of the eye, gather together again behind them, and after being thinned out are gathered together, going through the hole that is between the bones at the membrane of the brain and adhering to it. Under these two tunics, in the part where the pupil is, there is an empty space. Then below it again the tunic is most thin, which **Herophilus** named "cobweb-like."[36] 13C. This sinks in the middle, and contains in its hollow something that the Greeks call "glass-like"[37] from its similarity to glass. This is neither liquid nor dry, but is like a condensed fluid, from whose color derives the color of the pupil, whether this is black or bluish-gray, since the higher tunic is completely white. But a small membrane comes up from the internal part of the eye and encloses this fluid. Above these is a spot of fluid, similar to the white of an egg, from which proceeds the faculty of seeing. This is called "ice-like"[38] by the Greeks.

14A. Therefore, either from illness or a blow, the fluid condenses below the two tunics, in the place that I said was empty.[39] And this fluid as it hardens gradually makes itself an obstacle to the internal power of sight. There are many types of this problem. Some are curable, and some are untreatable. For if the cataract is small, if it is stationary, and truly has the color of sea water or of shining iron, and if there is still some sensation of brightness on the side, hope remains. If the cataract is big, if the black part of the eye has lost its natural shape and has turned into a different form, if the color of the cataract is blue or similar to gold, if it shakes and is moved from side to side, it is hardly ever helped. 14B. Generally the cataract is worse in cases where it derives from a more serious illness, from great pains in the head, or from a violent blow. Old age is not fit for treatment, since even without this problem old age has dull sight. But neither is childhood fit for treatment, but rather the ages between youth and old age. Neither a small nor a sunken eye is sufficiently fit for treatment. And there is a certain development within the cataract itself. Therefore one must wait until it is no longer fluid but seems to have condensed into some type of hardness. Before treatment the sick person should take little food, drink water for three days, and abstain from everything on the day before. 14C. After this the sick person must be seated in a chair facing forward, in a bright place, directly facing the light, with the physician sitting opposite and a little higher. An attendant should hold onto the upper part of the sick person's head that will

34. In Greek, *keratoeidēs:* the cornea.
35. In Greek, *chorioeidēs:* the chorioid membrane.
36. In Greek, *arachnoeidēs:* the arachnoid membrane, or retina.
37. In Greek, *haloeides:* the vitreous humor (see fig. 33).
38. In Greek, *krustalloeides.*
39. See Celsus, *On Medicine* 7.7.13.B above.

be treated, so that it remains motionless. For, with a small movement, sight can be snatched away permanently. So that the eye that will be treated may itself be made even more motionless, wool is placed over the other eye and tied up. The left eye must be treated with the right hand, and the right eye with the left hand. 14D. Then the needle must be applied, so sharp that it may pierce, but not too thin. And this should be inserted and guided through the upper two tunics in the middle place between the dark part of the eye and the adjacent angle closer to the temple, away from the middle region of the cataract so that no blood vessel may be injured. But the needle must not be inserted timidly, because it is admitted into the empty space. When it comes to this spot, not even someone moderately experienced can be mistaken, because nothing resists the needle's pressure. 14E. When it has come to this point, the needle is to be lowered against the cataract itself and should be gently rotated and gradually led below the area of the pupil. When the needle has gone over the pupil, it should be pressed on with greater force, so that it penetrates the lower part. If it sticks there, the treatment is completed. If it immediately comes back, the cataract must be cut up with the same needle and dispersed into many parts, which in single pieces are stowed away easily and obstruct vision less. 14F. After this the needle must be drawn straight out. The white of an egg soaked up in soft wool is to be applied, and above this something to limit inflammation. And it is thus to be bound up. After this there is need for rest, restraint, and anointing with light drugs. On the next day the sick person is given food at the right time, which should initially be liquid so the jaws need not be troubled. Then, once the inflammation has ended, food of the type proposed in the case of wounds[40] should be given. It is also necessary that water should be drunk for a considerably long time.

. . .

Book 7, Chapter 16. 1. Sometimes the belly is pierced by a stab of some sort, and it follows that the intestines roll out. When this happens, immediately there must be an examination of whether they are uninjured, then whether their color persists. If the smaller intestine has been pierced, as I have already said, nothing can be done.[41] The larger intestine can be stitched up, not with certain assurance, but because uncertain hope is better than certain hopelessness. For sometimes it closes up. Then if either intestine is bluish-gray or pale or black, it necessarily happens that it lacks sensation, and all medicine is futile. 2. If, however, the intestines to this point have their proper color, one must provide aid with great speed, for, when they are exposed to the external air, to which they are unaccustomed, they are changed in an instant. The person must be laid on his back with hips upright. And if the wound is too narrow for the intestines to be easily placed back, it must be cut open until it opens sufficiently. And if the intestines are already quite dry, they must be washed thoroughly with water, to which a small amount of oil has been added. Then the attendant must gently open the edges of the wounds with his hands or with two hooks inserted in the inner membrane. The physician must always first put back the intestines that prolapsed later in

40. Celsus, *On Medicine* 5.26.30.
41. See Text 12, Celsus, *On Medicine* 5.26.2.

such a way that he preserves the position of the individual coils.[42] 3. When all of these have been put back, the sick person must be shaken gently. In this way the intestines are brought individually into their own places and may settle in them. Once this is done, the peritoneum must also be examined, and if some part of it is black and dead, it should be cut out with forceps. What is uninjured should be brought gently in front of the intestines. Stitching of neither the highest layer of skin nor the inner membrane does enough on its own, but both must be stitched. 4. And two rows of stitching must be put in, thicker than in other places, because they can both be broken more easily with a movement of the belly, and because that part of the body is not especially susceptible to severe inflammations. Therefore the thread must be put into two needles, and held in two hands; and first the internal suture must be put into the membrane in such a way that the left hand is on the right edge of the wound, and the right hand on the left edge, from the beginning of the wound, sending the needle from the internal part to the exterior. This is done so that it is always the blunt part of the needles that is being put away from the intestines. 5. Once both parts have been crossed, the needles must be exchanged between the hands, so that the one that was in the left comes into the right hand, and the one that the right hand held comes into the left hand. And again in the same way they are inserted through the edges of the wound. And so when for a third and fourth time in succession the needles have been exchanged between the hands, the gash is to be closed. After this the same thread and the same needles are transferred to the skin, and stitching is also to be put into the skin with a similar method, always with the needles coming from the internal part, always being transferred between the hands. Then healing glue is applied. It is too obvious to say repeatedly that one must add either a sponge or juicy wool squeezed out with vinegar. When these things are applied, the belly should be lightly bandaged.

INCUBATION AND DREAM THERAPIES

We know of a few kinds of treatments in antiquity that involved dreams. The most common was a practice called "incubation," which involved sleeping in a temple or shrine dedicated to a deity, with the intention of receiving healing through a divine dream. The therapeutic practice developed in the ancient Greek world, related primarily to the healing god **Asclepius**, and continued into late antiquity and beyond in the shrines of Christian saints.

The Epidaurian miracle inscriptions included below (Text 30), which record the cures performed by Asclepius, give us a glimpse into the practice of incubation at one of the most famous temple complexes in ancient Greece (see fig. 49). Upon arrival, sick and suffering people would undergo purificatory rites, including a bath, and a change of clothing. They would make an offering to the god, as well as promising another offering if they received a cure. Finally, they offered anatomical votives, taking the shape of the body parts they hoped

42. Celsus is recommending that the part that came out last should be the first part to be put back in.

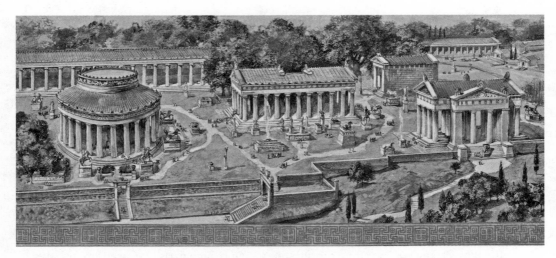

FIGURE 49 Illustrator's rendering of the temple complex of Asclepius in Epidaurus, Greece. The site looked different across its nearly 800-year history, with new buildings and amenities being constructed over time. The buildings shown in this illustration were part of the Classical/Hellenistic construction (fourth century BCE–second century CE). The temple of Asclepius is pictured in the center; the round building where songs and instrumental music were performed (called the *thumelē* or *tholos*) is pictured on the left; and the *abaton*, where people would sleep in hope that the god would visit them in their dreams, is the long colonnaded building pictured in the back left. Getty Images, Dea Picture Library, De Agostini collection.

the god would heal (e.g., arms, hands, legs, feet, ears, eyes, genitals, and viscera such as intestines, wombs, liver, and heart, see figs. 21, 32).

After making their vows, individuals would then sleep in a part of the temple complex called the *abaton*. Dream therapy worked in one of two ways. The god could heal the petitioner directly in their dreams. For example, a blind man—who was even reported to be missing one of his eyeballs from its socket—dreamed that the god prepared a **drug** and applied it to his eye; he awoke with the sight of both eyes restored. Another man who had the point of a spear stuck in his jaw for six years dreamed that the god extracted the spearhead, putting it in his hands; he awoke cured and holding the spearhead. Finally, a man who was ridiculed for going bald dreamed that the god anointed his head with a drug; thereafter his hair grew. Those who were cured in dreams were to return to the temple and, as a show of gratitude, make the offering they had promised when they arrived at the temple. These offerings could be as simple as a loaf of bread, coins, vessels, or utensils or as elaborate and expensive as jewelry, coins, or a dedicatory statue. Physicians who gave offerings to the god often dedicated medical instruments. It was important to fulfill one's vow; otherwise it was thought that the god might reverse the cure.

Alternatively, the god would prescribe a regimen or remedy in the dream that the sick person should follow upon waking. Sometimes the god instructed the person to engage in ritual acts, such as a sacrifice or libation. Other times, the god prescribed a regimen that

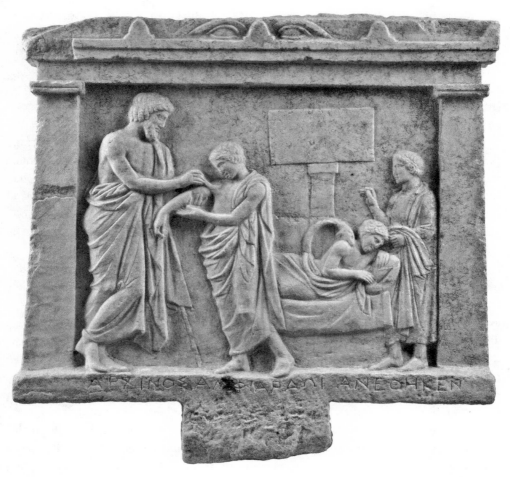

FIGURE 50 Relief from a fourth-century BCE dedication in Oropos, Greece, to Amphiaraos, who was a cult figure—hero and healer—akin to Asclepius. An extant inscription at the shrine gives us a sense of the incubation practices: "Whoever is in need of the god shall incubate . . . complying with the rules. The name of the incubant, as soon as he pays the money, is to be recorded by the *neokoros*—both of (the incubant) himself and of his city—and shall be displayed written up in the dormitory register, so that anyone who wishes may inspect it. In the dormitory men and women shall recline in separate places, the men to the east of the altar and the women to the west." This relief in particular depicts the cure of Archinos in two stages. On the left, Amphiaraos applies a treatment to the shoulder of the young man; on the right, a sacred snake bites his shoulder while his loved one or a temple attendant watches. Above the reclining man is a stele on which he has carved his inscription as instructed. Sculpture Collection, Athens National Archaeological Museum (inv. no. 3369). Photographer: Irini Miari. © Hellenic Ministry of Education and Religious Affairs, Culture and Sports/Hellenic Organisation of Cultural Resources Development.

closely resembled physicians' treatments. For example, in a dream Asclepius instructed a man who was spitting blood to eat the seeds of a pine cone mixed in honey. And, in a dream, the god gave a blind soldier, Valerius Aper, a recipe to make a salve to apply to his eyes. Other divine dream prescriptions were more complex. In order to cure one supplicant's dyspepsia, the god advised a multipronged regimen: the man was to eat a diet of cheese, bread, celery, lettuce, and milk with honey; to follow a bathing program that included hot water plunges; and engage in an exercise routine that included running, walking, and passive exercise. In the selections from **Artemidorus**, an ancient Roman dream interpreter, we see him offering explanations of more cryptic dream content. For instance, he records the dream of **Fronto**, teacher to the emperor Marcus Aurelius, who asked Asclepius for a cure for gout. The god advised him to take a walk in the suburbs, by which Artemidorus took Asclepius to mean that Fronto should use bee pollen as a drug (Text 32, *Interpretation of Dreams* 4.12). Artemidorus interprets the god to be playing on the Greek words *pro* (before) and *polis* (the city), indicating *propolis*, the Greek word for "pollen."

Thus there was much overlap between the boundaries of medicine and religion at Asclepian temples. Priests and temple attendants administered drugs, advised new regimens (dietetics, bathing, exercise), treated and bandaged wounds, and conducted surgery. Moreover, they worked in coordination with local pharmacists, who, as in Pergamum, had shops and stalls directly outside the temple entrance. And they sought assistance from local physicians to carry out the god's prescriptions from dreams. This relationship between physicians and Asclepius reminds us that most people in antiquity did not see religious and medical healing as at odds; rather, they thought that asking a god for assistance was part of a patient's treatment plan.

Moreover, physicians often recognized their place in the hierarchy of healers—understanding the gods to be the ultimate purveyors of health, and physicians to be their servants—and occasionally ceded treatment to the gods. For example, when **Aelius Aristides**, a Greek orator, was enduring a sickness that made him weak and rendered him homebound for months, he received a vision of the god Asclepius in a dream. Upon waking, Aristides informed his physician the remedy prescribed by the god, and even though the prescribed therapies were extreme and his physicians were tempted to object, they ultimately yielded to the god's recommendations.

In addition to cures and healing remedies, Asclepius also dispensed advice in dreams that had to do with a broader sense of well-being. For example, in his text *Sacred Tales,* Aristides describes 160 of his dreams, 70 of which relate to healing from the god, and the rest are advice from the god about how to conduct his professional life, or warnings of impending dangers. Similarly, **Galen** reports that Asclepius visited his father in a dream to tell him that his son should become a physician. In Galen's own dream, the god instructed him not to join the emperor Marcus Aurelius on a northern campaign, presumably to keep him out of harm's way.

We also know of incubation practiced among other religious communities, such as at Christian sites. For example, in late antiquity the sick and suffering were reported to have slept overnight at the shrine of the martyr Phocas hoping to receive dream-visions and healings, and just as they did at Asclepian temples, petitioners left votive offerings at the martyr's shrine. Similarly, the sick in Egypt sought dream oracles and healing at the shrine of the ascetic and martyr Menas in Abu Mina and the shrines of physician-saints Abbakyros and John at Menouthis. Finally, a side chapel in the church of Santa Maria Antiqua in Rome, which is decorated with images of Christian physician-saints, appears to have been an incubation room: paintings line the lower register of the room at the eye level of petitioners who were sitting or lying on the floor, and there is a niche low on the wall where they would have put devotional candles or votives before going to sleep.

Expecting healing or medical prescriptions in dreams reminds us that dreams were thought of differently in antiquity than today. In antiquity, many people believed that sleep was the time when the soul was able to rest from the work it did on behalf of the body—namely, processing information from the senses (such as sights, smells, etc.). When the soul withdrew from outer perceptions and focused inward it could receive other kinds of information, including messages from divine sources, and information about internal bodily states, such as its **humors**, current imbalances, and impending illness. We see this logic expressed most clearly in the selections from the Hippocratic text *On Regimen* (Text 31). The author provides multiple examples about the precise ways in which dream imagery signals bodily states, both healthy and unhealthy. For instance, the author notes that people who dream of a flooded landscape are likely experiencing an excess of moisture in their bodies and should seek out drying remedies (such as emetics, fasting, and exercise). On the other hand, people who dream of a parched and black environment are likely too dry and should avoid exercise and drying foods, with the goal of retaining moisture in the body. Hence, as part of the diagnostic process, physicians asked patients whether they were having any visions or dreams (see, for example, Text 6, **Rufus**, *On the Importance of Questioning the Sick Person* 28–33).

TEXT 30. INSCRIPTIONS FROM EPIDAURUS, SELECTIONS (FROM STELAI A AND B)

*Beginning in the late 1800s, archaeologists found pieces of inscribed stones at the site of a famous sanctuary to the god **Asclepius**, located in Epidaurus (central Greece). The slabs of stones, called* stelai *(singular:* stele*), recorded the miraculous healings experienced by people who came to the sanctuary. The stories were collected and edited by temple personnel, likely sometime in the fourth century BCE. The inscriptions below are selections from the* stelai.

SOURCE: Translated by Brent Arehart based on the Greek text from Rudolf Herzog, *Die Wunderheilungen von Epidauros: Ein Beitrag zur Geschichte der Medizin und der Religion*, Philologus Supplement 22.3 (Leipzig: Dieterich'sche verlagsbuchhandlung, 1931).

Stele A. 1. Cleo was pregnant for five years. Already pregnant for five years, she came to the god as a suppliant and slept in the sacred area. As soon as she came out of there and was outside the temple, she bore a son. Immediately after birth, he washed himself with the fountain waters and walked around together with his mother. Because she obtained these things, she inscribed on her dedication: "It is not the greatness of the tablet that should be marveled at but the divinity, since Cleo bore a burden in her belly for five years until she went to sleep inside and he made her well."

. . .

5. A voiceless boy. This boy came to the temple because of his voice. After he made the initial sacrifice and did the customary rites, the servant who carries around fire for the god looked over at the boy's father and ordered that he promise to give the thank-offering within a year if he got the things for which he came. The boy suddenly said, "I promise." His father was astonished and ordered him to speak again, and he spoke again. And after this he became well.

. . .

13. A man from Torone, leeches. This man saw a dream while sleeping inside. It seemed to him that the god ripped open his chest with a knife, took out the leeches, put them in his hands, and stitched his breast together. When morning came, he went outside holding the creatures in his hands and he became well. He swallowed them when he was tricked by his stepmother, who had tossed them into his barley drink while he was finishing it off.[43]

14. A man with a stone in his penis. This man saw a dream in his sleep. He seemed to be having intercourse with a beautiful boy. During the wet dream he ejected the stone. After picking it up, he left holding it in his hands.

. . .

17. A man's toe was healed by a serpent. Suffering terribly from a malignant sore on his toe during the day, he was carried out by the servants. He sat down on a bench. After sleep overcame him in this spot, a snake came out of the sacred area and cured his toe with its tongue, then retired back into the sacred area. When the man woke up, he became well and said that he saw a vision: it seemed like a handsome-looking young man sprinkled a drug on his toe.

Stele B. 21. Arata the Laconian, **dropsy.** Her mother slept inside on her behalf while she was in Lacedaemon and saw a dream. It seemed like the god cut off her daughter's head and hung up her body with the neck downwards. After liquids flowed out continuously, he untied her body and put her head back on her neck. After she had this vision and returned to Lacedaemon, she found her daughter healthy and learned that she had had the same vision.

. . .

25. Sostrata of Pherae was pregnant with creatures.[44] After she was carried all the way to the temple on a litter, she slept inside. But when she saw no clear dream in her sleep, she was carried back home. Later, around Kornoi, she and her attendants seemed to run into a handsome-looking man. After he learned about their misfortunes, he ordered them to set down the bed upon which they were carrying Sostrata. Then he cut up her belly and took out a great bunch of

---

43. The "barley drink" here might also be translated as "potion," referring to a drink believed to have magical or medicinal properties.

44. The inscribed stone is damaged here, and the text may actually be saying that Sostrata "had a false pregnancy."

creatures, two foot-basins worth. After he stitched her belly together and made the woman well, Asclepius revealed his presence and ordered her to send thank-offerings to Epidaurus.

26. A dog healed a boy from Aegina. This boy had a growth on his neck. After he came to the god, a dog from the sanctuary treated him with its tongue while he was awake and made him well.

. . .

30. Gorgias of Heracleia, pus. This man was wounded in some battle by an arrow to his lung, and for a year and six months it was festering so intensely that he filled up sixty-seven pots with pus. When he fell asleep inside, he saw a vision. It seemed to him that the god took the barb from his lung. When morning came, he went outside well, carrying the barb in his hands.

31. Andromache from Epirus, concerning children. When this woman was sleeping here she saw a dream. It seemed to her that a youthful boy uncovered her, and afterwards, that the god grasped her with his hand. From this, a son was born to Andromache by Arybbas.

. . .

33. Thesandrus from Halieis, **wasting.** When this man slept inside and did not see a vision, he was carried back to Halieis by wagon. A snake from the sanctuary was lying in the wagon, and it spent most of the journey wrapped around the axle. After they arrived at Halieis and Thesandrus lay down at home, the snake came down from the wagon and healed Thesandrus. When the city of Halieis investigated[45] what had happened and were at a loss as to whether they should carry the serpent back to Epidaurus or to leave it be, it seemed good to the city to send people to ask the oracle in Delphi what they should do. The god pronounced that the serpent should remain there, that they should dedicate space to Asclepius, and that they should make an image of him and set it up in the temple. Following the announcement of the oracle, the city of Halieis established a space for Asclepius and completed the things pronounced by the god.

TEXT 31. HIPPOCRATIC CORPUS, *ON REGIMEN* SELECTIONS (4.86, 4.90)

On Regimen *was attributed to* **Hippocrates***, but as with all the texts in the Hippocratic corpus, the authorship is uncertain. The text was likely written in the late fifth or early fourth century BCE. Its author was likely a physician, based on the references to personal experience and discoveries. In four books, the author provides a wide-ranging discussion of topics relating to regimen. The first three books discuss the human body and its composition, the impact of the environment and food on human health, and imbalances caused by too much or too little food or exercise. The selections below come from Book 4, where the author shifts the focus to dreams. The author explains how dreams should be taken into consideration when decisions about regimen are made,*

---

45. Another possible translation here is "announced."

since particular kinds of dreams suggest a need for people to change their regular patterns of diet or exercise.

SOURCE: Translated by Robert Nau based on the Greek text from Robert Joly and Simon Byl, *Hippocrate, Du regime,* 2nd ed., Corpus Medicorum Graecorum 1.2.4 (Berlin: Akademie Verlag, 2003).

Book 4, Chapter 86. The person who understands correctly the signs in dreams will find that they are very powerful in all matters. For the soul does not govern itself when it attends to the waking body and is divided up for many purposes. But the soul yields some portion of itself to each of the body's functions: hearing, seeing, touching, walking, and the actions of the whole body. The soul's own intelligence does not govern itself. But, when the body is at rest, the soul stirs itself and awakens, managing its own house and performing all the actions of the body. For the sleeping body is senseless. But the soul, since it is awake, knows all things. It sees sights, hears sounds, walks, touches, feels pain, and thinks deeply, though it resides in a small space. In sleep, the soul accomplishes all the functions of the body and soul. The person, therefore, who knows how to judge these things correctly knows a great part of wisdom.

. . .

Book 4, Chapter 90. The following also predict health: to see clearly and hear clearly the things on earth; to walk without falling and to run without falling and swiftly without fear; to see the earth level and well-worked, trees covered in leaves, rich in fruit and cultivated, rivers flowing normally with pure water no higher nor lower than appropriate, and springs and wells in similar condition. These all signify health for a person and that the body and its cycles, ingestions, and excretions are normal. If the dreamer sees anything contrary to these things, it signifies some impairment in the body.

If sight or hearing is impaired, it signifies an illness relating to the head, and so the dreamer must take longer walks early morning and after dinner in addition to their previous regimen. If the legs are impaired, there must be a drawing off by **emetics** and one must use more wrestling in addition to the former regimen. Rough land signifies that the **flesh** is impure; one must use longer walks after exercises. Fruitless trees reveal corruption of the person's seed. If the trees are shedding their leaves, the harm is from wet and cold but, if the trees have put forth leaves without fruit, the harm is from warmth and dryness. And so, for some cases one must warm and dry by their regimens and for other cases one must moisten and cool.

Rivers that are not normal signify aspects of the cycle of blood: if the water is high, there is too much blood, and if the water is low, there is too little blood. With a change in regimen, the first must be decreased and the second must be increased. If the rivers flow with impure water, they signify a disturbance. The impurities are purified by runs and walks which stir them up with frequent breath [*pneuma*]. Springs and wells signify something relating to the bladder; one must purify with diuretics. A troubled sea signals an illness of the **cavity;** one must purify with light and gentle laxatives. If the earth or a house shakes, it signifies for a healthy person, health for a sick person, and a change of the current circumstance. A person who is currently healthy benefits from a change in their regimen. First have the person vomit so that nourishment may be received again, for the entire body is being disturbed by the current nourishment. A sick person benefits from using their same regimen, for the body already is changing from its present condition.

To see the earth inundated by water or the sea signifies an illness arising from too much water in the body; one ought to use emetics, periods of fasting, exercises, and drying regimens and then adding nourishment little by little. It is not good to see the land black or burned up completely, rather there is a danger of meeting with a difficult and deadly illness, for it signifies an abundance of dryness in the flesh. One must remove their exercises and as much of their food as is dry, warm, bitter and diuretic. The regimen should include a boiled down decoction of barley-water, only small portions of light and soft foods, large quantities of diluted white wine, and many baths. The sick person should not bathe with an empty stomach. They should also lie in a soft bed, take things easily, and avoid cold and the sun. Pray to Gaia, Hermes, and Heroes.[46] If the person dreaming seems to dive into a lake, sea, or rivers, it is not good, for it signifies an abundance of moisture. In this case, it is beneficial to employ a drying regimen and more exercises. But a dream of this sort is good for the feverish, for the heat is being quenched by moisture.

TEXT 32. ARTEMIDORUS, *INTERPRETATION OF DREAMS* SELECTIONS (4.22, 5.9, 5.26, 5.59, 5.61, 5.66, 5.71–72, 5.79, 5.87, 5.89, 5.94)

Interpretation of Dreams, written by **Artemidorus** *(middle to late second century CE), is a manual on how dreams of all kinds should be interpreted and used to predict the future. As the selections below reveal, Artemidorus thought it necessary for dream interpreters to have some awareness of health and medicine. In the selections from Book 4, Artemidorus takes a firm stance that the gods, especially* **Asclepius**, *communicate about health and healing through dreams. Then the selections from Book 5 are examples of dream healings that provide empirical evidence in support of Artemidorus's argument.*

SOURCE: Translated by Martin Hammond based on the Greek text from Roger A. Pack, *Artemidori Daldiani Onirocriticon Libri V* (Leipzig: Teubner, 1963). First published in *Artemidorus: The Interpretation of Dreams*, Oxford World's Classics (Oxford: Oxford University Press, 2020). Reprinted with minor changes by permission of the Licensor through PLSclear.

Book 4, Chapter 22. As for divine prescriptions in dreams, it would be idle to question the fact that gods do prescribe cures for people. Many have been cured by prescriptions received

---

46. Gaia was the Greek goddess of the earth. Hermes was the god of messengers. "Heroes" refers to mortal or semidivine figures of the past who often had shrines dedicated to them.

at Pergamum and Alexandria[47] and elsewhere: and there are those who say that the art of medicine actually originated from such prescriptions.

. . .

But you will find that the gods' prescriptions are in fact straightforward and not at all enigmatic. They use the same terms as we do in prescribing ointments, **poultices,** food, or drink, and when they do send an allegorical dream the riddle in it is quite transparent. For example, a woman who had an inflammation of the breast dreamed that she was suckled by a sheep. She was cured by the application of a poultice compounded of plantain, because the name of the plant is a compound (*arno-glōsson*),[48] and explains both the tongue of the lamb in her dream and the herb itself, whose name literally means "lamb's tongue."

And if you look closely at any of these cures by divine prescription which you come across, whether you make the interpretation yourself or hear of their fulfillment at someone else's interpretation, you will find that they are completely consistent with medical practice and do not stray outside the science of medicine. For example, **Fronto,** who suffered from gout, asked the gods for a cure, and dreamed that he was walking about in the suburbs: he had a good measure of relief by rubbing himself with bee-glue.[49] This is why, as I have often advised you, you should make it your business as far as possible to get hold of medical treatises.

. . .

Book 5. 9. A man vowed in a prayer to Asclepius that he would sacrifice a cock to him if he got through the year without sickness. Then one day later he prayed again to Asclepius, vowing to sacrifice another cock if he did not suffer from ophthalmia. And indeed that night he dreamed that Asclepius said to him, "One cock is enough for me." The man did stay free of sickness, but suffered a severe bout of ophthalmia. The god was content with one vow, and turned down the other request.

. . .

26. A man dreamed that he had the name of Serapis[50] inscribed on a bronze tag hanging round his neck like an amulet. He contracted quinsy[51] and died in seven days. Serapis is considered a chthonic god[52] with the same significance as Pluto;[53] his name has seven letters; and the dreamer died of a disease affecting that part of him adjacent to the amulet.

. . .

47. Artemidorus is referring here to the temple of Asclepius in Pergamum (modern-day western Türkiye) and the temple of Serapis in Alexandria (Egypt).

48. There is a play on words in the original Greek here. The Greek word for "plantain" is a compound noun (two words combined into one), and a "compound" was also a word used to describe pharmaceutical cures.

49. There is another play on words here. The Greek word for "bee-glue" is *propolis*, which could also be interpreted as "in front of the city," hence a cure that took place in the suburbs.

50. Serapis was a god worshipped by Greeks and Egyptians, associated with the underworld but also with the sun, healing, and fertility.

51. Quinsy involves inflammation of the throat, and typically an abscess behind the tonsils.

52. Chthonic gods were associated with the underworld in Greek religion.

53. Pluto was the Greek god of the underworld.

59. A man dreamed that a javelin fell from the sky and wounded him in one of his feet. This man was bitten in the foot by a snake called the javelin-snake, contracted gangrene, and died.

. . .

61. A man dreamed that he had died after being struck in the stomach with a sword by Asclepius. He developed an abscess in the stomach, and Asclepius cured him with a surgical operation.

. . .

66. A man dreamed that someone said to him, "Sacrifice to Asclepius!" On the following day he met with a terrible accident. He was thrown from a vehicle which overturned, and his right hand was crushed. And so this was what the dream was telling him, that he should take precautions and make an apotropaic sacrifice to the god.

. . .

71. A man who was sick dreamed that he went into a temple of Zeus[54] and put his question to the god in these words, "Will I get better? Will I live?" Zeus spoke nothing in reply, but nodded with his head. The man died the next day, and this made complete sense: when the god nodded downwards he was looking at the earth. We could be confident from the next dream that there was nothing illogical in this outcome.

72. A sick woman dreamed that she asked Aphrodite[55] if she would live. The goddess indicated "No" with an upward nod, but nevertheless the woman did live. Aphrodite's gesture, looking up to the sky, was the opposite of that in the previous dream, and signified recovery.

. . .

79. A runner who was about to compete in the sacred games dreamed that he took a broom and cleared out a channel which was clogged with excrement and mud, then washed it through with a great deal of water, to leave it free-flowing and clean. On the next day, despite the imminence of the games, he gave himself an enema and removed the fecal matter from his intestines: this made him light and quick on his feet, and he won the crown.

. . .

87. A man dreamed that he was sexually penetrated by Ares.[56] He developed a condition in his anus and rectal passage which could not be cured by any other means, and he submitted to surgery to effect the cure. Ares signified the surgical knife, as we often refer metaphorically to a knife as an "Ares," and the pleasure the man took in the intercourse indicated that the surgery would not be fatal.

. . .

89. A man who had a stomach disorder and wanted a prescription from Asclepius dreamed that he entered the god's temple and the god held out the fingers of his right hand

54. Zeus was the Greek god of the sky and thunder, who was also king of the other gods.
55. Aphrodite was the Greek goddess of love, beauty, and sexuality.
56. Ares was the Greek god of war.

and invited him to eat them. The man ate five dates and was cured. The top-quality fruits of the date-palm are called "fingers."

. . .

94. A man who was due to have surgery on his scrotum prayed to Serapis about the operation and dreamed that the god told him, "Go ahead and have the operation: the surgery will cure you." He died: like a man cured, he was to have no more pain. And it made sense that this was how it turned out for him, because Serapis is not one of the Olympian or ethereal gods, but a chthonic god.[57]

THERAPIES OF TOUCH, WORD, AND SOUND

People suffering from illnesses in antiquity made use of various therapies involving touch, word, and sound, or therapies that combined the three. As treatments sometimes offered by physicians and other times by various other healers, these therapies are another example of the fluidity between the domains of medicine, religion, and so-called magic.

In the ancient Mediterranean, massage was the most common touch therapy prescribed by physicians, and implemented by professionals akin to our modern massage therapists. Massage involved a vigorous rubbing of the body often after anointing the body with oil. Physicians prescribed massage to treat a range of physical problems, considering carefully the different degrees of pressure necessary to produce the results they were after. For example, gentle touch was thought to soften **flesh**, open the channels in the body, dissolve and disperse illness-causing residues, break up solid matter trapped in the body, and liquify excrements that needed evacuation. Firm massage, on the contrary, was thought to have the effect of constricting, binding, toughening, and thickening. This tonifying kind of touch was also thought to create firm flesh or even to build flesh, both of which could prevent injuries (hence massage was important for athletes, gladiators, and soldiers).

In addition to treating ailments, massage therapy was also considered an important way to maintain health and thus was a key feature of many regimens, especially among the wealthy who could afford such treatments. For example, athletic trainers regularly massaged their clients before and after their workouts. And many bathing complexes, which were often attached to *gymnasia* or *palaestrae*, employed massage therapists to treat clients after their bathing routines. And, finally, infants—whose bodies were thought of as malleable and soft, in need of toning and shaping—were massaged from a young age in order to promote the formation of an ideal physique.

Beyond medical massage and massage that was part of one's customary regimen, we find a range of other touch therapies practiced by religious or ritual healers (see fig. 51). Although the logic of these therapies is not always explicitly articulated, it seems that a holy person (a person with a special relationship to divinity) or members of special communities

57. The Olympian gods were associated with the sky in Greek religion, in contrast to the chthonic gods, who inhabited the underworld.

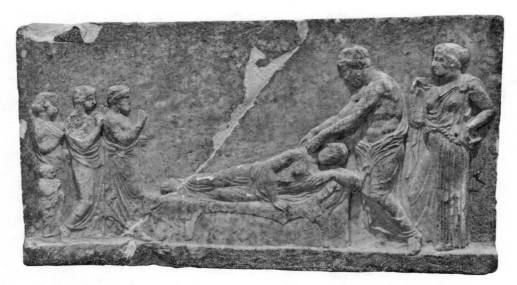

FIGURE 51 Fourth-century BCE marble relief from the temple of Asclepius in Piraeus, Greece, depicting a healer placing his hands on the neck and shoulder of a woman reclining on a couch, while a woman (presumably his assistant) stands behind him, and family, friends, or slaves look on from the other side of the scene. As the relief was found at a temple of Asclepius, the healer likely portrays Asclepius or a priest in his temple, and the assistant likely portrays Hygieia or a temple priestess. Archaeological Museum of Piraeus (acc. no. 405). Photo credit: George E. Koronaios, Wikimedia Commons, Creative Commons Attribution 4.0.

were thought to possess a potency of health that could transfer to the sick or injured person through body-to-body contact. For example, according to Jewish scriptures, when a child cried out about his head hurting and then died suddenly, the prophet Elisha stretched out his body atop the child, "putting his mouth upon his mouth, his eyes upon his eyes, and his hands upon his hands; and while he lay bent over him, the flesh of the child became warm" (2 Kings 4:34). Likewise, early Christian sources report that a hemorrhaging woman was healed by merely touching the garment of the holy man, Jesus (see fig. 52). Similarly, reports circulated that if someone was bitten by a certain kind of viper, one of the Psylli (members of an ancient Libyan people[58]) should lie upon the victim and they should rub their naked bodies together in order to counter the effects of the snake's venom.

Still other stories report that healing occurred when certain objects or substances were touched to the sick person. See, for example, remedies cited by **Pliny the Elder** for tooth inflammation, toothaches, and teething pain, which included attaching the tooth of a mole to a sick person's inflamed tooth or scraping a canine tooth of a dog on a tooth in pain. Given that moles and dogs were creatures known for their pronounced teeth and powerful

58. "Libyan" refers to people from any part of Africa other than Egypt (see fig. 17).

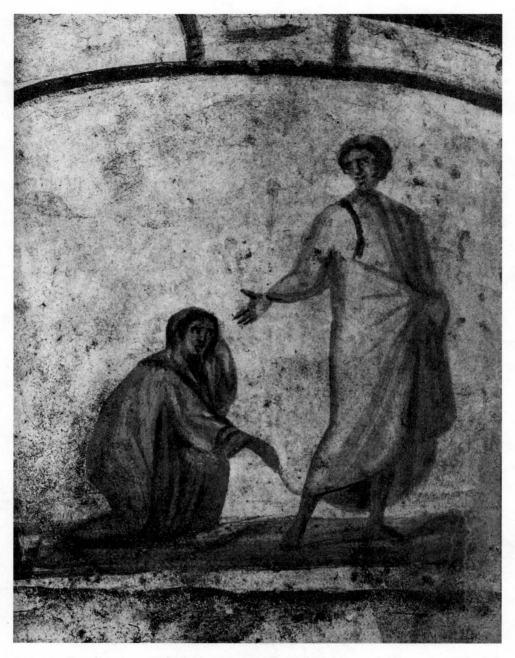

FIGURE 52 Fourth-century CE fresco depicting a scene in which a hemorrhaging woman is healed by merely touching the garment of the holy man Jesus. The accounts of this story in early Christian gospels do not provide any information about her condition (though our gynecological sources discuss the prevalence of hemorrhaging from the womb, particularly related to childbirth); rather, they focus on a transfer of healing power from Jesus to the woman. Catacombs of Marcellinus and Peter (Rome). Wikimedia Commons.

bites, it is likely that ancient people assumed these objects possessed a healthful potency that transferred to the sick body part through contact. Yet we also find remedies presumably based on the opposite logic: that sickness was attracted to sickness. For example, Pliny reports that placing a (kidney) stone evacuated from one person atop the pubic region of someone else who was similarly afflicted by stones resulted in healing, apparently because the sickness would be drawn out of the body to the object of like kind. Sometimes it is hard to disentangle the degree to which healing was thought to be enacted through the touch of a particularly powerful person or through medical reasoning. For example, the holy man Jesus was reported to have restored the sight of a blind man when he mixed his spit with dirt and applied the mixture to the blind man's eyes. The report does not say whether the healing was effective because of the medicinal properties of spit (see Text 28, Pliny, *Natural History* 35.28), the power of Jesus as a holy figure, or some combination of both.

In still other stories, touch therapy was paired with words, whether spoken or written. For example, Apollonius of Tyana resurrected a dead girl being carried in a funeral procession by touching her and whispering words in her ear. Based on this story and others like it, we find that words, especially of a formulaic sort (such as incantations or prayers), were thought to invoke the gods, other immortal beings, or nature to action. Knowing and using the name of a powerful being was a means by which one could access its powers. Many spells recorded in ancient papyrus handbooks, often referred to as the Greek Magical Papyri, include the use of divine, angelic, and daemonic names for overcoming different physical conditions. Similar invocations are recorded in amulets. See, for example, figure 2, which records a petition to the angels, the Holy Spirit, and the Lord for relief from headaches, gingivitis, and daemon possession.

The power of words is most clearly illustrated by the ritualized formulae (or "spells") found in these ancient "magical" handbooks. These spells relied on the power of words by invoking names, harnessing the power of a specific set of words to be spoken in a particular order, or through *voces magicae* (combinations of sounds that do not make sense in any language, such as strings of vowels in succession). For instance, part of an elaborate spell for the purpose of gaining divine knowledge of the cosmos, includes the following: "I invoke the immortal names, living and honored, which never pass into mortal nature and are not declared in articulate speech by human tongue or mortal speech / or mortal sound: ĒEŌ OĒEŌ IŌŌ OĒ ĒEŌ OĒ EŌ IŌŌ OĒĒE ŌĒE ŌOĒ IĒ ĒŌ OŌ OĒ" (*PGM* IV.605–15). These sounds were thought of as angelic or daemonic language.

These handbooks include curses to cause harm, love spells (also called "binding spells"), spells for success at business or in various forms of gambling and betting, and we find many spells for healing. Some of them incorporated objects (such as amulets—with or without writing on them—that one would attach to the body), and some involved elaborate rituals. But many healing spells were simple and short, in keeping with the kinds of emergency situations in which they were used (e.g., a fish bone caught in the throat, a scorpion bite, a fever, headache, and difficulty in childbirth). For instance, a ritual to cure fever with fits of shivering instructed the sufferer or healer to take oil and say "Sabaoth" (a Hebrew word referring to the host of heaven) seven times over the fever before rubbing the oil on the body from sacrum to feet.

Finally, some ancient sources inform us of sound therapies that were intended to heal the mind and body through music. For example, a late ancient biography of **Pythagoras** (c. 570–495 BCE) described the philosopher healing his students' physical and psychological suffering by playing music for them. He also played music for his students prior to bed and upon waking in order to rebalance their bodies and souls as they transitioned into and out of sleep. It seems that Pythagoras saw a connection between the harmony of music and the balance of body and mind (i.e., health). Furthermore, thinkers like him saw a connection between music, bodily health, and the cosmos. Cosmic bodies (planets and stars) were themselves thought to create an ethereal kind of music as they moved in their circular orbits in the supralunary realm. This ideal form of music was an expression of cosmic order and harmony. Thus human-made music—which mirrored the music, and thus also the order and harmony of the cosmos—could produce healing effects on a disorderly body. Interestingly, some of the circular buildings found at Asclepian temples may have been built with special acoustic properties meant to enhance hymns sung to **Apollo** and **Asclepius** as part of the healing program at the temple.

The foregoing examples demonstrate that people in the ancient Mediterranean world employed a rich diversity of healing practices that went beyond what we commonly think of as medical interventions today, many of these involving forms of touch, word, and sound.

ELEVEN

Physicians

Our sources indicate that early Greek medicine was a family affair. Families passed on medical knowledge and skills from one generation to the next, with certain families becoming recognized within their communities as expert healers. Some of these families enhanced their reputation by also claiming to draw their lineage from famous historical physicians or even from healing gods, such as the Ouliads and the Asclepiads, who claimed to descend from the medical writer Parmenides and the deified **Asclepius**, respectively.

Over time, the medical profession in Greece, and later in the Roman Empire, opened up to include nonfamilial apprentices who trained by shadowing their teachers. Apprentices accompanied physicians on house calls, learning how to give physical examinations, diagnose patients, administer various kinds of treatments, and embody an effective bedside manner. The Roman poet Martial reports that, when he fell ill, his physician invited his entourage of students to his bedside in order to master the intricacies of reading a pulse: "A hundred hands, frozen by the northern [wind], felt my pulse" (*Epigrams* 5.9). Apprenticeships afforded physicians-in-training experience and practice in the field. They also enabled physicians to take on more clients, since apprentices could be posted at patients' bedsides, to document every detail of their illnesses (see chapter 8 on case notes) and provide around-the-clock care (see Text 42, Hippocratic Corpus, *Decorum* 17), while their mentor made the rounds to visit other patients.

Beyond apprenticeships, physicians-in-training—especially those with some wealth—might also receive instruction at a handful of cities renowned as medical centers (e.g., Athens, Cos, Cnidus, Smyrna, Alexandria, and Rome). There they could listen to lectures by prominent physicians on a range of medical topics: from the theories of famous medical writers like **Hippocrates** to specialized lessons on joints, ophthalmology, or surgery.

(Scholars believe that some of our extant medical sources were originally lecture notes.) This training could expand or deepen the knowledge they acquired in practice, but physicians-in-training were warned not to rely on lectures and books alone. The Hippocratic author of *Joints* cautioned that instructions from books would be incomprehensible if readers did not already have hands-on experience with the body with which to compare what they were learning.

At these medical centers—especially in Alexandria, Egypt, during the Hellenistic period—one could also be trained in human anatomy, studying assembled bones of the human body (i.e., skeleton models), watching dissections of animals whose anatomy and physiology were similar to humans, and sometimes witnessing human dissection or vivisection (see fig. 53). Audiences at dissections learned about the underlying structures and the inner parts of the body that were not often visible to the naked eye. Thus, when later attempting to diagnose patients, the physician could visualize and imagine what might be happening inside their bodies. Arguing that the study of anatomy was essential to medical training, **Galen** insisted that students not only watch public dissections of animals, but also practice with their own hands (Text 34, *On Anatomical Procedures*).[1] He recommended an anatomical curriculum that started with the foundations of the body—the bones and muscles—and then moved on to more complicated structures, such as arteries and veins, nerves, and organs. For beginners, he recommended pigs and goats (probably because they were easy to acquire) and cattle (probably because they had large features that were easy for novices to work with). Galen himself preferred monkeys because they had the greatest anatomical similarity to humans.

Not everyone, however, approved of dissection. **Celsus** reports two objections: first, dissection did not in fact provide accurate information about the inner parts given that those parts necessarily changed once a person died or their body was cut open; and second, in the case of vivisection (the dissection of living bodies), the practice was cruel, even when performed on criminals (Text 4, *On Medicine*, Preface 23–26, 40–44).

Physicians-in-training who were averse to dissection or who did not have access to animal or human bodies were urged to take advantage of "anatomy by chance." They were advised to scrutinize the bodies of victims of crime who had been beaten and criminals who were flayed during execution or strung up in public places, and left to decompose in the sun and to be picked at by birds and animals. Physicians hired to accompany military troops could inspect the wounded bodies and corpses strewn about the battlefield, and physicians hired by gladiator troops learned anatomy from their clients' bodies, which were regularly torn open.

Beyond gaining anatomical expertise, working with the military or with a gladiatorial troop afforded some physicians specialized knowledge and skills in the field. For instance,

---

1. Public dissections of animals were not just for those undergoing medical training, but also appeared to be a form of entertainment for laypeople. This makes sense when we situate public dissections alongside the spectacles of animal fights in Roman arenas.

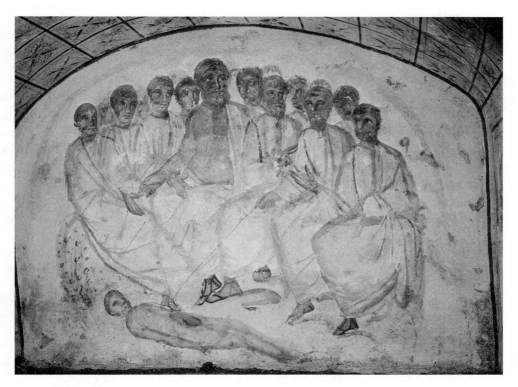

FIGURE 53 Fourth-century CE fresco from the Via Dino Compagni catacomb depicting a man gesturing toward a body with an open abdomen (a person who is presumably dead). Many scholars interpret this fresco as depicting a physician giving an anatomy lesson to the apprentices or students that surround him. Via Dino Compagni catacombs, Room I (Rome). Photo credit: Art Resource, NY.

Galen drew on his work with gladiators to write a commentary on the Hippocratic text *Fractures*. Furthermore, gladiator physicians appear to have developed top-notch skills, since bioarchaeologists who have examined gladiator remains have discovered fractured bones that had healed so well they are nearly imperceptible. Physicians hired to accompany military troops (such as Marcus Naevius Harmodius, Text 36) had an opportunity to learn about wound care from injured comrades, and also accumulated knowledge of plants and remedies in new locales (see Text 24, **Scribonius Largus**'s *Recipes*).

Physicians with considerable training and those who had a reputation for being successful found the highest-status positions. They were hired by wealthy clients, commanded the highest fees, and were awarded the highest honors (fame, a wide audience for their theories and writings, and official commendations). Yet their visibility also made high-status physicians targets of critique. When they were paid exorbitant fees, they could be accused of being greedy. Because of their proximity to the elite, they could be implicated in illicit household or court intrigue (such as adultery or political mischief). And when patients died under the care of these physicians, the powerful could accuse them of murder or even treason.

Employment of the highest status was found in the courts of kings or emperors, serving as their personal physicians (see, for example, the inscription for Tiberius Claudius Alcimus, Text 36). City physician was another high-status position. To ensure that a physician was available when needed, some local city councils paid a physician a salary to remain in residence in the city. Although city physicians were paid a retainer, it appears that most patients still paid fees for their individual medical bills. For that reason, we can imagine that city physicians likely gave preferential treatment to the wealthier members of the community. But occasionally city physicians were praised for having "treated all equally, poor and rich alike, slave and free" (*IG* V.1.1145, II.19–20) or for providing services to the poor without charging them fees (see, for example, the inscriptions honoring the city physicians Nicander, Antiochis, and Menophilus, Text 36).

These high-status physicians represented a small minority of those practicing medicine across Greek and Roman territories. Our evidence—the simple homes belonging to physicians, their modest funerary monuments, and requests to Galen to amend his drug recipes to include less expensive ingredients—suggests that most physicians enjoyed a more humble status and income. Most of these lower-status physicians practiced medicine on the road—they were what we call "itinerant physicians"—treating patients in one town or city before moving on to the next (see, for example, Lucius Sabinus Primigenius, Text 36).[2] On the one hand, itinerant physicians must have struggled with the challenges of not having a stable set of clients and having a limited number of instruments and drugs they could carry with them. On the other hand, their travels would have afforded them the opportunity to collect plants from various regions and to learn new remedies from local healers, broadening their experience and treatments.

When considering the status of physicians, we also must take into account differences across Greek and Roman territories. Most physicians in the Greek East were unable to amass great wealth, but they appear to have been predominantly freepersons. In the Roman West, on the contrary, most of the early physicians were slaves or prisoners procured through conquest of Greek territories in the last two centuries BCE, with other Greek physicians immigrating voluntarily thereafter. Moreover, big Roman estates trained slaves to provide medical care for their household, or to treat patients outside the household as an additional source of income. Thus we understand why medicine in the Roman Empire came to be regarded as low status: it was considered a servile occupation, and—because between 60 and 90 percent of physicians were of Greek origin—a profession of culturally inferior "foreigners." Even after the Roman leader Julius Caesar conferred Roman citizenship on all foreign physicians (46 BCE) and the emperor Antoninus Pius waived local taxes for physicians (sometime in the 140s CE), there remained two tiers of physicians: a small subset of high-status physi-

---

2. This is why texts like the Hippocratic *Airs, Waters, Places* (Text 2) were necessary: to guide the physician who was encountering different kinds of illnesses that arose from a variety of different environments.

cians, who treated elite patients and lived a comfortable life, and the greater majority of lower-status physicians, who eked out a living.

When it comes to the gender of physicians, our records suggest that, in its infancy, the field of medicine was dominated by men. Given the skepticism and criticisms surrounding the fledgling science and profession (discussed in chapter 5), it seems that one way to secure medicine's standing was to masculinize the field (leveraging the gender hierarchy of the time, which deemed all things associated with men as superior). Despite this, we can be sure that women were always involved in health care: growing medicinal plants in their kitchen gardens, applying home remedies, and—given modesty norms that made women reluctant to have their bodies examined by men—serving as the primary health-care providers for other women. Although some scholars assume that women healers treated only gynecological and reproductive issues, other scholars argue that they must have treated the full range of illnesses that befell women, who were reluctant to expose their bodies to men.

In the Hellenistic period, we find that the terms used for women health-care providers start to shift: they were no longer called only "**obstetrician**" (Greek *maia* or Latin *obstetrix*) but sometimes "obstetrician-physician" (*maia kai iatros* or *iatromaia;* see, for example, the inscription dedicated to Phanostrate in Text 36 and fig. 56) or simply "physician" (Greek *iatrinē* or Latin *medica*), the same terms used for male physicians, but with feminine endings. Scholars wonder whether this shift in title is an indication that women's medical practice was gradually expanding over time, or whether women were finally receiving the recognition and titles for work they had long been performing.[3]

When we look at women's medical training, it becomes clear that female physicians were educated in ways that were quite similar to the education of their male counterparts, and we find that women could earn the same level of renown as their male counterparts. For example, **Soranus** advised a curriculum for obstetricians that paralleled men's medical training, including medical theory, the full spectrum of therapeutic treatments (diet, drugs, and surgery), and medical ethics (Text 35). Soranus also expected obstetricians to exhibit the "manly" qualities that made a good physician: they should possess the endurance, rationality, and equanimity of men.

---

3. In his collection of myths, etymologies, and genealogies, the Latin author Hyginus reported that women were disallowed from practicing medicine in Athens until a woman, **Agnodice**, disrupted the system: she cross-dressed as a man in order to receive a medical education and then she began treating women who, out of modesty, refused to be examined by male physicians. When she was found out, the women of Athens purportedly revolted, demanding health care, thus opening the door for women to become obstetricians. Some scholars regard Hyginus's story as an accurate reflection of how the gendered division of labor was negotiated in Athens during the classical period: women could attend to women's reproductive care (holding the title "obstetrician"), whereas the higher-status, masculinized role of professional physician was reserved for men (holding the title "physician"). Other scholars, however, suspect that Hyginus's story was fabricated and rather served to push back on the expanding roles for women health-care providers of his own time: leveraging an origins story to put women in their place and limit their activities within the field.

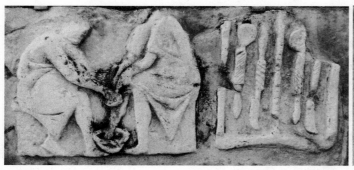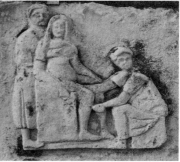

FIGURES 54 and 55 Circa 140 CE terracotta reliefs from the tomb of a medical couple. In the Isola Sacra necropolis near the harbor of ancient Rome, there is a brick enclosure tomb that belonged to a medical couple, Scribonia Attice and Marcus Ulpius Amerimnus. Above the entrance to the tomb there is an inscription and two terracotta reliefs on either side (that presumably depict the wife and husband). The inscription indicates the authority of the wife, Scribonia, who built the monument for herself, for her husband, for her mother, and for her freedmen and their descendants. The relief on the right depicts a woman (crouched) and her assistant (standing) delivering the baby of a woman seated in a birthing chair. The relief on the left depicts a seated man treating the leg of another seated figure, as well as several medical instruments. Tomb 100, Isola Sacra necropolis (Portus, Italy). Photo credit: Kristi Upson-Saia.

And women physicians could achieve the same acclaim as their male counterparts. Take, for example, Antiochis of Tlos, who learned medicine from her father, the physician Diodotus. Antiochis eventually became the city physician of Tlos (see the honorary inscription, Text 36), a role that would have required her to treat the full range of illnesses experienced by all patients in the city. Not only did Antiochis earn the commendation of her city, but her fame spread far and wide: Galen cited her remedies, and **Heraclides** dedicated one of his books to her. We have over fifty attestations of women physicians like Antiochis in inscriptions and monuments that praise women's medical skill and success (we include a handful below, in Text 36). Moreover, within medical literature, male authors credit women's contributions to medical knowledge. For example, in his collection of remedies, **Pliny the Elder** cited Sotira's remedies for fevers and epilepsy, **Salpe's** remedies for mad dog bites and fevers, and the abortifacients used by Lais and Elephantis. So too Galen credited Aquillia Secundilla with his favorite recipe to treat lumbago, and **Aëtius of Amida** cited the medical ideas of **Aspasia** more than those of the prominent male physician Soranus.

Physicians—regardless of gender—depended on each other and often collaborated. When in need of remedies, they shared recipes or ingredients. Galen, for example, mentioned how physician colleagues helped him with drug trials, testing the efficacy of his drugs on their patients. Physicians might call in a colleague to help with a difficult case or to offer a second opinion (see Text 42, Hippocratic Corpus, *Decorum*). Some husband-and-wife teams worked collaboratively (see, for example, figs. 54 and 55). In cities with a critical mass of medical professionals, physicians sometimes formed guilds (*collegia*), with their own clubhouses. These groups gathered for social events, honored their members with statues and plaques. provided proper burial for and regular remembrances of deceased members, and built goodwill within the city by pooling their money to fund public improvements, such as rebuilding the lighthouse at Smyrna. There are some indications that physicians in guilds also might have engaged in profit-sharing mechanisms that ensured the financial security of all members.

Yet, despite this evidence of collaboration, we also know that competition between physicians could be fierce, especially when physicians fought to acquire customers. We hear of bitter disputes in which one physician publicly assailed a colleague's treatment or spread rumors about a colleague's incompetence. And these disputes carried weight. Competing physicians' critiques—coupled with the death of a patient or two—could end a physician's career or force a physician to relocate their medical practice.

Given that there were no standardized educational programs, no centralized medical association that licensed physicians, and no system by which physicians were regularly assessed, it could be hard for sick and suffering people to discriminate between well-trained and experienced physicians, inexperienced novices, "armchair" intellectuals who had no clinical experience, and charlatans who intended to collect fees and then flee town. Patients were forced to rely on word-of-mouth commendations and critiques from family, friends, or trusted professionals. Or, much to the chagrin of physicians like Galen, they might hire physicians based solely on the way they carried themselves. Galen urged patients to be more discriminating, outlining steps they could take to examine physicians before hiring them (Text 33). Only by doing so, Galen stressed, could the sick be sure they were choosing the best physician in a marketplace populated by healers with widely disparate skills.

TEXT 33. GALEN, *ON EXAMINATIONS BY WHICH THE BEST PHYSICIANS ARE RECOGNIZED* SELECTIONS (1–3, 5, 9)

*In addition to his medical texts written for fellow physicians, **Galen** (c. 129–c. 216 CE) wrote a text for sick and suffering people, offering advice on how to select the best physician. The text takes for granted that readers had the time, money, and education to know a fair amount about medicine themselves, meaning that it would have been most relevant for wealthy members of the Roman upper classes. Galen's advice is riddled with his usual criticisms of other physicians of his time—complaining that they were not as well educated and as skilled as he was—complaints that were not likely an entirely accurate reflection of medical practice at Rome in the second century. The original Greek version of this text does not survive, but an Arabic translation made by Ḥunayn ibn Isḥaq (809–873 CE) is likely an accurate rendering of the original Greek, preserving the text's contents.*

SOURCE: Translation by Albert Z. Iskandar based on the Arabic text from Albert Z. Iskandar, *Galen, On Examinations by Which the Best Physicians Are Recognized*, Corpus Medicorum Graecorum Supplementum Orientale 4 (Berlin: Akademie-Verlag, 1988). Reprinted with permission from Akademie-Verlag.

Chapter 1. 1. Galen said: Most people, through ignorance, are so remiss as to neglect matters about the virtues of the soul and what is of advantage to it. If they were also so remiss as to neglect the preservation of the health of their body, either through ignorance or from under-estimating its importance, my amazement would have been less. Yet, I have found that health is so exalted that some orators compose poems in praise or invocation to God. To all the bless-ings, they prefer that of good health for which they ask before all other requests. (Orators) have not been blamed for so doing, people praise them and accept their poems which they recite in temples: and our predecessors conducted their recitals in the temple of **Asclepius**. 2. I am therefore extremely amazed that, although (health) is (highly) valued, men are so remiss as to neglect it: they refrain from seeking instruction in an art by which they will regain (health), and (consequently) they fail to distinguish between the best and the worst among those who take up this art. 3. In ancient times, when men were not yet obsessed, as they are (now), with the pursuit of luxury, students of this art: the virtuous kings and the sons of divine kings and their kinsmen, were worthy of this (art) on account of their superior innate virtues. Those kings educated their sons in this (art), and, at that time, none of them had ever thought that it was shameful to take up this art of **Apollo** and Asclepius. 4. At present, its sta-tus has declined; it is suitable (only) for slaves and despicable men. Kings are now ashamed of being instructed in this art, and nowadays they seek recovery through divine medicine. We never find any country, or any city, without places where recovery is sought through divine medicine, some named after Asclepius, others after Apollo. None of the rich men of our time thinks it worth-while to be instructed in this art: they all look upon it with disdain.

5. In addition to their aversion to studying medicine, they do not consider it their duty to distinguish between the best and the worst physicians. But some, when burdened with dis-ease, will seek out physicians, hoping to find relief. Some patients refrain from seeking out doctors and put themselves in the hands of those to whom they are accustomed, as if all those who take up this art were equally learned. 6. Others will think and agree in the end that men who take up this art may differ in merit, but they distinguish between them and examine their skill by things remote from and irrelevant to the practice of medicine. Wealthy physicians, they believe, are better than poor and needy (physicians), and those who are accepted by many great and rich citizens are better than those who are not. 7. Furthermore, patients do not investigate the reasons why some physicians are particularly favored and honored by those (rich citizens) we have (just) mentioned. Has their choice of physicians to honor been based on testing them, and on knowledge of the distinction between the best and the worst physicians? Or have they been misled by praise from servants or viziers? Or has a physician been accepted without examination, merely on the intercession of an inter-mediary? Most of our contemporaries rely on other people in examining physicians: they themselves shun this matter because they realize, and personally feel that they are without any erudition or knowledge which would enable them to recognize such distinctions; though ignorant, in this (matter) they are justified.

8. When wicked men realized how stupid others could be, they found it unnecessary to obtain any medical instruction in order to acquire skill and dexterity. They resorted to hunt-

ing rich men, each in the way, in their opinion, he would be easily led: this is an approach to the hunting of beasts. If they thought that "women" were the obsession of a rich man whose fortune they sought, they would introduce the subject of women; and if they thought that "slaves" were his obsession, the subject of slaves would be brought forward. 9. We also come across many rich men who have been cheated by the tricks of charlatans and those who claim to be diviners. Most of the rich are accustomed to flattery from those who visit them frequently: they listen and act with one purpose, to seek pleasure. Wicked men who take up medicine are aware of this, and by coaxing the rich seek—among other things—to deceive them and to extort money. 10. Should a rich man fall ill, those practitioners, aware of the desire of their client for pleasure, would not administer the treatment most conducive to good health, but, instead, they would prescribe a most desirable and pleasurable regimen. In any case, they would be unable to correctly administer the most appropriate treatment, should they wish to do so. This is because it has never been their intention to apply the art of medicine properly. Their only aim is to gain money, power, and position. 11. They do not seek the most protective methods for patients, but pursue those which offer the best safeguard for their personal desires. For, if someone proceeds in this way and his patient is saved from a disease, he will say to him, "Let my reward be generous." But should his patient die, he would be untroubled, and would be relieved of someone whom he feared might blame him and lodge a complaint against him.

12. One peculiarity of Rome, which is not shared by other cities is that not even neighbors, let alone other inhabitants, know how a patient has died, or by whom he has been treated. This is because the city is great and populous: its inhabitants are very eager for, and occupied in, the pursuit of money and prestige. 13. I have not written this book of mine for people whose way is like this: being constantly occupied, they cannot devote any time to reading or to anything else. I have written it for those who think that their body is better and more important than all their possessions; or who, if they do not think that the body is better and more important, (at least) do not consider it to be too inferior (to their possessions).

Chapter 2. 1. I begin my discourse with a statement by **Hippocrates**: in the past, this man was considered eminent, among the divine men, although in our time he no longer holds this rank. A summary of his statement is that a practitioner should be able to know beforehand what will happen to the patient later. To quote him literally, "If a physician knows beforehand, declares the present and the past, foretells the future, and expresses on behalf of the patients whatever they may fail to express (themselves), he will be taken into their confidence as a man of experience and insight, thus relieving the patients from anxiety: they would willingly put themselves in his hands; and his treatment will be conducted in the best way, since he can know beforehand from the present illness what will take place later."

2. Nobody doubts that he who has an adequate knowledge of the complaints of patients is the best person to be entrusted with confidence, not just on account of his knowledge, but also because, at the same time, he will be ready to meet any impending occurrences long before they happen. Just as a skilled helmsman is not, in our opinion, one who can diligently manage his ship amidst disturbed seas; he could not be safeguarded against defeat by strong

winds and violent disturbances at sea: but, in our opinion, a skilled (helmsman) is one who can predict such disturbances long before their time from (certain) indicative signs, and will anchor immediately if he finds a harbor nearby. Should deep water prevent him from anchoring, he would apply every means to guard and protect his ship against damage and without haste, before the onset of terror and confusion. 3. Similarly, the best physicians should be able to foresee whatever is likely to happen to their patients. They should take precautionary measures, a long time in advance, by getting ready and by preparing everything that might be needed against whatever might occur.

4. I know of many practitioners who happen to be short of essential **drugs** and instruments when confronted with symptoms suddenly appearing in patients. Frequently, many patients suffer suddenly from failing strength as a result of bleeding which occurs from the nose or elsewhere. This may also be caused by severe diarrhea, sweating, vomiting or intense pain. Without any forewarning by attendant physicians, many patients may be suddenly stricken with a deep coma, convulsion or delirium. A patient, while having a meal, may unexpectedly suffer an outbreak of fever without any rigor; yet, none of the physicians attending him could have forewarned of this. 5. Should these things occur, how necessary it would be for their physicians to run away and to be swallowed up in the earth for attending patients, without knowing (beforehand) that such occurrences will happen later. If they are not ready in advance and do not have to hand all that is required, they will endanger the lives of patients. Furthermore, patients may suddenly suffer from debility, from paleness, arrest of the pulse, and intense coldness of the body, while physicians, knowing nothing of (all) this, remain unequipped with all that is required.

6. Practitioners should not be merely equipped with all the necessary drugs, foods, drinks, and instruments to meet anything that might happen to the patient: it is their duty, should they foresee that anything might happen, to seek to eliminate the cause of such occurrences, thus, whenever possible, preventing them altogether. If such (attempts) are impossible, they should try to break up the adverse (effects) of the occurrences and decrease their intensity. As to my statement that physicians should be ready in advance to meet whatever might happen to (their) patients, these (precautions) should follow prognosis, by which they might gradually foresee future eventualities.

Chapter 3. 1. I have found (doctors) who fail in diagnosis: I have often come across patients who suffer from failing strength, as well as showing other symptoms similar to prostration, while practitioners are ignorant of the causes of such signs. Hippocrates also made a statement about this matter, as I will here describe to you. It is as follows, "I have also found physicians to be inexperienced in diagnosis of the debility they encounter among patients, and (not to know) whether it is caused by the decline of strength, or an upsurge of severe pain and an acute disease, and other additional symptoms relating to the patient's physical constitution and his condition, in all their varieties." 2. The majority of practitioners who neglect this matter also ridicule its proponents. They do not praise those who investigate the cause of any accident that may happen to a patient; instead, they are eager to scoff at them, to rebuke and slander them, claiming that they pursue frivolous matters and impose on themselves superfluous and unnecessary tasks. Should they be required to understand the arguments on this matter, they would say, "We are neither sophists nor logicians; but we are content with therapy by way of empiricism." 3. And when their therapy is exposed, you will find some who, when disgraced, will behave impudently and contentiously towards their opponents in debate; and you will find others who keep silent at the time, yet spy on those who expose them, employing deceitful tricks in conspiring against their opponents until they suffer misfortune; like those practitioners in the time of **Quintus** who conspired against him, causing him to be banished. We find it necessary, however, to describe the way in which their therapy can be exposed, for this is our intention and purpose in writing this book of ours.

4. I say: some practitioners, who disregard Hippocrates and the Ancients, might attend a patient whom they believe to be suffering from failing strength. Thereupon they would wish to strengthen him by filling his belly with eggs, bread soaked in wine, and similar foods. Another practitioner who might attend the same patient might say that he did not need any of these (foods), nor did he need the small amount which he used to have. He would then order the patient to abstain from food altogether. Upon obeying his order the patient's health would be invigorated and restored. Those who attended the patient would realize clearly that he would have been stifled had he followed the first diet. This (case) would bring disgrace upon the (practitioner) who prescribed food and would indicate skill on the part of the one who ordered a restricted diet.

. . .

Chapter 5. 1. If you wish primarily to examine the matter whether a physician knows or does not know about medicine, you should begin first by asking him questions on those things which I have described: "Where and how did Hippocrates mention them, and what evidence has he provided to prove them?" You will find many famous physicians in our time, of whom people speak favorably, ignorant of any books in which Hippocrates mentioned these (precepts) and unaware of the reasoning behind them. If you attain this (end) you will have distinguished between the best and the worst physicians, and furthermore, will have recognized leading and skilled doctors. 2. Should you put questions on such matters to anyone who could let you know, by informing you of the source-books, you should further ask him: "Did **Erasistratus** approve or disapprove of Hippocrates' precepts about treatment of patients? Did he disapprove of one thing or many things or all of his precepts? Or did he give contrary instructions?" Moreover, you should ask questions about the opinions of all other famous physicians; these are: **Diocles, Pleistonicus, Phylotimus, Praxagoras, Dieuches, Herophilus,** and **Asclepiades.** 3. (A student) who has followed the right course of instruction will be able to describe the doctrines of each of these. If he is really perfect, he will be able to describe to you the doctrines of the Ancients, together with those of their successors, outlining their differences and agreements. Furthermore, he will be able to inform you of his own judgment on their differences, justifying correct doctrines and exposing those which are erroneous. 4. Nevertheless, this method demands training in the demonstrative science, on the part of the examiners of physicians who apply it. This is because nobody can understand demonstration unless he has had previous instruction and has become knowledgeable in it: in the same way that nobody can calculate without having been previously taught arithmetic. If rich dignitaries and men of power were able to distinguish the correct demonstration from false doctrines, they would be able to examine every physician by means of disputation, without finding it necessary to test him in therapy. 5. But since they would accept anything more readily than to be trained in demonstration, then the least they could do is to seek out (physicians) and examine them in therapy in order to assess each one, finding out how far he falls below the complete physician. The complete physician foretells the nature of the disease at its onset, when it will reach the culmination, and the occurrence of its **crisis**. As to the one who is not so (accomplished), the more errors he makes on each of these (points), the more he will fall below the complete physician.

. . .

Chapter 9. 14. You now know that it is not difficult to apply tests to the practice of this art, if you are resolved to do so. If you are too proud to examine physicians, because you are a wealthy man or a hero, you will be the first to be punished. Unlike the fact that it is up to you whether you accept or reject the (idea of) examining physicians and studying medicine, it is not up to you when it comes to needing medicine.

TEXT 34. GALEN, *ON ANATOMICAL PROCEDURES* SELECTIONS (1.1–3, 3.1–2)

Galen's (c. 129–c. 216 CE) On Anatomical Procedures is a practical guide by which a reader could learn anatomy and physiology. As Galen explains, the information in the handbook derived largely from dissections and vivisections of animals (a proxy for the human body, given taboos about human dissection; see Text 4). Although Galen's dependence on animal bodies led him to make some errors in his claims about human anatomy and physiology, his investigations were based on the use of a rigorous experimental method. In the selections below, Galen directs readers in how to conduct dissections to familiarize themselves with bones, muscles, tendons, blood vessels, and nerves. He asserts that practice in dissection is essential for accurate diagnosis and for proper surgical techniques that do not cause more harm in the attempt to heal. As is usual for Galen, he devotes considerable energy to explaining how his text is superior to other physicians, and he references other texts that he has written on related topics.

SOURCE: Translation by Jessica Wright based on the Greek text from Ivan Garofalo, *Galeni anatomicarum administrationum libri qui supersunt novem: Earundem interpretatio arabica Hunaino Isaaci filio ascripta*, vol. 1 (Naples: Lugduni Batavorum, 1986).

Book 1, Chapter 1. I wrote *Practical Anatomy* earlier, at the time when I first arrived at Rome, just as Antoninus,[4] our present ruler, was beginning to govern. Nonetheless, it seemed fitting to write this additional work for two reasons. The first is this: that Flavius Boethus, a

---

4. Marcus Aurelius, Roman emperor from 161 to 180 CE.

man who was Roman consul, on departing from Rome for his own homeland, Ptolemais,[5] urged me to write that handbook for him, who had developed as keen a love for anatomical theory as anyone else who has ever lived. On his departure, I also gave other treatises to this Boethus, together with *Practical Anatomy in Two Books*. For, since he observed a great deal at my hands in a short time and was afraid that he might forget what he had seen, he wanted a reminder via books of this sort. Since this man has now died and I have no copies of the former books to give to friends, those which I held onto having been destroyed in Rome, and at the encouragement of these friends, I decided to write other books. The second reason is that the treatise that I am now about to publish will be far better than the earlier one, in part because it is extended across a greater number of volumes for the sake of clarity, and in part because it is more accurate than the previous treatise, since I had conducted many anatomical investigations in the meantime.

For while Boethus was still living in the city of Rome, the following texts were written: *On the Anatomy of **Hippocrates** and **Erasistratus**, On the Anatomy of Living Creatures*, and, further, *On the Anatomy of Dead Creatures,* together with *On the Causes of Breathing* and *On the Voice*. On his departure, I wrote a long treatise, *On the Usefulness of the Parts,* which I completed in 17 books and sent to Boethus while he was still alive.

I wrote a three-book work, *On the Movement of the Thorax and Lung,* a very long time ago, when I was still a youth, as a gift for a fellow student. He was returning to his homeland after a long time and wished to make a display of his abilities in public, but was unable to compose orations. When that man died, these books came to be made public, because many possessed copies of them, despite the fact that they were not written for publication. For I wrote them while I was still living in Smyrna on account of **Pelops,** who was my second teacher after **Satyrus,** the student of **Quintus,** and I had not yet made any significant or original discovery. Later, I was in Corinth for the sake of studying with **Numisianus,** who was famous among the students of Quintus, and then in Alexandria and several other regions where I found a student of Quintus who was more famous than Numisianus. Then, returning to my homeland and remaining there a short time, I came to Rome, where I performed many dissections for Boethus and those who were always present with him—Eudemus the Peripatetic and Alexander the Damascene, whom the Athenians have now deemed worthy to teach Peripatetic philosophy at public expense, and frequently other men in office also, such as the prefect of the city of Rome, Sergius Paulus the Consul, a man foremost in all things, both in actions and in words, in relation to philosophy. It was at that time that I composed *Practical Anatomy* for Boethus, a work that falls far short of what I will write in the present work, not only in clarity, but also in accuracy. And so, if you would, turn your attention to the beginning of the work.

Chapter 2. Just as so-called poles are to tents and walls are to houses, so is the nature of bones in living creatures. For the other parts of the body are naturally disposed to assimilate to them and change shape with them. That is to say, if a creature's cranium is spherical, then

5. Ptolemais was located in the Roman province of Syria.

the brain must be too, and if it is elongated, the creature's brain is also elongated. If the jaws are small and the whole face is somewhat round, the jaw muscles must also be small. And again, if the jaws are big, then the whole face of such a creature will be big and broad, and the muscles will be similarly large. Therefore, indeed, the monkey is—of all living creatures—most similar to the human being in viscera, muscles, arteries, veins, and nerves, because it is similar in the shape of its bones. Through the nature of its bones, the monkey walks on two legs and uses its front limbs like hands, and has the flattest sternum of all quadrupeds, a collar bone just like that of a human, and a round face and small neck. Since these things are similar, the muscles could not be arranged otherwise, since they are stretched over the outside of the bones, such that they mimic their size and shape. The arteries accompany the muscles, as do the veins and nerves, and these, therefore, are similar to the similar bones.

Since, indeed, the shape of the body conforms to the bones, and the nature of the other parts follows them, I consider it of utmost importance before everything else that you gain accurate expertise in human bones, not through incidental observation, nor only by reading about them in a book, which some people title *Ostologia,* some *Skeletons,* some simply *About Bones,* such as my own, which I am convinced surpasses all earlier works in the accuracy of the material, in the brevity of the explanation, and in clarity. Let it be your task and pursuit not only to learn accurately the shape of each bone from a book, but also to make yourself an attentive witness of human bones with your own eyes. This is very easy in Alexandria, insofar as the physicians there teach students about the bones through visual examination. And if for no other reason, then on this account alone you should try to visit Alexandria.

For those who are unable to do this, however, it is possible to observe human bones some other way. I myself have seen them quite often, indeed, whenever a grave or tomb has been broken open. Once, also, a river entered a tomb that had been constructed in makeshift fashion a few months earlier, destroyed it easily, and by the force of its onslaught dragged out the entire corpse. The **flesh** was already rotted, and the bones still attached to one another in proper arrangement, it was carried and dragged for a **stade** downhill. When the outskirts of flat marshland received the body of the dead man, it became stranded there, and it was then possible to see the kind of thing a physician might intentionally prepare for the instruction of young men. Once we also saw the skeleton of a robber lying on a mountain a short distance from the road. A traveler, who had first traveled with a robber, had killed him when the robber attacked. No one who lived in that land intended to bury the robber, but out of hatred they rejoiced at his body being eaten by carrion birds, which devoured its flesh at sunset and left the skeleton as a lesson for those who wished to examine it.

If, however, you do not have the good fortune to observe such things, then dissect a monkey, remove the flesh, and observe each of its bones closely. Select those monkeys that are most like the human being;[6] they do not have long jaws, and their so-called canine teeth are not big. In this kind of monkey, you will find the other parts arranged as in human

6. Galen was likely working with rhesus monkeys.

beings, on account of which they walk and run on two legs. Whichever ones are similar to the dog-faced baboon, however, have projecting jaws and large canine teeth. These can scarcely stand upright on two limbs, such that they avoid walking or running. Monkeys that are most similar to the human being depart a little from a genuine upright posture: this is because the head of the femur supports the socket in the hip joint at a more slanting angle, and also because some of the muscles that are fitted to the calf advance further. Both of these features prevent and impair upright stature, as do the feet themselves, which have narrower heels and toes that are significantly separated from one another. But these differences are small, and the monkey only loses a little in terms of uprightness on this account. Those monkeys that are similar to the dog-faced baboons, diverging more obviously from the human form, also possess obvious dissimilarity in their bones.

Once you have selected, then, the most humanoid of the monkeys, learn the nature of bones accurately upon these as you read through my writings. For it will be possible for you to become immediately accustomed to their names, and these will be useful for the study of the anatomy of the other parts. In this way, if you should happen upon a human skeleton at some point later on, you will easily observe and remember what you have learned.

If you trust in reading alone, however, and do not become accustomed to observation of monkey bones, then you will not accurately observe the human skeleton if you suddenly come across it, and you will not remember what you have learned. For the recall of perceptible things requires continuous practice. For this reason also, we recognize those human beings most clearly whom we have met frequently, and we pass by those we have seen once or twice across a long time, neither recognizing them at all, nor remembering what we saw before. Thus, the notorious "anatomy by chance experience,"[7] which some physicians consider best, is not sufficient to teach the nature of things that have been observed. For, in order to know all of the parts immediately upon seeing them, one must examine each at great length, preferably in humans themselves, but if not, then in animals that are close to the human being. For example, many people had parts stripped of skin, and some even of flesh, by certain pustules that spread widely in many of the cities in Asia.[8] At the time I was still living in my homeland, studying under Satyrus, who was in his fourth year of living in Pergamum with Cuspius Rufinus, who was constructing a temple of the god **Asclepius** for us. Quintus, the teacher of Satyrus, had died not long before. Those of us who had observed Satyrus readily recognized the exposed parts when we dissected them, and made a precise diagnosis, commanding the sick people to make a particular movement, which we knew was carried out through a certain muscle, and sometimes slightly contracting and turning aside the muscles for the purpose of observing a large artery, nerve, or blood vessel that lay adjacent. But we saw all the others, ignorant to the point of blindness of the revealed parts, necessarily suffer one of two things: either they raised up and turned aside many parts of

7. "Anatomy by chance experience" is a critique directed at Empiricists.
8. For Greek authors, "Asia" referred primarily to Asia Minor, which is roughly equivalent to modern-day Türkiye.

the exposed muscles, on which account they became troublesome and annoyed the sick for no reason, or they did not even attempt to begin such an observation. Others knew better through practice how to instruct the sick person in moving the part appropriately. I learned clearly from this, therefore, that for those who had been taught in advance, the observation of wounds corroborated what they had learned, while for those who had no foreknowledge, it was impossible for them to learn anything.

But we must get to the matter at hand. As I have said, one must examine the nature of all the bones, if possible either in the human body or in the monkey, and preferably in both; then it is necessary to come in turn to the dissection of the muscles. For these both lie beneath all the rest, like the foundations of a building. After these, you will be equipped to first learn your preference of the following: the arteries, the blood vessels, or the nerves. Recognition of the nature of the viscera will come to you as you familiarize yourself with the dissection of these parts, as will knowledge of the guts, the fat, and the glands, which it is appropriate for you to examine closely and individually. It is fitting, therefore, to train in this order.

The person who is making a demonstration to another must prepare the part he proposes for study as quickly as possible, and to display it in many different ways, sometimes from a different approach, as I will explain. And it is a good idea to prepare to dismember the bodies of other animals whenever you lack monkeys, quickly distinguishing how they differ from the monkey, as I will make clear.

Chapter 3. As I said, I have written an account of bones separately. Read this book first to have at hand the recollection not only of things, but also the names for them, so that I should not now need to explain anything incidental during the argument. *On the Dissection of Muscles* was written not long ago, when others demanded it, in order that they might have reminders while abroad. They urged me to write this *Dissection* separately and for its own sake in particular because I had received a book by **Lycus**, which extended a few lines short of five thousand, erring in most of them, even so far as to have left out several muscles. The book in which I dealt with this anatomy is perhaps a third of the size, teaches all the muscles, and beyond this also makes mention of Lycus, a man ignorant of the functions of many muscles and entirely neglectful of others. Anyone who desires may use that book to train himself, by dissecting a monkey. Yet, still more from this book he will learn how it is appropriate to attempt the dissection of the muscles in each part.

First, you must practice on a dead body in order to observe the beginning and end of each muscle, as well as its fibers—whether they are all similar to one another throughout the length of the muscle or are variously composed. For you will find that the fibers of some muscles have a single nature, and others a double, such that they appear like many muscles layered on top of one another, but with fibers further lying crosswise to the length. All of this is useful to you for surgery, and also for the identification of functions. For in surgery we sometimes need to cut the muscles themselves because of deep abscesses, necrosis, or putrefaction. But the most useful purpose is to recognize what function is destroyed so that major wounds may be predicted in advance, where the whole muscle has been cut obliquely. If you predict the function that will be destroyed, you will be blameless even to critics who are likely to blame the loss on the physician's therapy rather than the pre-existing injury. Moreover, it is absolutely essential for accuracy in surgery to know the functions of the muscles, for the work of some parts is so important that the whole part becomes useless if it is deprived of this particular function, while other parts govern less important functions. Foreknowledge of such things is preferable, therefore, in order to cut the former muscles with caution, and the latter freely.

It is also preferable for incisions to be made along the fibers of the muscle, since incisions that are oblique to the fibers paralyze the function. (I call "oblique" those incisions that come at a right angle to the fibers.) Sometimes, though, oblique incisions are necessary, in order to access parts that have deep, narrow wounds, and at other times for other purposes. With regard to piercing wounds in the sinewy part, especially at the head or origin of the tendon, where, with the whole wound being narrow, there is a risk that the surface may be knit back together while the depths remain unhealed, we undertake to cut muscles for the sake of drainage. It is often the case, furthermore, that because of the position of the wound, the depth of the cut disappears and is concealed. For example, if a wound happens to be received when the arm is extended, it is impossible for a person to hold this position for the entire duration of the treatment, and one must take the most painless of positions at this time. Yet, in changing the position of the wound toward that which is more convenient in the present moment, the depth of the cut sometimes becomes invisible and is completely hidden, such that no **drug** can be applied to it and the serous fluid cannot flow out. In such cases, therefore, one must open up the wound, whether you wish to draw it open breadthwise or to join it back together. For this task it is essential to know both the arrangement of the fibers and the functions of the muscles.

The student of anatomy must do everything carefully [himself], even as far as skinning [the animal] [. . .].[9] My predecessors, for instance, were ignorant of eight muscles, since they entrusted the skinning of monkeys to others, as I did also at the beginning. Of these eight muscles, two have been provided by nature for the movement of the jaw, and two others attach the arms to the ribs.

They were absolutely ignorant of these muscles, therefore, and they were also ignorant about the use and tendons of the other four muscles. For each of these culminates in a tendon that is perfectly round, and this tendon finally comes to flatness with the delicacy of a membrane when it has been unfurled. The one associated with the foot is inserted under the sole, and that associated with the hand is inserted beneath the hairless palm. All anatomists plainly declare that the tendons in the hands bend the fingers, while those in the shin draw back the heel, and this is reasonably the case. For in the feet there is no single muscle that has been set apart from the outset by nature for the origin of this tendon. Rather, there is one bipartite muscle beginning in the calf, and one portion of this produces the tendon in question. With regard to the hands, the origin of the tendon is clear, but in skinning the

9. Some words from the Greek text are missing here.

animal it is torn away, since it is impossible to separate it from the smooth palm of the hand. Finding, therefore, that the tendon clearly grows from the muscle, and then seeing its lower end has been torn away, they carefully attempted to make inferences rather than conduct anatomy and thought that this was because it flexes the fingers, just like the muscles that lie beneath it.

Many things of this sort have been discovered throughout the entire animal, although neglected by the anatomists through their reluctance to dissect in detail, while they proclaimed the most plausible of opinions to themselves. One must not, then, wonder at the multitude of things that were unknown to them, given that the animal remained alive. For when those who are neglectful pass over what can be observed only through careful dissection, would they really make it their business then to cut or ligate parts of the animal while it is still living in order to learn which function is harmed?

At first, then, one of my attendants skinned the monkeys, a task that I avoided as clearly beneath me. But when one day I found a small piece of flesh by the armpit, being carried by and joined with the muscles there, and could not find a way to attach it to any of them, I decided that it would be better to skin another monkey with precision. I drowned it in water as I was accustomed to do in order to avoid bruising the parts in the neck, and tried to remove the skin alone from the surface, touching nothing of what lay beneath. In this way, I discovered a fine, membranous muscle that was stretched under the whole rib cage, having its origin from below, where it was extended beneath all the skin that covers the flanks. This muscle was continuous with the covering of the spine at the loin, which grew outward from the bone of the spine, having the nature of a "ligament"—as I call all such outgrowths from bones, just as I call those that grow from the brain and spinal marrow "nerves," and the tendinous ends of muscles "tendons." When once I had found this muscle, the nature of which will be described completely in proper sequence—I was all the more keen always to skin the animal myself. From this, therefore, I discovered that all those muscles I named a short while earlier had been brought into being by nature for significant purposes.

. . .

Book 3, Chapter 1. Whoever neglects the hard work of the art and shows more enthusiasm for the reasoning of sophists, therefore, has little interest in accurately recognizing the nature of the limbs. For they do not attempt to heal dislocations (with or without wounds), fractures, or mortification of the bones resulting from these cases. It goes without saying that those who do not show even enough interest to open a vein correctly also do not safely incise abscesses, cut out mortification, or remove projectiles and thorns. But I consider it valuable for beginners to train first in all such practices, because I see that their purpose is necessary, and that if the knowledge is trivial, as they think, then the shame of ignorance is worse.

The whole nature of the limbs is put together out of bones, ligaments, muscles, both arteries and veins, nerves, and, further, the covering that is common to all of these things, what is called the skin. The most celebrated anatomists have been tripped up with regard to the nature of the skin, as well as other parts, including both the innermost part of the hand and the underside of the foot, which they call the sole. On account of this ignorance, a man who had a considerable reputation for surgery, when excising the bone from a mortified wrist, robbed the palm of sensation. Not long ago, when I was with another surgeon who was operating on this very part of the body, I showed him the place where the tendon that grows beneath the hairless part of the hand first begins to widen and suggested that he guard against cutting through it. Because of this, the sensory power of the person being operated upon was preserved. But if the tendon should mortify and be destroyed, you will be blameless so long as you predicted the inevitable loss of sensation that would follow. In the same way also, if the whole tendon should be cut through by some sharp object from outside, as indeed happened to one individual, the physician will be without blame, so long as he has foretold how the matter will end.

It is appropriate, therefore, to learn these facts regarding the inside of the hand and the underside of the foot, and no few facts about the arteries, the veins, and the nerves. First, the sensory and motor powers of each digit do not all come from the same nerves. Second, of all the nerves going to these parts, whether in the arm through the upper arm and forearm, or in the leg through the thigh and calf, when they cut the nerve in the thigh or in the calf [. . .] they render some of the digits at the extremity of the foot and hand insensitive and immobile.[10] These things happen to them through their ignorance of the nerves.

Countless other accidents happen through ignorance of the arteries and veins, which some physicians are not sufficiently familiar with to protect against damaging them in surgery. Because of this, they sometimes cut through significant veins when excising bones or lancing abscesses, and at other times, by severing major arteries, they meet with unstoppable hemorrhage. Others, when engaged in bloodletting, cut into an artery, since they do not know which of the veins in the limbs have arteries lying underneath.

No one is ignorant—given his fame as a sophist—of the man I treated who had been deprived of sensation in his little finger and half of the middle finger. While the physicians from the Third Sect[11] who were taking care of him worried over his fingers, as though it was the fingers that had suffered injury, the bodily condition was located where the nerve first grows out of the spinal marrow. The Methodists, then, applied drugs—first those called "slackening," then those called "compound"—to the fingers, and did not bother themselves with the antecedent causes, but knew only that numbness and low sensitivity had come about of its own accord in the fingers and was progressing little by little.

The sick person, who was not benefitting from the drugs, shared the details of the treatment with me. I asked him, then, if there had not been some prior blow to his upper arm or forearm. Since he said that there was none, I asked the same question with regard to the upper part of his back. He said that he had fallen from a carriage three or four months earlier, and that when he was thrown to the ground he hit a projecting rock, which struck the upper part of his back. After intense suffering, he became pain free within seven days. Fifteen days after the initial blow, however, a slight sensation of insensitivity and numbness

10. Some words in the middle of the sentence are missing from the Greek text.
11. "Third Sect" refers to the Methodist school of medicine.

began in his fingers, and this kept growing right up to the present moment, not helped by the drugs. I reasoned, therefore, that a remnant of the swelling at the root of the nerve that went to the damaged fingers had hardened, and that while this itself was painless, it had become the underlying cause of the loss of sensitivity in the fingers to which it ran. And indeed, when I moved the application of drugs from the fingers to the area originally struck, I brought about a cure for the condition.

The day would run out if I narrated all the injuries I have seen happen to both feet and hands—soldiers wounded in battle, so-called single-combat fighters,[12] and many other private individuals—through the many chance upheavals of life, because of all those who disgrace themselves through ignorance of anatomy. Either they undertake surgery and sever a nerve that, while small, has significant power—because of which an underlying part loses sensation or movement, or sometimes both. Or, when someone is wounded through chance circumstances, they hold responsibility for the emergence of sickness, since they do not predict what will come about.

Observing, then, that knowledge of the limbs is most necessary—as is the anatomy of all the outer parts—but has been completely neglected, I judged it valuable to build on my existing anatomy of the muscles in the limbs by successively adding that of the arteries, veins, and nerves, and to encourage young people who are practicing dissection to train on those parts first. Every day they witness physicians who are educated as to the number and kind of cardiac valves, and the muscles of the tongue, and many other such things, but who, being ignorant of external anatomy, make serious mistakes in prognosis of—as well as in surgery on—conditions arising here, while those familiar with external anatomy, although ignorant of the rest, enjoy daily success.

Chapter 2. Let us next describe the appropriate manner to handle the dissection of vessels and nerves in the limbs . . .[13]

To begin the undertaking, strip the skin in a circle from the underlying tissues—not, indeed, however it happens to come off, as the leather dressers do, simultaneously removing the underlying membrane, through which the veins that nourish the skin travel. Instead, leave the membrane in place on the body, and cut away only the skin [that is wrapped around the underlying muscles],[14] using a sharp knife from the very beginning to separate the skin from the membrane. Having taken hold of any one part of the limb, remove the hair from a sufficiently large area for making the first incision. It will be easier to cut if you strip it of hair. It is probable that on the first try you will either leave some part of the skin uncut, or you will cut through the underlying membrane. Attempting a second and third time—and

---

12. I.e., gladiators. Early in his career, Galen served as a physician to the gladiators in his native city of Pergamum.

13. We have omitted a short section here where Galen discusses a few specialized points of Greek anatomical terminology.

14. The text in square brackets was likely added by a later scribe who copied the text.

having increased or lessened the depth of the cut—you will quickly learn the appropriate proportion of the incision from this experimentation. (Obviously, I am calling "proportionate" the incision that neither leaves behind any part of the skin, nor cuts the underlying membrane . . .[15])

In order to separate the skin from the membrane, press the knife hard against the skin because if you incline the knife toward the membrane, you will injure it. But if, scraping the membrane from the skin, you should at some point injure the skin, you will not have compromised the task ahead. Indeed, applying substantial force will not cause injury to the skin, but only a superficial scratch. This task requires quite a bit of time. Whenever you demonstrate the parts of the arm to someone who is eager to learn, therefore, peel the membrane from the skin in advance, as instructed above, before the spectator arrives. If, however, you wish to share the process of dissection with an associate who himself wishes to demonstrate it to others at some later time, then make the attempt in his presence. It is a task that requires a great deal of accuracy and is suitable for a man who loves hard work and learning. I myself have often entrusted the task to an associate and found the membrane torn in many places, and elsewhere still clinging to the skin. Whenever a part is in such a condition, it is no longer possible to see the blood vessels and small nerves beneath the skin, above all in monkeys. They do not disappear in horses, donkeys, mules, and cows, on account of their size, but if the membrane is torn from the continuous tissue underneath, then it is no longer possible to make a clear investigation. In small animals, meanwhile, everything is destroyed if any of the events described above happen to the membrane.

Strip the whole arm of skin, therefore, while the entire membrane, which comes after the skin, remains wrapped around the underlying tissues. Examine the surface blood vessels and nerves in this arm immediately, before the membrane dries out. These do not appear equally in every instance, since the nerves are by nature thinner in some monkeys, as in some humans, and also because some animals have fat, while others do not. The nerves, then, can be seen more clearly in thin bodies, and are hidden in those that have fat. The blood vessels directly beneath the skin are most visible when the monkey has a large quantity of blood, but become difficult to see when the animal's blood is scarce. Regardless, however, let these parts be examined in all cases, and try to memorize the roots and passage of the surface nerves, so that whenever you need to make an incision, you can situate the cut along their length. In this way you will sever at most one nerve, and perhaps none at all. If you thrust the knife crosswise, meanwhile, you will cut across many of them at the same time. And try above all to keep away from the roots, knowing that, just as it is in the case of trees—where, in cutting a few branches or boughs, you might injure the plant, while if you cut through the crown of the root, then you destroy the whole—so it is also with regard to nerves. If you cut toward the root, you will render insensitive the whole region that received

15. We have omitted another short section here where Galen discusses specialized points regarding Greek anatomical terminology.

its sensory power from the nerve that has been split. If, indeed, you remember the anatomy of the muscles, which I went through in Book One, you will learn now how easily to locate the source of the nerves that spread through the skin.

TEXT 35. SORANUS, *WOMEN'S HEALTH*[16] SELECTION (1.2–3)

In Women's Health, **Soranus of Ephesus** *(second century CE) is guided by two main concerns: protecting women's health and managing pregnancy and childbirth. In the selection below, Soranus offers advice on the ideal features of a* maia *(a word often translated as "midwife," but that we think is best translated as "**obstetrician**").*

SOURCE: Translation by Molly Jones-Lewis based on the Greek text from Paul Burguière, Danielle Gourevitch, and Yves Malinas, *Soranus d'Éphèse, Maladies des femmes, Livre 2* (Paris: Les Belles Lettres, 1990).

Book 1, Chapter 2. Who is a fitting candidate to become an **obstetrician?**
At this point, a reckoning is worthwhile of the sort of people who are best suited to be taught, so as not to expend effort pointlessly. The ideal candidate is a woman who is literate, sharp of mind with a good memory, fond of hard work, regular in her habits and, as a general rule, unimpaired in her senses, with straight limbs, strong, and, as some say, with long, slender fingers on her hands and fingernails trimmed short.

She should be literate so she can take up the art through theory. She should be sharp of mind so she can easily follow what is being said and what is happening around her. She should have a good memory so that she will retain the knowledge passed down to her (for knowledge comes with memory's grasp). And she should be fond of hard work to persevere in the face of the eventualities that happen (for a man's endurance is needed if she intends to take up such knowledge). And she should be regular in her habits since she is going to be entrusted with household matters and the secrets of life, and because less reputable women have a tendency to use their medical profession as a cover for aiding and abetting unethical conspiracies.

She should also be unimpaired in her senses since she needs to be able to see things, hear the responses to her questions, and identify some objects through her sense of touch. She should have straight limbs so as to perform necessary tasks unimpaired, and she should be strong because she manages a double burden in her labors. And she should have long, slender fingers on her hands and fingernails trimmed short to help her reach the recesses of the body to examine inflammations. However, this result can be achieved by more extensive practice and training in those procedures.

16. This text has previously been translated with the title *Gynecology,* but this traditional title may give the misleading impression that the text is only concerned with women's reproductive system, and not with women's health more generally.

Book 1, Chapter 3. Who is the best obstetrician?

One must now speak to the qualities that make for the best obstetrician, so that those who are best at this can recognize themselves, and beginners can look at them as role models, and the general public can know which ones to call when they need to.

In general, we call an obstetrician competent if she performs the essential tasks of the medical profession, but we call her best when she has also gained mastery of medical theory to support her authority. And we would have even better grounds for calling her the best obstetrician for being well practiced in all the branches of treatment (because she must treat some cases with regimen, some with surgery, and some with **drugs**), for being able to give advice, to observe both common and specific features of cases, and from this understanding what is useful, not from causes or repeated observation of general symptoms or anything like that.

More specifically, she does not change course at each shift of the manifestations of the condition, but explains what is happening during the course of the condition; is unflappable, and unflustered in dangerous circumstances; is well able to provide clear reasons for her remedies, offering advice to women who are ill; and is sympathetic. And it is not essential, as some claim, that she has given birth herself in the past, so that she will be able to empathize with the suffering of women giving birth. Women are not more sympathetic just because they have given birth.

She must be in good physical shape because of the nature of her job and need not, as some say, necessarily be young, because some young women are also out of shape and, conversely, some who are not young are in good physical shape. She must also be self-possessed and sober at all times because it is never certain when she will be called on to treat women who are in danger. She needs to have a calm personality since she is destined to share in many of the secrets of life. She should not be greedy and, therefore, will not give an abortifacient unethically, for money. She is not overly intimidated by the supernatural, and so will not pass over an appropriate treatment because of a dream, omen, customary rite, or common superstition.

Additionally, she must maintain the softness of her hands, protecting them also from wool-working, which can toughen the skin, and cultivating this level of softness with balms if they are not naturally soft. The best obstetrician must be like this.

TEXT 36. INSCRIPTIONS RELATED TO PHYSICIANS

Hundreds of thousands of inscriptions—stones and monuments inscribed with a textual message—survive from the ancient Greek and Roman worlds. Many of these carved texts were epitaphs written to memorialize the dead (like inscriptions in modern-day cemeteries) or found on public monuments honoring a person who contributed to the well-being of the community. The inscriptions below are a selection of funerary epitaphs or honorary inscriptions for ancient medical professionals. Several of the inscriptions were written as original poems, while others are full of commonplace phrases and standard abbreviations.

Square brackets in the translation indicate spots where portions of an inscription are missing because the inscription has been damaged or where one or more words are implied. In many cases, editors have been able to hypothesize or restore missing sections of the inscriptions.[17]

SOURCE: Translation by Jared Secord based on the Greek and Latin.

Funerary monument dedicated to Phanostrate. Mainland Greece. c. 350 BCE. IG II².6873. Greek. (See fig. 56.)

Phanos[trate]
of Melite[18]
Phanostrate, obstetrician and physician (*maia kai iatros*), lies here,
Causing pain to no one and missed by everyone when she died.

Honorary decree for Nicander of Halicarnassus. Delos (Greek island in the Aegean Sea). 2nd century BCE. IG XI.4.775. Greek.

It was resolved by the council and people, as Telemnestus, son of Aristides, said: since the physician Nicander of Halicarnassus,[19] son of Parmeniscus, continues to be a good man concerning the temple and people of Delos and provides service both in public and private to the Delians who meet him in [ ][20] [and] has shown himself to be honorable to those who have need of him, it has been resolved by the council and people that Nicander of Halicarnassus, son of Parmeniscus, shall be a public guest and benefactor of the temple and the Delians, both himself and his descendants. They shall have the right of owning land and buildings in Delos, and the privilege of having the front seats[21] and first access to the council and people after sacred matters. They shall be given by the people . . .[22]

Funerary monument dedicated to Gaius and Naevia Clara. Rome. 1st century BCE. AE 2001, 263. Latin.

Gaius Naevius Philippus, physician and surgeon, freedman of Gaius.

Naevia Clara, freedwoman of Gaius, physician and a learned woman. 11.5 feet wide, 16 feet long.[23]

17. The inscriptions are identified by their standard abbreviations. Readers seeking to identify these abbreviations should consult the following list: https://antiquite.ens.psl.eu/IMG/file/pdf_guide_epi/abreviations_guide.pdf.
18. Melite was a neighborhood located in the center of Athens.
19. Halicarnassus is modern-day Bodrum in southwestern Türkiye.
20. Something is missing from the inscription here.
21. This privilege gave Nicander and his descendants the right to sit at the front at the theater, in assembly meetings, and at similar public events.
22. The damaged inscription breaks off here.
23. These measurements are the dimensions of the tomb.

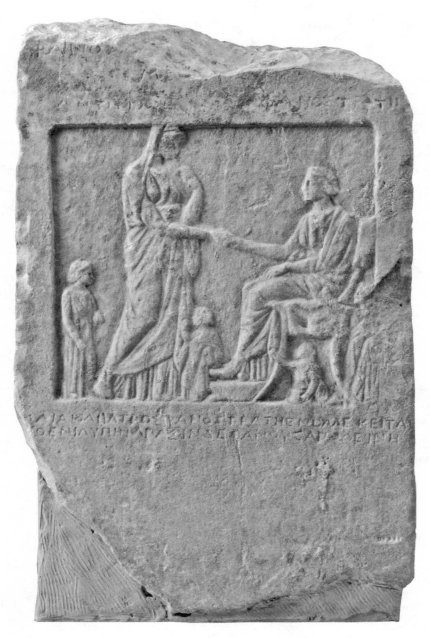

FIGURE 56 Fourth-century BCE relief from the grave stele of the obstetrician-physician Phanostrate. The seated Phanostrate greets a woman named Antiphile, with smaller figures (who could be children, or their smaller stature could denote their status as slaves or assistants) surrounding the two women. Sculpture Collection, National Archaeological Museum, Athens (inv. no. 993). Photo credit: Irini Miari. © Hellenic Ministry of Education and Religious Affairs, Culture and Sports/Hellenic Organisation of Cultural Resources Development.

Honorary inscription for Antiochis. Tlos (modern-day southwestern Türkiye). 1st
century BCE. TAM II, 595. Greek.

Antiochis, daughter of Diodotus of Tlos, who was recognized by the council and people of
Tlos for her experience in the medical art, set up her own statue.

Commemorative inscription for Publius Decimius Eros Merula.
Modern-day Assisi (central Italy). c. 1–50 CE. CIL XI.5400. Latin.

Publius Decimius Eros Merula, freedman of Publius,[24] clinical physician, surgeon, eye doctor, *sevir*.[25] He gave 50,000 sesterces for his freedom.[26] For his position as a *sevir* he gave
2,000 sesterces. For putting up statues in the temple of Hercules he gave 30,000 sesterces.
For paving roads he gave 37,000 sesterces to the public treasury. On the day before he died,
he left an inheritance of 800,000 (?) sesterces . . .[27]

Honorary inscription to Tiberius Claudius Alcimus erected by his
student Restituta. Rome. 1st century CE. IG XIV.1751. Greek.

To Tiberius Claudius Alcimus, physician of Caesar. Restituta made [this monument] for her
patron and teacher, a good and worthy man. He lived 82 years.

Funerary monument dedicated to Marcus Naevius Harmodius.
Rome. c. 100 CE. CIL III.2887. Latin.

To the spirits of the dead. To Marcus Naevius Harmodius, physician of the 10th Praetorian
cohort,[28] who lived 55 years. His children Marcus Naevius Naevianus and Naevia Harmodia
and his freedwoman wife Naevia Gluconis made [this monument] for a most dutiful father
and themselves and their freedmen and freedwomen and their descendants. Well deserving.
They made [this monument]. 10 feet wide, 10 feet long.[29]

24. The four names listed here for Publius Decimius Eros Merula show that he was a Greek
slave who took on the name of his former owner when he received his freedom.

25. A *sevir* was literally "someone who was part of a group of six men" (the Latin word in the
inscription is written as VIvir, which combines the Roman numeral for six [VI] with the Latin word
for "man" [*vir*]). The status of the *sevir* was between a regular person and the higher decurian or
equestrian classes. As this inscription suggests, the title of a *sevir* could be given to wealthy
freedmen (former slaves) who received recognition for the financial contributions they made to
their community.

26. Sesterces were Roman coins. The sums mentioned here are large, demonstrating that Publius Decimius Eros Merula was likely as wealthy as some members of the Roman upper classes.

27. The damaged inscription breaks off here, and the amount of money that Publius Decimius
Eros Merula left to the town is unclear.

28. The Praetorian Guard was an elite unit of the Roman army charged with protecting the
emperor and members of his family.

29. These measurements are the dimensions of the tomb.

Funerary monument dedicated to Julia Saturnia. Modern-day Spain.
c. 150–225 CE. CIL II.497; ILS 7802. Latin.

A sacred rite to the spirits of the dead. To Julia Saturnia, aged 45, an incomparable wife, the best physician, and most pious woman. Cassius Philippus, her husband, [made this monument] in honor of her merits. She is buried here. May the earth be light upon you.

Funerary monument dedicated to Pantheia. Pergamum (modern-day Bergama in western Türkiye). c. 100–200 CE. H. W. Pleket, Epigraphica, vol. II: Texts on the Social History of the Greek World (Leiden: Brill, 1969), no. 20. Greek.

Farewell, lady Pantheia, from your husband. After your fate, I have inconsolable grief for your destructive death. For Hera, goddess of marriage, never saw such a wife: your beauty, wisdom, and self-control. You gave birth to children completely like me, you cared for your husband and children, and you guided the rudder of life in the house and raised up our shared fame in healing, and though you were a woman you were not inferior to my skill. For this reason your husband Glycon has built this tomb for you, who also buried here the body of the immortal Philadelphus.[30] And I myself will also lie here when I die, since I shared my bed with you only when I was alive, so I may also cover myself in shared earth.

Honorary inscription for city physician Menophilus. Cadyanda.
c. 100–200 CE. TAM II, 663. Greek.

The council and the people of Cadyanda[31] honored with a gold crown and a bronze statue Menophilus, son of Dositheus, of Cadyanda, of the tribe Apollonias, for his benefactions, a good and noble man distinguished with all the virtue of his ancestors who lives wisely and faithfully and who practices medicine nobly, successfully, and blamelessly with the greatest experience. He was chief city official voluntarily and took on many expenses with his own money.

Funerary monument dedicated to Domnina. North-central Asia Minor (modern-day Türkiye). Between 100 and 300 CE. H. W. Pleket, Epigraphica, vol. II: Texts on the Social History of the Greek World (Leiden: Brill, 1969), no. 26. Greek.

You have hurried off to be among the immortals, Domnina, and neglected your husband. You have raised up your body to the heavenly stars. No one among humankind will say that you died, but that the immortals snatched you up because you saved your homeland from illnesses. Farewell and rejoice in the Elysian Fields.[32] But you have left behind pains and endless laments for your loved ones.

---

30. Philadelphus was Glycon's father, and also a physician. An epitaph for Philadelphus is inscribed on the same monument for Pantheia.

31. Cadyanda is now called Üzümlü in modern-day southwestern Türkiye.

32. The Elysian Fields were a place of paradise where especially virtuous people were thought to go after they died.

Funerary monument dedicated to Geminia. Northern Africa.
3rd century CE. CIL VIII.806. Latin.

Savior of everyone through medicine. Geminia . . .[33]

Funerary poem dedicated to Lucius Sabinus Primigenius. Iguvium (central Italy).
Uncertain date from the Roman imperial period. CIL XI.5836; ILS 7794. Latin.

Lucius Sabinus Primigenius, freedman of Lucius.
Born from Iguvium, a physician who visited many city forums
Reputed for my knowledge of the art, and my more famous honesty.
In the strength of my youth while I was still maturing Fortune
Abandoned me and inflicted a sudden funeral pyre.
The ashes of the flame went to a grave in Clusium,[34]
And my patron restored my bones to my ancestral land.

33. The damaged inscription breaks off after mentioning Geminia, the woman physician to whom the funerary monument seems to have been dedicated.
34. Clusium is modern-day Chiusi in central Italy.

TWELVE

Patients

When reading medical sources, we only occasionally hear the voices of patients. **Galen** sometimes reported his patients' descriptions of their symptoms—for example, "His fingers were difficult to move and numb and [were] making a crackling noise, as he himself called it," and "Recently someone said, when he was stung by a scorpion, that he felt as if pelted by hailstones" (*On the Affected Parts* 3.11 [8.195K]). Most of the time, however, medical sources privileged the perspectives of physicians. In this chapter, therefore, we turn to letters, inscriptions, and other sources that highlight the perspectives of sick and suffering people (see Texts 37–39).

Letters give us a unique window into ancient people's experience of sickness and suffering. In a set of letters between the Roman rhetorician Marcus Cornelius **Fronto** and the Roman emperors Marcus Aurelius and Antoninus Pius, for instance, the men trade complaints about chronic knee pain, stiff necks, bouts of fever, diarrhea, and a close encounter with a scorpion, while also expressing concern about family members' ailments. So prevalent were these experiences that the Stoic philosopher **Seneca** asserted that suffering and sickness were the inescapable and normal conditions of life. Writing to a friend with a bladder ailment, Seneca reminded him that such illnesses were to be expected, since they were built into the very structure of human life: "A long life includes all these troubles, just as a long journey includes dust and mud and rain" (*Letter* 96). In another letter, Seneca again noted the precarity of health, illustrated by the fact that his friend Cornelius Senecio, in the course of a single day, felt well enough in the morning to sit bedside with a sick companion and then suddenly took ill and died later that night. Finally, letters also reveal the toll precarious health could take on friends and family. We read, for example, that Seneca's wife Paulina worried about his health and urged him to take better care of himself because "her very life-breath comes and goes with [his] own" (*Letter* 104).

Constantly battling sickness, injury, impairment, and pain might explain why some ancient people sought help from all the resources at their disposal. Extant inscriptions indicate that sometimes people went to both the gods and physicians in search of healing. Proclus of Sinope and the unknown dedicator of an inscription from Laodicea, for example, extend gratitude to the gods Fortune (Tuche/Tyche), **Asclepius,** and **Hygieia,** as well as to their physicians (Text 39). Perhaps this was a strategy to maximize their chances of recovery or because they understood the gods and physicians to work in concert with one another.

Yet other sources revealing the perspectives of sick and suffering people indicate that many feared and distrusted physicians. What specifically were patients worried about? Many sick and suffering people recoiled at the painful treatments their physicians recommended, calling them "cruel" and "wicked torture." The Ionian philosopher Heraclitus, for example, argued that treatments such as **cautery** and surgery "torment the sick . . . having the same effects [on patients] as the illness itself" (F81 Graham). Similarly, the North African bishop Augustine told a story about his friend Innocentius, who was so traumatized by an unsuccessful operation to remove an anal fistula that he was reluctant to undergo the procedure a second time, despite the fact that the condition was excruciatingly painful. While it might have been worthwhile to endure medical treatments if they worked, patients could never be sure they would recover. Take, for instance, the treatment of Socles, who, "promising to set Diodorus' crooked back straight, piled three solid stones, each four feet square, on the hunchback's spine. As a result, Diodorus did in fact become straight as a ruler, but [in the process] he was crushed and died" (*Greek Anthology* 4.129). And in cases when the physician did more harm than good, patients and their families had no legal recourse because the profession of medicine was immune from prosecution. Hence many came to liken physicians to "murderers" and "undertakers."

Beyond the painful treatments and bad outcomes, patients were not sure they could trust physicians who were unreliable and self-interested. We hear numerous accounts of physicians who abandoned their patients midtreatment or who refused to treat certain ailments (likely because the physician regarded the illness as terminal or chronic, thus falling outside the purview of medicine as explained in Text 3, Hippocratic Corpus, *On the Art of Medicine* 8). For example, in an inscription by Felix Asinianus, he reports that he was forced to seek help from the temple of Bona Dea because he was abandoned by his physicians (Text 39). Patients were likewise distrustful of physicians who appeared to be motivated by fame and money more so than healing. In his travels, a fourth-century writer called Pliny (not to be confused with Pliny the Elder) reported witnessing many physicians selling useless remedies at outrageous prices, and also prescribing treatments they knew would prolong an illness so they could earn more money. Additionally, Pliny reported that these physicians engaged in showy debates that revealed them to be more concerned with proving their superior knowledge than arriving at a diagnosis and treatment that would benefit the patient.

Given these fears, we better understand why some sick and suffering people turned to religious figures. We have, for example, a record of a man petitioning the god Priapus for help because "when my penis was injured I feared the surgeon's hand" (*Carmina Priapea*

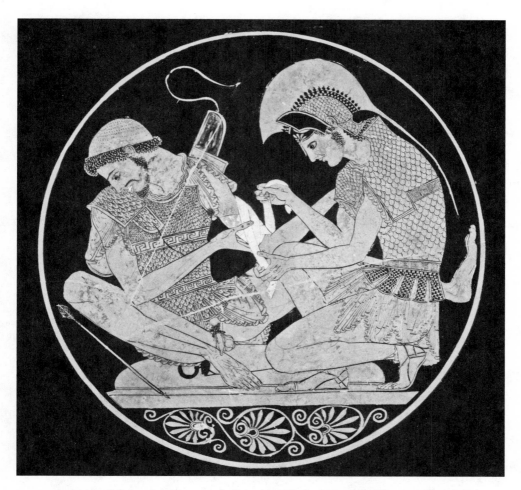

FIGURE 57 Attic red-figure drinking cup (kylix), 550 BCE, depicting Achilles wrapping a bandage around the arm of Patroclus, who clenches his teeth in pain. The arrow to the left suggests that Patroclus may have been struck by an arrowhead. (The painting presumably depicts a scene in the Trojan War, but it is not a recognizable scene in the Homeric epic *The Iliad*.) The depiction here highlights the fact that soldiers sometimes would have tended to each other's injuries when a medic was not available or when there were too many injuries for medics to handle. From Vulci, Italy. © Antikensammlung, Staatliche Museen zu Berlin—Preußischer Kulturbesitz (inv. no. F 2278). Photo credit: Johannes Laurentius. Art Resource, NY.

XXXVII). An inscription by the freedwoman Prepousa indicates that she chose to petition the gods in order to avoid the high costs of physicians (see Text 39). Others turned to religious healing after physicians failed them. For example, a woman who had been suffering from hemorrhages for twelve years and who "had endured much under many physicians and had spent all that she had and was no better, but rather grew worse" (Mark 5:26) eventually decided to turn to the Jewish holy man, Jesus (see fig. 52).

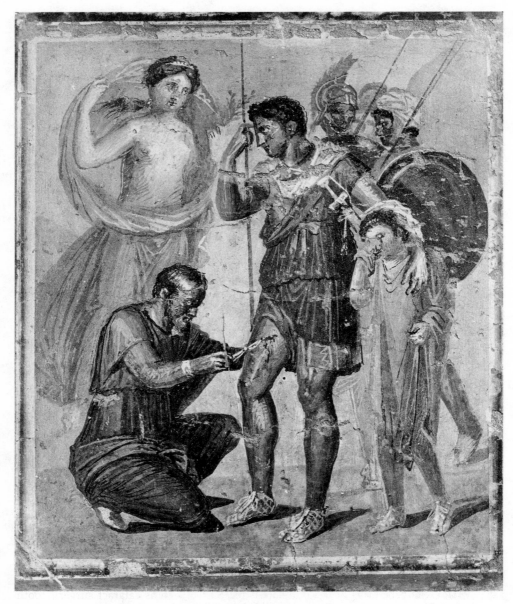

FIGURE 58 First-century CE fresco depicting the physician Iapyx attempting to extract an arrowhead from the thigh of Aeneas using forceps. As in Virgil's *Aeneid* 12.383, from which this scene is drawn, Aeneas is "unmoved by tears" as he endures the "cruel pain" of the injury and of the procedure. House of Siricus (VII 1,25), Pompeii. Naples Archaeological Museum (inv. no 9009). Wellcome Collection. Attribution 4.0 International (CC BY 4.0).

Many sick people also opted to be treated at home, with the women or a slave medic of the household being tasked with such work. Household caregivers grew medicinal plants in home gardens, courtyards, or on windowsills (see fig. 9). Neighbors swapped medicinal recipes and ingredients and consulted collections of remedies, such as the recipes Pliny compiled from his travels (Text 28) or the recipe books stored in the spice warehouse in Rome.

Our sources occasionally give us glimpses into the kinds of care and assistance provided by family, slaves, and friends (see fig. 57). For example, in his will, Domitius Tullus, who was "crippled and deformed in every limb," commended his young and healthy wife and his slaves who hand-fed him, cleaned his teeth, and turned him in his bed. Their dedication and care, Tullus remarked, sustained his will to live (Pliny the Younger, *Letter* 8.18). For people with chronic mobility or visual impairments, we hear about accommodations provided by slaves or friends who would carry the impaired to business appointments or who would read aloud to them. We even hear of members of the household engaging in complicated procedures. For instance, when a woman was suffering from severe pain, another woman inserted her hand into the opening of her womb and withdrew a large, rough stone (see Text 8, Hippocratic Corpus, *On Epidemics* 5.25).

Even when sick and suffering people called on physicians to treat their loved ones, they still appear to be deeply engaged in the care provided. Our sources describe the bedsides of the sick populated with family, slaves, and friends. They informed the physician about the patients' symptoms, what brought on the illness, and the course the illness had taken. They weighed in about the course of treatment. For example, when Seneca felt a fever coming on, he considered the advice of his elder brother alongside that of his physician (see Text 38, Letter 104). And they assisted the physician—who might visit only once a day—in providing care. Galen tells us of friends who "busied themselves applying wet dressings to [their loved one's] head" when he had a fever and was delirious (*On the Affected Parts* 4.2 [8.227K]). With respect to his own patients, Galen regularly describes members of households and friends feeding, bathing, and administering medicine, as well as keeping careful watch over them throughout the night. Even when family and friends are not mentioned in medical sources, it is easy to imagine ways in which they would have been called upon to assist. For instance, when we read about the symptoms associated with spinal injury—including incontinence, weakness in the lower limbs, or loss of control over the full body—we surmise that such symptoms would have required around-the-clock care to clean the patient and to assist with lost functions. Additionally, as we read about treatments such as cataract surgery, tooth extraction, and bloodletting, we presume that members of the household would have been required to assist in holding down the patient to keep them still during the procedures.

While the patient, family, and friends sometimes assisted the physician, they also pushed back when they disagreed with the physician's judgment or were unhappy with the care given to their loved ones. Galen recounts that members of a household who found his physician friend incompetent refused to allow him to finish his treatment or even to touch the patient again. Galen mentions another physician who worried that if his patient didn't recover, he "risked being torn apart" by the patient's friends (*A Method of Medicine to*

Glaucon 10.3 [10.676K]). Such violence was likely rare, and antagonism with one's physician was more likely expressed as simple disobedience. For example, Galen tells a story of a patient who agreed to comply, but as soon as the physician left, the patient and his friends erupted in laughter and disdain, with no intention of following his instructions. Our extant medical literature is replete with physicians' complaints about their patients' refusal to take medicine they found distasteful, patients who did not rest as long as they should have when recovering from an injury, and patients who, when confronted about their disobedience, lied (see, for example, Text 42, Hippocratic Corpus, *Decorum* 14). Thus ancient physicians prized patients who showed proper submission to and reverence for the expertise of physicians, as well as patients who mustered the courage and fortitude necessary to endure painful or distasteful medical treatments. In fact, the term "patient" refers to such idealized qualities (the Latin *patiens* meaning "one who suffers," "one who endures suffering with forbearance and courage," and "one who is submissive"). These qualities were illustrated, for example, in how the hero Aeneas positioned his body to best assist the physician Iapyx as he attempted to extract an arrowhead from his thigh: he submits his body to his physician and endures the painful treatment without flinching, groaning, or tears (see fig. 58).

In antiquity there was a recognition that patients had power and agency, whether in their ability to provide home health care, their process of choosing and hiring a physician, or their acquiescence or disobedience of the physician's instructions. As made clear in the **Hippocratic** "triangle of medicine," the patient, the illness, and the physician were equally important. For that reason, physicians were required to appease, satisfy, collaborate, and negotiate with their clients, necessitating that physicians hone their relational skills (on some of these strategies, see Text 42).

TEXT 37. FRONTO, *LETTERS* (SELECTIONS OF LETTERS TO MARCUS AURELIUS AND ANTONINUS PIUS)

*Marcus Cornelius **Fronto** (c. 95–166 CE) was a lawyer and advocate, and the tutor of Marcus Aurelius, who was the Roman emperor from 161 to 180 CE. The two men exchanged letters in which they discussed philosophy, their families, and mundane aspects of day-to-day life. The letters below focus on the health complaints that Fronto and Marcus (as well as their relatives) suffered over a period of about fifteen years. The final letter included below is from Fronto to the adoptive father of Marcus Aurelius, Antoninus Pius, who was emperor from 138 to 161 CE.*

SOURCE: Translation by Christopher Lougheed based on the Latin text from Michael P. J. van den Hout, *M. Cornelius Frontonis Epistulae* (Leipzig: Teubner, 1988).

4.11. Marcus Aurelius to Fronto. 148 CE
By the gods' will, we seem to have obtained reason to hope for health: flowing of the bowel has stopped, the minor fevers are beaten back. Nonetheless, there is leanness, and something of a minor cough remains. You understand immediately that I am writing this to you

about our dear little Faustina,[1] on whose behalf I have been occupied enough. As to whether your health settles itself in accordance with my wish, let me know, my teacher.

5.21. Fronto to Marcus Aurelius. Between 147 and 156 CE
To my lord.

After you were gone, I was seized by a pain in the knee, though indeed one so moderate that I could both walk tentatively and make use of a carriage. This night, a more violent pain came on, but in such a way that I can easily bear it lying down, unless something further should assail me. I hear that your Augusta[2] is afflicted. I, for my part, entrust her health to the gods. Farewell, sweetest lord. Greet the lady.[3]

5.23. Marcus Aurelius to Fronto. Between 139 and 152 CE
To my teacher.

I spent the last days like this: my sister was suddenly seized by such pain in her female parts that her face was terrible for me to see. My mother, in turn, in that moment of anxiety, was careless and banged a rib on a corner of a wall. With that blow she seriously affected both herself and us. I myself, when I went to lie down, came upon a scorpion in my bed. I took care, however, to kill it before I lay down on top of it. As for you, if you are in properly good health, it is a consolation. My mother is now in less serious condition, by the gods' will. Farewell, my best, most pleasant teacher. My lady greets you.

5.25. Fronto to Marcus Aurelius. Between 145 and 161 CE
To my lord.

Just now, Victorinus[4] reveals to me that your lady is more feverishly hot than yesterday. Cratia[5] was announcing that everything was less serious. I, for my part, have not seen you for this reason, that I am weak from a head cold. Tomorrow morning, however, I will come to you at home. At the same time, if it is opportune, I will also visit the lady.

5.26. Marcus Aurelius to Fronto. Between 145 and 161 CE
To my teacher.

Faustina[6] was feverishly hot today as well, and indeed it seems to me that I have perceived it more today. But, with the gods' help, she herself puts my mind more at ease, because she adapts herself so compliantly to us. As for you, if you had been able, naturally, you would

1. Marcus's daughter Faustina, who was born the year prior.
2. Marcus's wife Faustina, who held the title Augusta.
3. References to "the lady" in the letters are to one of three women, depending on the date of the letter: Marcus's birth mother, his adoptive mother, or his wife.
4. Aufidius Victorinus, a Roman senator who was one of Fronto's students, and eventually his son-in-law.
5. Cratia was Fronto's daughter, and the wife of Victorinus.
6. This Faustina was Marcus's wife.

have come. I take pleasure, my teacher, that now you are able and that you promise that you will come. Farewell, my most pleasant teacher.

5.28. Marcus Aurelius to Fronto. Between 139 and 156 CE
To my teacher, greetings.

I seem to have passed through the night without a fever. I took food not unwillingly, and now I am doing very well. What the night may bring, we will find out. But, my teacher, from your own recent anxiety, you certainly appreciate how I felt when I learned that you were seized with pain in your neck. Farewell, my most pleasant teacher. My mother greets you.

5.55. Fronto to Marcus Aurelius. Between 139 and 156 CE
To my lord.

I was stricken with an ailment of the bowels to the point that I was losing my voice, I was gasping, then I was choked by shortness of breath, finally my veins gave out, and without any pulse in my veins, I lost consciousness. Finally, I was mourned as dead by the people closest to me, and I had no sensation for a while. No time or opportunity was granted to the physicians for restoring or soothing me with a warm bath, cold water, or food, except that, after evening, I swallowed the smallest of crumbs moistened with wine. Thus, I was completely revived. After this, I did not receive my voice back for three whole days. But now, with the help of the gods, I am very pleased with my health, I move about easily, I shout out clearly. Finally, if the gods lend their help, I intend to be transported in a carriage tomorrow. If I bear the flint pavement easily, I will hurry to you as best I can. When I see you I will truly be alive. I will set out from Rome on the 7th day before the Kalends,[7] if the gods grant their help. Farewell, sweetest, most desired lord, best reason for my life. Greet the lady.

5.59. Fronto to Marcus Aurelius. Between 147 and 156 CE
While my slave boys were carrying me from the baths in a sedan-chair as they are accustomed to do, they carelessly struck me against the burning-hot entrance of the bath. Thus, my knee was at the same time scraped and burnt. Afterwards, a swelling emerged from the sore. The physicians saw to it that I kept to my bed. This matter, if it seems appropriate to you, you will relay to the lord your father, only if it seems appropriate. Also, tomorrow it will be necessary for me to stand by a friend in court. Therefore it is with today's leisure and quiet that I will prepare myself for tomorrow's work. Our Victorinus will plead in court, so you should not suppose that I will. Farewell, sweetest lord. Greet the lady.

5.60. Marcus Aurelius to Fronto. Between 147 and 156 CE
To my teacher, greetings.

You have increased my worries, which I hope that you will alleviate as soon as possible once the pains in your knee and in the swelling are settled. As for me, however, the poor health of the lady my mother does not allow me to rest. Added to this, there is the approach-

7. In the Roman calendar, the Kalends was the first day of each month.

ing prospect of childbirth for Faustina. But we ought to trust in the gods. Farewell, my teacher most pleasant to me. My mother greets you.

5.69. Fronto to Marcus Aurelius. Between 139 and 156 CE
To my lord.

It is the third day that, through the night, I am suffering a biting in my stomach with diarrhea. Indeed, this past night I was so troubled that I was not able to go out, but rather I kept to my bed. The physicians recommend that I make use of a bath. I pray to the gods that you may celebrate many birthdays. Farewell, lord. Greet the lady.

5.71. Fronto to Marcus Aurelius. Between 139 and 156 CE
To my lord.

I have a wretched throat, due to which I have also been feverishly hot all night. The pain in my knee is moderate. Farewell, lord. Greet the lady.

5. Fronto to Antoninus Pius. 161 CE

I wish to bargain away a part of my life, emperor, so that I might embrace you on the most happy and most welcome day of the beginning of your reign, a day which I consider the birthday of my health, honor, and freedom from care. But serious pain in my shoulder and, much more serious, in my neck, has so stricken me that until now I can barely lower or raise or turn myself, so immobile I find my neck to be. But, among my Lares and Penates and my personal gods,[8] I have both repaid and taken up vows and I have prayed that next year I might embrace you twice on this day, that twice I might kiss your chest and hand, performing at the same time the function for the past and the present year.

TEXT 38. SENECA, *LETTERS* (LETTERS 54, 104.1–3, 6)

*Lucius Annaeus **Seneca** (c. 4 BCE–65 CE) was a Roman philosopher and politician. He served as a tutor and adviser to the emperor Nero (who reigned from 54 to 68 CE) until he was ordered to commit suicide for suspected treason. Seneca subscribed to the Stoic school of philosophy, advocating that people should accept with equanimity and live in harmony with whatever circumstances fate dealt them. The two letters below, written to Seneca's friend Lucilius, provide a window into Seneca's philosophical outlook with respect to his own health issues. In Letter 54 Seneca followed the Stoic approach to adversity, accepting a chronic ailment that seems to have been something like asthma attacks. In Letter 104 (the start of which is included here), however, Seneca deliberates about actions he can take to ward off a fever in deference to his wife's fears for his life.*

SOURCE: Translation by Margaret Graver and A. A. Long based on the Latin text from L. D. Reynolds, *Seneca, Ad Lucilium Epistulae morales*, vols. 1–2 (Oxford: Clarendon Press, 1965). Latin. First published in *Seneca: Letters on Ethics, To Lucilius* (Chicago: University of Chicago

---

8. The Lares and Penates were Roman household gods.

Letter 54: From Seneca to Lucilius

Greetings

1. Ill health had given me a long respite; then suddenly it assailed me again. "What was the trouble?" you ask—and well you may, for there is no illness with which I am unacquainted. But there is one that has me in its charge, so to speak. Why should I use its Greek name?[9] I can call it wheezing; that fits well enough.

Its attack is quite brief, like a squall; it is usually over within the hour. No one can be at last gasp for very long! 2. Every bodily discomfort, every peril, has passed through me; and nothing, I think, is harder to bear. How could it not be? Anything else is just being sick; this is pushing out one's life breath. For this reason doctors call it "the rehearsal for death": the constriction sometimes achieves what it has so often attempted. 3. Do you think that I am glad to be writing these things to you, glad that I escaped? If I delight in this cessation as if it were a return to health, I am as laughable as the person who thinks he has won his case just because his hearing has been postponed.

Yet even as I was suffocating, I did not fail to find peace in cheerful and brave reflections. 4. "What is this?" said I. "Does death make trial of me so many times? Let it—I have made trial of it as well," long ago. "When?" you ask. Before I was born. Death is just nonexistence. I know already what that is like: what will exist after me is the same as existed before me. If there is any torment in this thing, then there must have been torment also before we saw the light of day. Yet we did not feel any discomfort at that time.

5. I ask you this: wouldn't you say a person was quite stupid if he thought that a lamp was worse off after it was extinguished than before it was lighted? We too are extinguished; we too are lighted. Betweentimes there is something that we feel; on either side is complete lack of concern. Unless I am wrong, dear Lucilius, our mistake is that we think death comes after; in fact, it comes both before and after. Whatever was before us is death. What difference is there between ending and simply not beginning? Both have the same result: nonexistence.

6. With these encouragements, and others in the same vein, I did not cease to encourage myself—without speaking, of course, since I had no breath to spare. Then, gradually, my wheezing, which had already given way to panting, began to come at greater intervals, then slowed and finally steadied. Even yet, though the attack is over, my breathing does not come naturally; I feel a kind of catch in it, a hesitation.

So be it, as long as I am not sighing on purpose! 7. Here is my pledge to you: I shall not tremble at the end; I am already prepared; I am not thinking at all about my overall span of life. The person you should praise—and imitate—is the one who enjoys living and yet is not

9. The Greek word Seneca has in mind is presumably *asthma* (which means "gasping").

reluctant to die. For what virtue is there in departing only when you are cast out? Yet there is virtue here too: I am indeed being cast out, and yet it is as if I am making my departure.

For that reason, the wise person too is never cast out, for being cast out is being driven away from a place you are unwilling to leave. The sage does nothing unwillingly: he escapes necessity in that he wishes to do what necessity will in any case require.

Farewell.

Selections from Letter 104: From Seneca to Lucilius

Greetings

1. I have run away to my villa at Nomentum.[10] Why, do you think? To escape the city? No, I wanted to avoid a fever that was creeping up and had already cast its hold on me. My doctor was saying that it had started with a rapid and irregular pulse. So I gave orders for my carriage to be made ready at once. I insisted on leaving in spite of my dear Paulina's attempts to stop me.[11] All I could say was what my mentor Gallio had said when he was on the point of starting to have a fever in Greece. He immediately boarded a ship, and kept insisting that his sickness was due to the location and not to his body. 2. I told this to Paulina. She is very anxious about my health. In fact, realizing that her soul is completely bound up with mine, I am beginning, in my concern for her, to be concerned about myself. Getting on in years has made me more resolute in facing lots of things, but here I am losing the benefit of age. I have come to think that within this old man there's a young person who needs indulgence. Since I can't prevail on her to show more courage in loving me, she prevails on me to love myself more carefully.

3. One has to give in, you see, to honorable feelings. There are times when, to honor a family member, one has to summon back one's dying breath, however painfully, and actually hold it in one's mouth. A good man should live not as long as it pleases him but as long as he ought to. The person who does not think enough of his wife or his friend to prolong his life—who insists on dying—is thoroughly self-indulgent. When the interest of loved ones demands it, the mind should require even this of itself: even if one not only wants to die but has actually begun to do so, one should interrupt the process and give oneself over to their needs . . .

6. I suppose you are curious to know how my travel project has worked out. As soon as I got away from the city's heavy atmosphere and the smell that smoking kitchens make when they discharge their accumulation of noxious fumes and dust, I felt an immediate change in my health. Can you imagine how much my strength increased once I reached my vineyards? Like an animal let out to pasture, I really attacked my food. The result is that I am fully

10. Nomentum was located about eighteen miles northeast of Rome.
11. Pompeia Paulina was Seneca's wife.

myself again now, without a trace of physical unsteadiness and mental weakness. I'm beginning to concentrate completely on my studies.

TEXT 39. INSCRIPTIONS RELATED TO PATIENTS

Hundreds of thousands of inscriptions—stones and monuments inscribed with a textual message—survive from the ancient Greek and Roman worlds. Many of these carved texts were epitaphs written to memorialize the dead (like inscriptions in modern-day cemeteries) or inscriptions at religious sites that either ask or express gratitude for divine help. The inscriptions below are a selection of funerary epitaphs or temple inscriptions that give us the perspective of sick and suffering people. Several of the inscriptions were written as original poems, while others are full of commonplace phrases and standard abbreviations.

Square brackets in the translation indicate spots where portions of the inscriptions are missing because the inscription has been damaged or where one or more words are implied. In many cases, editors have been able to hypothesize or restore missing sections of the inscriptions.[12]

SOURCE: Translation by Jared Secord based on the Greek and Latin.

Temple inscription of Hermodicus. Epidaurus (southern Greece).
3rd century BCE. IG IV².1.125. Greek.

Hermodicus of Lampsacus.[13]

As an example of your virtue, **Asclepius**, I set up this stone that I had lifted up, visible for everyone to see, a record of your art. For before I arrived into your hands and those of your children I lay sick with a hateful illness, with an abscess on my chest and paralyzed in my hands. But you, Paean,[14] by persuading me to lift this rock caused me to live free from illness.

Temple inscription of Prepousa. Lydia (modern-day western Türkiye).
c. 85 BCE. SEG 39.1276. Greek.

To Men Axiottenos[15] and his power. Because Prepousa, the freedwoman of the priestess, prayed on behalf of her son Philemon, that if he should be whole without spending money on physicians, she would inscribe an account of this on stone. And the prayer was fulfilled, but she did not pay what was due, so the god demanded the prayer and punished the father

---

12. The inscriptions are identified by their standard abbreviations. Readers seeking to identify these abbreviations should consult the following list: https://antiquite.ens.psl.eu/IMG/file/pdf_guide_epi/abreviations_guide.pdf.

13. Lampsacus was a Greek city on the western coast of modern-day Türkiye.

14. Paean is a title given to the gods Asclepius and **Apollo** that was also associated with physicians.

15. Men Axiottenos was a local Phrygian god who shows up in many inscriptions from the region. Axiottenos comes from the place-name Axiotta.

Philemon.[16] Thus Prepousa fulfills the prayer on her son's behalf and from now on praises [the god.]

Dedicatory inscription by Felix Asianus. Rome. Late first century BCE. CIL VI.68; ILS 3513. Latin.

Felix Asianus, public slave of the high priests,[17] discharged his vow to Bona Dea Agrestis Felicula,[18] freely and with good cause, [sacrificing] a white heifer on account of the restoration of his eyesight. Abandoned by physicians, he was healed after ten months by taking medicines, by the aid of the Mistress.[19] Through her, all things were restored during the term of office of Cannia Fortunata.[20]

Temple inscription of Diophantus. Athens. c. 150 CE. IG II².4514. Greek.

Diophantus of Sphettus:[21] I, a beloved temple attendant, say these things to you, Asclepius, the son of Leto's son.[22] How will I reach your golden house, O blessed longed-for divine head, since I do not have the feet with which I previously came to the shrine, unless you graciously wish to lead me back again after healing me, so that I may look at you, my god, brighter than the earth in springtime.

So I, Diophantus, pray to you: save me, blessed and mightiest, by healing my pernicious gout in the name of your father, to whom I offer a great prayer. For no one among the mortals on earth could bring deliverance from such pains. Only you, blessed divine one, have the power. For the supreme gods brought you, the compassionate one, as a great gift to mortals, deliverance from pains.

Three-times blessed Paean Asclepius, by your art Diophantus was healed of the incurable pernicious wound. No longer does he look crab-footed[23] nor as if he walks on thorns, but sure-footed, just as you promised.

16. Because Prepousa did not fulfill her vow to the god for restoring her son's health, the god punished the boy's father (who shared the same name as the son).

17. "High priests" translates the Latin word *pontifex* (plural, *pontifices*), referring to the most distinguished group of priests in Rome.

18. Bona Dea, literally "Good Goddess," was the Roman goddess of fertility and chastity for women and was also associated with healing. The title Agrestis Felicula may be linked to the Latin words for "field" (*ager*) and "fruitful" (*felix*). Bona Dea's sanctuary in Rome likely supplied medications to people seeking healing.

19. The Mistress appears to be an official related to the cult of Bona Dea.

20. Cannia Fortunata appears to be an official in the cult of Bona Dea.

21. Sphettus was a village in rural Attica.

22. Leto was the father of Apollo, who was the father of Asclepius.

23. The meaning seems to be that Diophantus previously walked with difficulty, like a crab, before he was healed.

*Dedication to physician and Asclepius. Lycia (modern-day
southwestern Türkiye). Between the first and third centuries CE. Thomas Corsten,
Die Inschriften von Kibyra (Bonn: Habelt, 2002), no. 83. Greek.*

[I? . . .[24]] from Laodicea,[25] thank the god[26] that I was saved, and the Fortune[27] of the city, and the physician Dionysius, son of Dionysius, who treated me.

*Dedicatory inscription of Marcus Ulpius Honoratus. Rome.
c. 150 CE. CIL VI.19; ILS 2194. Latin.*

Marcus Ulpius Honoratus, decurion of the singular equestrian class of our emperor,[28] [set up this memorial] to Asclepius and **Hygieia,** in return for his own health and that of his family and his physician, Lucius Julius Helix, who took diligent care of me, along with the gods. He is happy to discharge the vow freely, as is deserved.

*Temple inscription of Proclus of Sinope. Pontus (modern-day north-
central Türkiye). Between 100 and 300 CE. Studia Pontica III 25. Greek.[29]*

Proclus of Sinope,[30] cured in the nose, gives thanks to Asclepius and the nymphs[31] and Gordianus the chief physician, who is a friend to everyone and who always says that "it is fitting to prosper." Gordianus also healed many other conditions of Proclus and of his sons Symphorus and Proclianus. Chrestus of Sinope the stone-cutter, Proclus' brother, made [this dedication.]

*Funerary monument dedicated to Lucius Minicius Anthimianus.
Rome. 3rd century CE. IGUR IV 1702. Greek.*

To the spirits of the dead.[32] Lucius Minicius Anthimus and Scribonia Felicissima, unfortunate parents, for Lucius Minicius Anthimianus, the sweetest child and for their own god, who listens to prayers. He lived 4 years, 5 months, and 20 days.

---

24. The name of the person making this dedication is lost in a damaged part of the inscription.

25. Laodicea was located near the modern-day city of Denizli in southwestern Türkiye.

26. The god referenced here is likely Asclepius, since this inscription was found with another inscription that mentioned him.

27. "Fortune" (Greek *Tuche*) referred to the personification of destiny, good or bad fate.

28. The titles "decurion" and "equestrian" here indicate that Marcus Ulpius Honoratus was a member of one of the more privileged classes of Roman society.

29. The right side of this inscription is damaged, but scholars and this translation have been able to reconstruct the parts of the words that are missing. Because the missing letters in Greek do not correlate with the letters supplied in the English words, we are not using square brackets in this translation to indicate places where damaged words have been restored.

30. Sinope was a Greek city located in modern-day north-central Türkiye.

31. The Nymphs were minor Greek goddesses typically associated with nature.

32. Though a poem written in Greek, this inscription includes the conventional invocation that begins many Latin epitaphs, *Dis Manibus.*

Traveler, I am an infant who has reached this tomb. When you come across my rocky gravestone, you will immediately cry about what I suffered in the short time of my life.

When the Hours[33] brought me into the light from the birthing pains of my mother, my father rejoiced to take me up from the earth in his hands and washed me clean of the blood of the womb and himself placed me in the swaddling clothes. He offered prayers to the immortals which were destined not to be, for the Fates[34] were the first to have made all the judgments about me. And my father picked my mother as nurse and reared me. Immediately I sprouted and bloomed and was dear to everyone.

But in a few seasons the mark of the Fates came upon me, who afflicted me with a terrible illness around the testicles. But the long-suffering father who begat me healed my dread illness, thinking to save my fate with medicine. And then another illness seized me, most pernicious and many times worse than the previous illness. For the metatarsus of my left foot had decay in its bones. And so the friends of my father cut me and took out my bones, which gave grief and wailing to my parents. And in this way I was healed again, just as before.

My awful birth was still unsatisfied, but Fate brought me again another illness, this one of the belly, swelling up my insides and wasting away the other parts, to the point when the hands of my mother took my life from my eyes. I suffered these things in the short span of my life, stranger, and left behind the hateful wasting away for those who bore me. Doomed to a sad end, I leave behind three unmarried siblings.

33. In Greek mythology the Hours—or Horae—were goddesses linked with time and the seasons of the year.
34. In Greek mythology the Fates—or Morae—were goddesses linked with destiny, often depicted as three women who measured out with string how long humans would live.

THIRTEEN

Ethics and Professional Conduct

Some ancient sources stressed that the best physicians were those who entered the profession already possessing innate virtue, whereas other ancient sources suggested that virtue was something that could be learned and, in fact, something one needed to practice in order to master. For example, the Hippocratic *Oath* and the Hippocratic text *Decorum* (Texts 40 and 42) asserted that ethical and professional conduct were skills physicians acquired in their training, alongside technical clinical skills. Regardless of what view one held, it appears that the act of swearing a medical oath compelled physicians to a higher standard of virtue and, moreover, to uphold more vigorously the moral duties, responsibilities, and obligations of their profession. Oaths, which were sworn to the gods—for example, the Hippocratic *Oath* to **Apollo, Asclepius,** and **Hygieia** (Text 40; fig. 59); and the *Oath of Asaph and Yoḥanan* (Text 41) invoking the Jewish god—heightened the stakes of their professional behavior by introducing consequences: if physicians failed to fulfill the promises made in their vow, they would accept punishment from the gods.

Most ancient oaths and ethical texts proposed a guiding ethical principle that governed physicians' decision-making and behavior, such as the pledge to "do no harm." Ethical principles like these might appear straightforward, but when we take a closer look we quickly realize that general principles could lead to a range of applications in practice. For instance, how was "harm" to be construed? Many of the treatments physicians applied—such as cutting, probing, **cauterizing**—were painful and regarded by many patients as "harmful." But surely the short-term "harm" a physician was forced to inflict for the sake of recovery was distinct from the "harm" physicians pledged to avoid. Additionally, was harm to be understood as active or passive? Could physicians be blamed for a death that resulted from withholding treatment as much as they could be blamed for a death that resulted from acts of their own hands? And, finally, harm to whom? To the sick individual, the well-being of the household, the flourishing of society? The query about whose harm was privileged is best illustrated by the pledge in the Hippocratic *Oath* not to provide abortifacients. As **Soranus** reported, some physicians—acknowledging the high death rates of women in childbirth or of postpartum infections—chose to help abort a fetus when women's lives were in danger—that is, when harm would come to the woman. Yet we can imagine that other physicians withheld abortifacients because of the harm it would cause to households in need of heirs or societies facing perennial demographic instability. Thus in the case of abortifacients alone, we can see how physicians might use the same ethical principle but end up taking different stances depending on their interpretation of harm.

Another example of the difficulty of interpreting "do no harm" was the debate about whether or not to administer lethal **drugs**. The Hippocratic *Oath* asks physicians to pledge that they will refrain from causing harm to their patients' physical health by prescribing drugs. That said, a deadly drug might be seen as a welcome kindness to one facing prolonged suffering with no hope of recovery. Additionally, those sentenced to die might prefer the harm of a deadly drug over a more gruesome death such as torture in the arena, both because it would be comparatively quick and painless and because it preserved their dignity.

"Do no harm" was not the only ethical principle proposed in our ancient sources on medical ethics. **Scribonius Largus** alternatively asserted that physicians should be guided by compassion (*misericordia*) for their patients: feelings of empathy that produced a spirit of human kindness (*humanitas*). The physician who was guided by this ethic of compassion, Scribonius contends, would provide treatment even for hopeless cases (disagreeing with the Hippocratic stance to refuse treatment to the terminally ill in Text 3, *On the Art of Medicine* 8). The fourth-century CE Greek teacher Libanius adopted a similar guideline, namely, a "love for humanity." He made an impassioned appeal to medical professionals: "When you are summoned, run [to your patient]. Upon arriving, examine the sick person with all your intelligence. Sympathize with the distressed; rejoice with them when they recover; consider yourself as being a partner in their illnesses. Bring everything that you know to bear on this struggle" (*Progymnasmata* 7.3.7).

Beyond general ethical principles, there are a handful of specific ethical issues that come up repeatedly in our medical sources. One issue has to do with the cost of medical care, which could cause anxiety or could be altogether prohibitive for those living at subsistence levels. For this reason, the Hippocratic author of *Precepts* warned physicians never to discuss fees at the outset, since it only exacerbated patients' worry, in turn aggravating their illness. He implored physicians to offer their services for free to those without the means to pay because a sick person could improve through the mere act of receiving care: "For some sick people, though conscious that their condition is perilous, recover their health simply through their contentment with the goodness of the physician" (*Precepts* 6). (Yet he also remarked that the patients who survived would feel more obliged to pay a seemingly selfless physician.)

It is unclear how many physicians heeded this call. **Galen** reportedly bragged that he did not require payment from his patients. "In fact, I offer to my patients, as long as they need

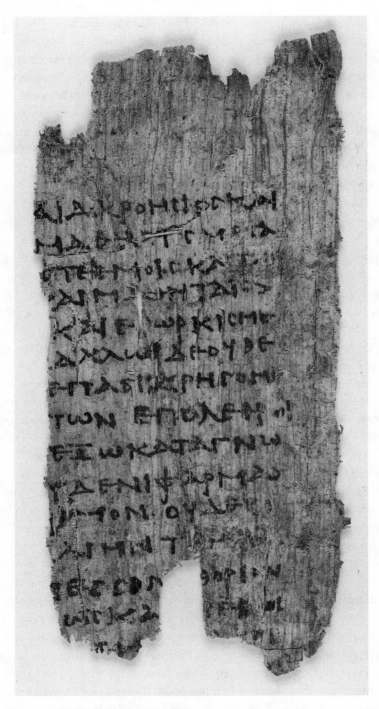

FIGURE 59 Third-century CE papyrus fragment of the Hippocratic
Oath. Papyrus Oxyrhynchus 2547. Wellcome Collection. Attribution 4.0
International (CC BY 4.0).

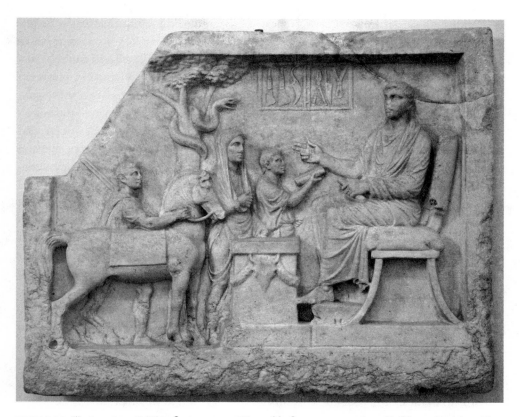

FIGURE 60 First-century BCE to first-century CE marble funerary or votive relief for a physician. The seated physician is depicted as larger than the other figures in the scene, suggesting his elevated prestige. The scroll in his hand suggests his learned nature, and the case of medical instruments near his head identifies him more specifically as a physician. Given that there are two scalpels and two knives, it is possible he was a surgeon. From Greece. © Antikensammlung, Staatliche Museen zu Berlin—Preußischer Kulturbesitz (inv. no. Sk 804). Photo credit: Johannes Laurentius.

it, not only medicines, drinks, massages and similar things, but I even provide them with nurses if they do not have servants, and besides I have food prepared for them" (Galen, *That the Best Profit from Their Enemies*, from Meyerhof, *Sudhoffs Archiv* 22 [1929]: 84). Subsidized or free care might have been more common among Jewish and Christian physicians whose religious traditions stressed the importance of care for the poor and needy. For example, the Jewish *Oath of Asaph and Yohanan* (Text 41), which dates from the third to sixth century CE, admonished physicians to provide care to the poor and needy out of a feeling of pity. By late antiquity a category of Christian healers—the *anargyroi*—came to be known for the practice of not charging fees, and from the fourth century CE onward Christians opened "hospitals" that provided free, in-patient care for the poor, needy, and vulnerable. The fact that some physicians were praised for providing free or subsidized health care, however, suggests that they might have been an exception to the norm.

Another ethical issue that comes up repeatedly in our medical sources has to do with privacy and confidentiality during treatment. Because many consultations took place in patients' homes, physicians might observe private household affairs (such as business transactions) or they might overhear household gossip or witness indiscretions. The physician became privy to sensitive information about the household, information that, if made public, could undermine the reputation of the family, especially the leading men of the household. To allay patients' fears that their private matters might be divulged, physicians pledged confidentiality about what they witnessed or overheard (see Text 40, Hippocratic *Oath*) and promised not to sell the household's secrets (see Text 41, *Oath of Asaph and Yoḥanan*). Physicians also pledged to refrain from misconduct, such as sexual impropriety with or violence against members of the household that might be easier to enact if the man of the household was weak or bedridden.

Just as physicians were motivated to follow ethical and professional codes to avoid drawing the ire of the gods and to put to rest the fears and anxieties of patients, so too they had more self-serving interests. At a time when it was hard to discriminate between competent health-care providers and charlatans, ethical and professional clinical conduct was one way to demonstrate one's professionalism, to cultivate one's reputation, and to attract clients. For example, the Hippocratic author of *Decorum* (Text 42) asserted that physicians' professional behavior—such as their preparation (including premixed drugs and an organized medical case; see fig. 44); their graceful and adept handling of the body, bandages, and instruments; their attention to detail; and their demonstrated knowledge of drugs—made them appear trustworthy in the eyes of patients. The calm and decisive way in which physicians conveyed their judgments, their reassuring yet serious manner of speaking, and even the way they comported their body and dress inspired patients' confidence that they were in good hands (see figs. 19, 31, 50, 56, 60). And the frequency of their visits, leaving apprentices behind to monitor patients between check-ups, assured patients that they would not be abandoned midtreatment and that the physician was committed to seeing them through to recovery.

TEXT 40. HIPPOCRATIC *OATH*

The Hippocratic Oath, *easily the most famous text of ancient Greco-Roman medicine, was attributed to* **Hippocrates,** *but as with all the texts in the Hippocratic corpus, the authorship is uncertain. Some scholars date it to the late fifth or early fourth century BCE, but the oath has affinities to other Hippocratic texts from the Hellenistic period, and our first direct reference to the oath comes from the first century CE, so other scholars believe it was written centuries later. The first paragraph is the private contract where new physicians outline the responsibilities and duties they have to fulfill for their teacher and other physicians. The remainder of the document focuses on physicians' obligations to the sick, including a list of procedures that they promise not to perform.*

SOURCE: Translation by Robert Nau based on the Greek text from I. L. Heiberg, *Hippocratis Opera*, vol. 1.1, Corpus Medicorum Graecorum 1.1 (Leipzig: Teubner, 1927).

1. I swear by **Apollo** the Physician, **Asclepius, Hygieia** and Panacea, and all gods and goddesses, making them witnesses, that I will fulfill this oath and this contract to the best of my ability and judgment. To consider my teacher of this art equal to my parents; to have him as a partner in my livelihood; if he cannot repay his debts, to contribute a share; to consider his sons equal to my brothers; to teach them this art without a fee or contract, should they wish to learn; to share written and spoken instruction and all other knowledge with my own sons and my teacher's sons, and to students bound by the contract and sworn as is customary for physicians, but with no one else.

2. To the best of my ability and judgment, I will use a regimen that is for the benefit of the sick, and I will keep them from a regimen that is wrong and causes injury and wrong.

3. I will neither give a deadly drug to anyone, even if asked to, nor will I guide such a plan; likewise, I will not give an abortifacient **pessary** to a woman.

4. But I will faithfully keep my life and my art undefiled and pure.

5. I will not cut, not even those who suffer from stones, but will yield to the men who practice this trade.

6. Into whatever houses I enter, I will come for the benefit of the sick, remaining free from all willful wrong-doing and corruption, and especially from sexual acts on the bodies of women and men, free and slave.

7. And, while I treat the sick and in the course of my interactions with people while I am not treating the sick, whatever I see or hear, which must never be divulged, I will keep silent and deem such things as not to be spoken.

8. And so, if I fulfill this oath and do not break it, may I reap the fruits, being held in honor before all people for my life and my art for all time; but if I transgress and break the oath, may the opposite happen.

TEXT 41. *OATH OF ASAPH AND YOḤANAN*

The Oath of Asaph and Yoḥanan *is found in the medical compendium called the* Book of Remedies *attributed to Asaph the Jew. The book, which includes sections on anatomy, physiology, pulse and urine diagnosis, pharmacology, and regimen, in addition to medical ethics, purports to be a collection of medical knowledge conveyed to Noah by an angel and then subsequently passed down and expanded over generations. So although scholars date the* Book of Remedies *to the third–sixth century CE or even later, and despite the fact that the book clearly borrowed from and adapted earlier Hippocratic texts (including the Hippocratic* Oath), *the book itself makes the case that Greek medicine is the heir to Jewish medical knowledge.*

SOURCE: Translation of the Hebrew text by Shlomo Pines from "The Oath of Asaph the Physician and Yoḥanan Ben Zabda—Its Relation to the Hippocratic Oath and the Doctrina Duarum Viarum of the Didachē," originally published in *Proceedings of the Israel Academy of Sciences and Humanities*, vol. V, no. 9 (Jerusalem: The Israel Academy of Sciences and

Humanities, 1975), pp. 224–226. © The Israel Academy of Sciences and Humanities. Reprinted by permission.

[1] This is the pact which Asaph ben Berakhyahu and Yoḥanan ben Zabda made with their pupils, and they adjured them with the following words:

[2] Do not attempt to kill any soul by means of a potion of herbs,[1] [3] Do not make a woman [who is] pregnant [as a result] of whoring take a drink with a view to causing abortion, [4] Do not covet beauty of form in women with a view to fornicating with them, [5] Do not divulge the secret of a man who has trusted you, [6] Do not take any reward [which may be offered in order to induce you] to destroy and to ruin, [7] Do not harden your heart [and turn it away] from pitying the poor and healing the needy, [8] Do not say of [what is] good; it is bad, nor of [what is] bad: it is good, [9] Do not adopt the ways of the sorcerers using [as they do] charms, augury and sorcery in order to separate a man from the wife of his bosom or a woman from the companion of her youth, [10] You shall not covet any wealth or reward [which may be offered in order to induce you] to help in a lustful desire, [11] You shall not seek help in any idolatrous [worship] so as to heal through [a recourse to idols], and you shall not heal with anything [pertaining] to their worship, [12] But on the contrary detest and abhor and hate all those who worship them, put their trust in them, and give assurance [referring] to them, [13] For they are all naught, useless, for they are nothing, demons, spirits of the dead; they cannot help their own corpses, how then could they help those who live?

[14] Now [then] put your trust in the Lord, your God, [who is] a true God, a living God, [15] For [it is] He who kills and makes alive, who wounds and heals, [16] Who teaches men knowledge and also to profit, [17] Who wounds with justice and righteousness, and who heals with pity and compassion, [18] No designs of [His] sagacity are beyond His [power]. [19] And nothing is hidden from His eyes.

[20] Who causes curative plants to grow, [21] Who puts sagacity into the hearts of the wise in order that they should heal through the abundance of His loving-kindness, and that they should recount wonders in the congregation of many; so that every living [being] knows that He made him and that there is no savior [other] than He. [22] For the nations trust in their idols, who [are supposed] to save them from their distress and will not deliver them from their misfortunes [23] For their trust and hope is in the dead. [24] For this [reason] it is fitting to keep yourselves separate from them; to remove yourselves and keep far away from all the abominations of their idols, [25] And to cleave to the name of the Lord God of spirits for all **flesh**, [26] And the soul of every living being is in His hand to kill and to make live, [27] And there is none that can deliver out of His hand.

1. Literally: "root."

[28] Remember Him always and seek Him in truth, in righteousness in an upright way, in order that you should prosper in all your works [29] And He will give you help to make you prosper in [what you are doing[2]], and you shall be [said to be] happy in the mouth of all flesh. [30] And the nations will abandon their idols and images and will desire to worship God like you, [31] For they will know that their trust is in vain and their endeavor fruitless, [32] For they implore a god, who will not do good [to them], who will not save [them].

[33] As for you, be strong, do not let your hands be weak, for your work shall be rewarded, [34] The Lord is with you, while you are with Him, [35] If you keep His pact, follow His commandments, cleaving to them, [36] You will be regarded as His saints by all men,[3] and they will say: [37] Happy the people whose [lot] is such, happy the people whose God is the Lord.

[38] Their pupils answered saying: [39] We will do all that you exhorted and ordered us [to do], [40] For it is a commandment of the Torah, [41] And we must do it with all our heart, with all our soul and with all our might. [42] To do, and to obey. [43] Not to swerve or turn aside to the right hand or the left. [44] And they[4] blessed them in the name of God most high, maker of heaven and earth.

[45] And they continued to charge them, and said: [46] The Lord God, His saints and His Torah [bear] witness, that you should fear Him, that you should not turn aside from His commandments, and that you should follow His laws with an upright heart, [47] You shall not incline after lucre [so as] to help a godless [man in shedding] innocent blood. [48] You shall not mix a deadly **drug** for any man or woman so that he [or she] should kill their fellow-man. [49] You shall not speak of the herbs [out of which such drugs are made]. You shall not hand them over to any man, [50] And you shall not talk about any matter [connected] with this, [51] You shall not use blood in any work of medicine, [52] You shall not attempt to provoke an ailment in a human soul through [the use of] iron instruments or searing with fire before making an examination two or three times; then [only] you should give your advice. [53] You shall not be ruled—your eyes and your heart being lifted up—by a haughty spirit. [54] Do not keep [in your hearts] the vindictiveness of hatred with regard to a sick man, [55] You shall not change your words in anything, [56] The Lord our God hates [?] [this?] being done, [57] But keep His orders and commandments, and follow all His ways, in order to please Him, [and] to be pure, true and upright.

[58] Thus did Asaph and Yoḥanan exhort and adjure their pupils.

TEXT 42. HIPPOCRATIC CORPUS, *DECORUM* SELECTIONS (5, 7–18)

Decorum *was attributed to* **Hippocrates,** *but as with all the texts in the Hippocratic corpus, the authorship is uncertain. Some scholars believe it may have been written as early as the fourth or*

2. Literally: "in your hand."
3. Literally: "in the eyes of all flesh."
4. Asaph and Yoḥanan.

third century BCE, but other scholars have suggested it could be as late as the first or second century CE. The text is roughly divided into two parts, beginning with a discussion of wisdom as the foundation of medicine: that wisdom derives from equal parts education and experience, science and art. The remainder of the text, the selections below, focuses on questions about how physicians should behave in their interactions with patients. "Decorum" refers to the etiquette and appropriate behavior that the text recommends.

Translation of some parts of the text is difficult because of serious corruptions in its Greek text, as well as some unusual grammar and phrases. Corrupt sections of the text are marked in the text with the symbol †.

SOURCE: Translation by Robert Nau based on the Greek text from I. L. Heiberg, *Hippocratis Opera*, vol. 1.1, Corpus Medicorum Graecorum 1.1 (Leipzig: Teubner, 1927).

5. And above all, on account of this, as you undertake each of the goals just mentioned,[5] transfer wisdom into medicine and medicine into wisdom. For a physician philosopher is godlike. For there is [not] much difference[6] between medicine and wisdom, and in fact everything in medicine pertains to elements in wisdom. For all the features of wisdom are in medicine. It possesses freedom from greed, reverence, a sense of shame, modesty in dress, good repute, judgment, conviction, quiet, cleanliness, thoughtfulness, knowledge of the things that are useful and necessary for life: the absence of impurity, freedom from superstition, and divine dignity. For the features they have in the face of licentiousness, quackery, greed, lust, thievery, and shamelessness. This is the knowledge of incomes and use of resources with friendship in mind, and how and in what manner to conduct oneself towards children and money.[7] And so a type of wisdom is a partner to medicine, since the physician has these qualities and even most other things.

. . .

7. Since all the things just mentioned are true, the physician must have a certain quick wit, for severity is unappealing to both the healthy and the sick. And the physician must guard himself from exposing too much of his body and from gossiping at length to laypeople, but converse only about necessary matters. †For the physician judges that gossip will bring criticism for his treatment.[8] † He must especially do none of these things in a fastidious or ostentatious way. All these things should be considered so that you may prepare them ahead of time for convenience, as may be necessary. If not, you will always lack what is required.

8. In medicine, one must practice these things with all reserve: in the matter of palpation, anointing, and washing; to ensure delicacy in moving the hands in the matter of linen,

5. The "goals" refer to the discussion in chapters 1 through 4 on how to use wisdom.
6. Some manuscripts of the Greek text here omit "not," which does not make sense in terms of the author's position. The omission was likely a scribal error introduced when copying the manuscript.
7. This sentence seems out of place here, and its meaning is unclear.
8. The Greek text is corrupt here.

compresses, bandages, putting things back into place; in the matter of **drugs** for wounds and for the eyes, and for things of this sort; in order that you may prepare in advance tools, devices, metal instruments; and so on. For a deficiency in these matters leads to helplessness and harm. Also, there should be a second and simpler case for traveling[9] that you can carry by hand. The most manageable case is methodically arranged, for the physician cannot go through everything.

9. Remember well your drugs and their properties, both simple ones and those compound, since the healing of sicknesses also exists in the mind. Also remember well the character of these drugs, the many ways in which they may be used for each sickness. For in medicine, this is the start, middle, and end.

10. Prepare in advance your emollients in categories according to the uses of each. Chop up plants for powerful medicinal drinks prepared from a formula according to their different kinds. Also, prepare in advance ingredients (taken from suitable places) for purges, prepared in the necessary way in their various categories and sizes, with some left to age, others kept fresh for immediate use, and similarly for the rest.

11. After making these preparations, when you enter into the house of the sick, know what must be done before entering so that you will not be at a loss, with each and everything arranged well for what will be done. For many cases do not need reasoning but rather help through actions. Thus one must forecast, from experience, what will happen. Truly this brings fame and is easy to learn.

12. When you pay your visit, be mindful of how you sit, modesty, adornment, authoritativeness, concise speech, perfect composure in actions, bedside manner, attention to details, responsiveness to counter objections and the troubles that arise, your own vigor, rebuke against disturbances, and readiness for services. In addition to these considerations, be mindful of your initial preparation. And if not, † one must be faultless in the other matters, which include directions on readiness. †

13. Pay frequent visits. Think carefully about instances where you have been deceived regarding the changes of all things.[10] You will understand the situation more easily and at the same time be more at your ease. For the elements in **humors** are unstable, and so they are also easily altered by nature and chance. Not seeing the right time for medical treatment allows the condition to get a head start and kill, for there was no help provided. For when many things acting together produce an effect, it is difficult. What happens one at a time is more manageable and, with skill, can be handled.

14. Also look out for the faults that the sick make, which often lead them to lie about the prescribed foods. They die when they do not take unpleasant medicinal drinks, whether these are purgative or for treatment. When they do not confess what was done, people blame the physician.

9. The "second and simpler case" refers to a medical case in which physicians kept their instruments, drugs, and other equipment necessary for their practice (see fig. 44).

10. The "changes" refer to an illness passing from one phase to another.

15. Also consider matters relating to the person's position in bed. Some concerns here relate to seasons and some to types of sicknesses. For some of the sick are to be in well ventilated places, some in underground or dark places. Also consider sounds, smells, and especially the smell of wine. This is by far the worst; one must avoid or change it.

16. During treatment, do all these things calmly and with appropriate manners while keeping most things secret from the sick person. Dictate what must be done in a friendly and gentle way, while turning the person away from their circumstances. At the same time, rebuke sharply and strictly. With attention and care soften what details you must while revealing nothing of what will happen next or what threatens them. For because of this, namely because of the disclosure just mentioned of what threatens or what will be next, many people have taken a poor turn.

17. Have one of your students be left in charge of applying your instructions without being harsh, and of implementing the prescribed treatment. Of these students, choose those who have already been admitted into the art of medicine to provide anything additional as required or to employ treatments safely, so that in the meantime nothing escapes you. Never give decision-making power to laypeople. †If not, what has been poorly done, blame will advance on you. If you have no doubts about those from whom your treatment will advance,[11]† neither will they hang blame upon you. Instead, what has been done will add to your fame. Announce in advance to those who should know more all these matters as they are done.

18. This being how things are with reputation and decorum in wisdom, in medicine, and in all other arts, the physician must, after he has marked off the parts we have discussed, while at all times wrapping himself in the other parts,[12] watch over it as he keeps it and employ it as he transmits it. For glorious things are guarded well by all people, and those who make their way through them are held in honor by parents and children, and if some of them do not know many things, they are brought into understanding through practice.

---

11. Exact meaning is uncertain, but the general idea is that the physician will be blamed for the faults of those he puts in charge and therefore must be careful.

12. The author does not identify what the "other" is here. It might refer to "theory" as opposed to "practice."

FOURTEEN

Life Stages

Ancient medical writers believed that the body changed over the course of a lifetime, changes that accounted for the main signs of aging. **Herophilus,** for example, thought that the pulse differed according to age, with a child's pulse being naturally quicker and an older person's being slower. The main change thought to take place across one's lifetime, though, was that the body went from a hotter and wetter state as an infant to a drier and colder state in old age (see Text 48, **Galen,** *On Hygiene* 5.3). The "prime of life" was thought to be the age at which people were in a state of balance with regard to the four qualities (wet, dry, hot, cold) and thus prone to be most healthy.

These overarching principles about the varying states of the body at different ages served as the basis for understanding the particular kinds of ailments that people were susceptible to at different life stages. These principles also informed the different regimens endorsed for people at different ages. For example, one Hippocratic author recommended drying regimens for younger people to offset their characteristic moistness, and regimens that induced moisture for older people to offset their characteristic dryness (see Text 20, *Regimen in Health* 2 and 6).

When diagnosing patients of different ages, therefore, it was important for physicians to consider the bodily state associated with their patient's age. For example, Herophilus was concerned if an older person's pulse rate was observed in a child (which indicated chilling and possibly death), just as a faster pulse in an older patient was also an alarming sign. And the Hippocratic author of *On the Sacred Illness* warned that one should be watchful for moist residues in very young children, which needed to be shed in order to avoid seizures in early life (see Text 17). Physicians were also to consider how their patients' bodily states interacted with other factors to influence their health. For example, in the selection from *On Medicine* below, **Celsus** discussed the way in which the seasons of the year affected the body differently at different life stages (Text 43, following Hippocratic ideas found in Text 2, *Airs, Waters, Places* 1). Winter, the cold season, is a hard time for older people, who are already predisposed to being cold, while summer, the hot season, is difficult for children, who are already predisposed to being hot.

Using age as a diagnostic variable became even more complicated when combined with gender. As we have seen, most medical thinkers believed women's bodies to be colder and moister than men's hot, dry bodies (see the section on women's illnesses in chapter 9). Thus when physicians attempted to figure out how a patient's bodily state might be contributing to an illness, they had to account for age and gender together. Medical thinkers also devised gender-specific regimens that sought to ensure the maintenance of health across various stages of men's and women's lives, regimens that were also tailored to their gender-specific societal roles. For example, regimens for boys and men sought to promote the physical and psychological characteristics best suited to their participation in work and civic life. Of even greater importance to society were the regimens for women of childbearing age. Their habits were carefully monitored and regimens designed to promote their ability to become pregnant and to bear children (see below).

Starting with the Hippocratic corpus, most medical writers categorized life stages using roughly the same age ranges. (It is notable that most were interested mainly in men's life stages, although some writers, like Galen, also identified similar stages for women.) Infancy, according to Galen, lasted for the first seven years of life (see Text 47, *On Hygiene* 1.12). This stage was followed by childhood proper, which lasted another seven years. Then came the stage of puberty and adolescence. According to Galen, puberty was the time in life when boys and girls grew pubic hair, when semen was produced in boys' bodies, when girls' breasts developed, and when menstruation began. Adulthood—often called "youth" and regarded as the "prime of life"—lasted a relatively long time: from about twenty until forty years of age. Finally, the last stage of life was old age, a time when men were thought to be past their prime.

TEXT 43. CELSUS, *ON MEDICINE* SELECTION (2.1)

On Medicine, *written by Aulus Cornelius **Celsus** (first centuries BCE and CE), was originally part of an encyclopedia that covered a range of topics, including agriculture, medicine, rhetoric, philosophy, and military science. The section on medicine, the only one to survive, is organized around the three major divisions of ancient medicine: regimen, pharmacology, and surgery. Scholars debate whether Celsus was himself a practicing physician, but his text offers hints of real experience, especially in the sections on surgery. In the selection below, Celsus discusses the conditions and illnesses that people might expect to experience as they progressed through the stages of life, from infancy to old age.*

SOURCE: Translation by Jared Secord based on the Latin text from Guy Serbat, *Celse, De la médicine*, vol. 1 (Paris: Les Belles Lettres, 1995).

Book 2, Chapter 1. 17. As relates to the ages of life, children and those near to them in age are in their best condition in the spring and are safest at the beginning of summer. Old people are in their best condition in the summer and the first part of autumn, and youths and those who are between youth and old age are in their best condition in the winter. Winter is more harmful to old people, and summer is more harmful to young adults. 18. At that time, if some weakness arises, it is likely that infants and children still of a young age will be troubled by crawling sores of the mouth (which the Greeks call "thrush"[1]), vomiting, insomnia, discharges from the ears, and inflammations around the navel. Those teething have ulceration of the gums, feverishness, sometimes spasms of the tendons, and attacks of diarrhea; teething children fare especially badly when the canine teeth are coming in. Those who are the plumpest and those who are constipated are especially in danger. 19. But for those who are a little older, there arise inflammations in the tonsils, some spinal curvatures, swelling in the lymph nodes of the neck, a painful type of wart that the Greeks call "acrochordons,"[2] and many other swellings. When puberty begins, in addition to many of these same conditions, there are also chronic fevers, and nosebleeds. 20. All childhood is especially subject to danger, first around the fortieth day, then in the seventh month, then the seventh year, and afterwards around puberty. Also, if some types of illnesses happen during childhood, and have not come to an end during puberty or at the time of the first sexual experiences, or the first menstruations for women, they are generally chronic. More often, however, childhood illnesses that have lasted for a rather long time come to an end. 21. Adolescence is liable to acute illnesses and also seizures, and especially by the **wasting ailment**; almost all who spit blood are youths. After this age there are pains of the sides and lungs, lethargy, ailments of the bowels, madness, and the discharge of blood through, as it were, certain mouths of veins (the Greeks call these "hemorrhoids"[3]). 22. In old age, there is difficulty breathing and urinating, coldness in the head, pains of the joints and kidneys, paralysis of the tendons, the bad state of the body that the Greeks call a "bad bodily condition,"[4] insomnia, long-lasting problems of the ears, eyes, and nostrils, and especially looseness of the bowels and all that accompanies it: sharp pains or excessive lubrication of the intestines and the other harms of a lax belly.

PREGNANCY AND OBSTETRIC CARE

Although ancient medical writers often categorized the stages of men's and women's lives similarly, women's lives were also segmented according to their primary role in society: the conception, birthing, and rearing of children. Up to the point of puberty, the suggested regimen for girls and boys tended to be the same. But, after the onset of menses, medical

1. In Greek, *aphthas.*
2. In Greek, *akrochordonas.*
3. In Greek, *haimorroidas.*
4. In Greek, *kachexian.*

writers created gender-specific regimens for young women that focused on ensuring healthy pregnancies and childbirth. They also focused on the dangers involved in giving birth. Many women (and infants) did not survive the experience, whether dying during childbirth or from postpartum infections. The selections in this section reflect the reproductive priorities of medical writers and give us a vivid glimpse into the health risks faced by women during and after childbirth.

Ancient gynecological texts sought to understand how menstruation was linked to conception and how to deal with problems that hindered reproduction. Hippocratic writers understood the onset of menses to be the result of an accumulation of blood that needed to be expelled. When a woman's vaginal channel was opened wide enough, it allowed for the outflow of menstrual blood, and this evacuation would rebalance the body in terms of both heat and moisture (recall that blood was characterized by both of these qualities). According to the Hippocratic *Diseases of Women*, women with the best chances to conceive were those who menstruated at regular intervals and evacuated an appropriate amount of blood, neither too much nor too little. **Soranus** suggested that women's ability to conceive was not only related to the uterus being in a state of balance between wetness and dryness, but also a balanced state between looseness and constriction (these latter qualities were emphasized by those, like Soranus, who subscribed to the Methodist school of medicine).

Physicians were also concerned about a number of problems related to menstruation that might afflict young women. On the one hand, they worried about the retention of menses (or "backed-up blood"), which could pool to form abscesses or collect around organs, disrupting their proper functioning (see chapter 9, on women's illnesses). On the other hand, they worried about scant menstruation, which they thought interfered with conception. Physicians recommended several treatments for these disorders. Some prescribed sexual intercourse to widen narrow passages, allowing the blood to flow. Others prescribed pharmacological remedies, that could involve the ingestion of herbs and **drugs**, or the **fumigation** of the vagina and uterus with smoke from burning substances, or the irrigation of the uterus with infusions of wine, water, vinegar, and other liquids, or the insertion of vaginal suppositories, wool or wax soaked with simple or compound drugs.

Medical writers also observed that young girls at this stage of life were beginning to feel sexual desire; writers such as Soranus advised physicians and parents on how to keep young girls' desires under control and prevent them from engaging in sexual activity before they were safely married. Their main recommendations had to do with adjusting young girls' regimens: requiring them to take moderate exercise regularly and to bathe daily.

Among the medical debates centered on the care and health of young women, the most significant was whether it was healthy for them to bear children as soon as they were physically able or whether they ought to wait to develop more fully physically and psychologically. Since, for example, in Roman society girls could marry as young as twelve years of age, medical writers considered the health concerns that could arise with early pregnancy, concerns that had to be weighed against the social and familial advantages of early marriages. Another

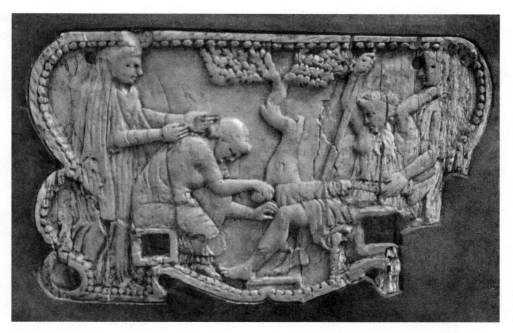

FIGURE 61 First-century CE ivory carving of a birthing scene, from Pompeii. The carving depicts a woman grasping the head of the child being delivered. The woman giving birth grabs the neck of the assistant standing behind her with her left hand and grasps a staff with her right hand, presumably for leverage. Another assistant stands with arms open and ready to assist. Naples Archaeological Museum (inv. no. 109905). Photo credit: Kristi Upson-Saia.

debate had to do more generally with whether it was healthier for women to avoid pregnancy and childbirth altogether (an inference many—especially women—made after witnessing the deaths of their mothers, sisters, and friends in childbirth) or if pregnancy and childbirth were healthful, in fact curing women's ailments (for the main arguments in favor of this position, see chapter 9). On these questions, the second-century CE physician Soranus took the stance that pregnancy—especially too soon after the onset of menses—could be damaging to a young woman's health. He also acknowledged the ways in which pregnancy and childbirth at any stage of life exhausted women and put them in mortal danger. He, therefore, disagreed with Hippocratic writers, concluding that pregnancy and childbirth were not healthy for women, despite being necessary evils in the service of societal needs for reproduction (Text 44, *Women's Health* 1.13).

Ancient gynecological sources discuss other interesting ideas related to conception. For instance, writers debated whether women, just as men, contributed seed (*semen*) in the conception of a fetus. Therefore they debated whether it was necessary for a woman to experience pleasure in order to ejaculate her seed, just as a man must orgasm to ejaculate his. Medical writers also discussed the time in the menstrual cycle when women were most likely to become pregnant. Some also wondered whether the time of year and the stage of the moon in its cycle contributed to the likelihood of conception (though some thinkers like Soranus were generally dismissive of these views as merely popular folklore). They also talked about the impact of the conditions of conception—namely, the physical and emotional states of the sexual partners—on the character of the fetus. For example, in the selections below, Soranus expressed a widely held assumption in his day: that the sensory experiences of the mother during conception (and during pregnancy) impressed themselves on the developing embryo (Text 44, *Women's Health* 1.12). Ancient biologists and medical writers appealed to this idea of imprinting via the faculties of perception and *phantasia* (roughly, "imagination") to explain the appearance of children upon birth and their nature as they grew up. For instance, some thought that if a woman imagined a horse while engaged in sex, she ran the risk of bearing a child with horse-like features, or if she gazed on a painting of a drinking party in her bedroom when having intercourse, the child conceived could turn out to be a drunkard. Hence, mothers were urged to have in view or mind images of beautiful and noble things when engaging in sex and throughout their pregnancy to assure the development of well-formed and well-behaved offspring.

Once conception was successful, Soranus devised a detailed regimen for pregnant women that was divided into three stages. The first stage focused on retaining the seed by avoiding disturbances of any kind, both physical and emotional, since sudden movements could inadvertently discharge the seed. Soranus also advised against activities that relaxed and loosened the body too much, such as an overly warm bath, since the body needed a certain amount of constriction to retain the seed. Although most medical texts expressed strong injunctions against abortions, women who did not want to be pregnant merely followed the opposite advice, exercising vigorously and taking hot baths. And women wishing to terminate an unwanted pregnancy could also turn to friends with experience or to a variety of professionals (such as pharmacists, **obstetricians**, and sex workers) for advice about practices and drugs that worked as abortifacients.

Soranus's second stage of pregnancy focused on managing symptoms of nausea, vomiting, and strange cravings, especially for substances such as dirt or charcoal (a set of symptoms called **kissa** or **pica**). **Aëtius of Amida** prescribed a wide variety of treatments for *pica* depending on the cause of a particular craving. For some women, he prescribed purslane and endive, for others pickled fish and radishes in vinegar (see Text 45, 16.10).

Soranus identified the third stage of pregnancy as preparation for giving birth. He advised a regimen that would both strengthen and relax women to facilitate delivery: they were to eat more fortifying foods, engage in strengthening exercises, and take frequent baths to relax the womb. In addition to following this medical advice, pregnant women also prepared for a safe and easy childbirth by petitioning the gods and goddesses for support. Women also availed themselves of protection in the form of amulets (such as carved gemstones they wore on their bodies during pregnancy and delivery), and they used spells for further protection. For instance, one extant Greek spell instructed that a woman should use the phrase "Come out of your tomb, Christ is calling you" while placing a potsherd on her right thigh (*PGM* CXXIII a, 50–55).

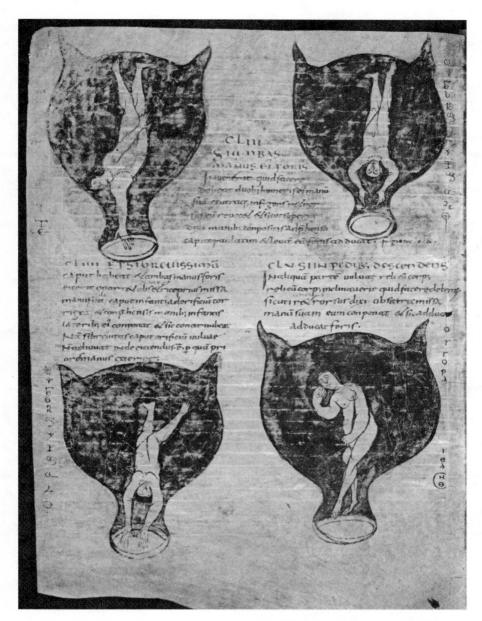

FIGURE 62 Illustration from a medieval manuscript of Muscio's sixth-century CE treatise on gynecology depicting various positions of the fetus in the uterus, some of which would lead to a difficult childbirth. This illustration also portrays the typical parts of the uterus (such as its mouth, neck, and fundus; see fig. 21), and what came to be called the uterine "horns," "tentacles," or "suckers." Medical writers like Diocles asserted that these protuberances of the uterus were similar to breasts—broad at the base, and tapering at the end—and were providentially created by nature so that the fetus formed the habit of sucking in preparation for breastfeeding. Brussels Koninklijke Bibliotheek van België— Bibliothèque royale de Belgique (ms. 3701–15). Wikimedia Commons.

When the day finally came to give birth, babies were generally delivered by obstetricians (see Text 35, Soranus, *Women's Health* 1.2–3, for a description of the ideal obstetrician; see figs. 55, 61). Soranus provides an in-depth discussion of the proper preparation of the birthing room, the necessary equipment and supplies that should be on hand, how to deliver babies in various positions (see fig. 62), and the ways obstetricians and their assistants ought to facilitate a healthy and safe delivery. The selections below from Aëtius describe situations when the birthing process did not proceed in an easy manner and the mother's life was in danger (Text 45, 16.22–23). These descriptions of fetal dismemberment and concerns about retained uterine material give us a window into the perils of delivery in the ancient world. Still more, in the Hippocratic collection of case histories, we hear about a number of postpartum complications, including death (see Text 8, *On Epidemics* 1.4 and 1.8).

We do not have extensive discussions about postpartum care of mothers, though some ancient medical texts advise a regimen for nursing women. Instead, medical texts tended to focus on care for the newborn infant, a topic we will take up in the next section.

Finally, another important life stage for women was when menses ceased and women were no longer able to conceive children (what we call "menopause"). This transition was understood in terms of the gradual drying and cooling process of aging. This time in life did not receive a lot of attention from medical writers, but given how frequently women gave birth, it is likely that many women would have experienced pelvic organ prolapse, a condition that ancient physicians treated in a variety of ways, but mainly through the insertion of **pessaries.**

TEXT 44. SORANUS, *WOMEN'S HEALTH*[5] SELECTIONS (1.10–13, 1.16, 1.22, 2.1)

In Women's Health, **Soranus of Ephesus** *(second century CE) is guided by two main concerns: protecting women's health and managing pregnancy and childbirth. In the selections below, Soranus discusses the conditions that will most likely lead to conception, including the age of the woman, her body type and physical state, and the timing of sexual intercourse. Soranus also provides detailed instructions on caring for pregnant women and assisting with labor and childbirth.*

The Greek text is incomplete in several of these selections, but an adapted translation of the text into Latin survives, which gives us a sense of the missing text. We include these sections of the text in the footnotes.

SOURCE: Translation by Molly Jones-Lewis based on the Greek text from Paul Burguière, Danielle Gourevitch, and Yves Malinas, *Soranus d'Éphèse, Maladies des femmes* (Paris: Les Belles Lettres, 1990).

5. This text has previously been translated with the title *Gynecology,* but this traditional title may give the misleading impression that the text is only concerned with women's reproductive system, and not with women's health more generally.

Book 1, Chapter 10. Up to what age a female should be kept from sexual activity.

Since the male only emits seed, he is in no danger from his first act of sexual intercourse. But the female both receives the seed and gestates it into the substance of a living being, and she is found to run a greater risk from this either from being led too quickly or too slowly into sexual activity, so it makes sense that we investigate the matter at hand.

Some people suggest that it is a good idea for the female to continue in her virginity as long as she does not yet have the urge for sexual activity. For nature itself, in unspeaking animals just as in humans, has developed passions and has put urges into motion at the time for sex, and that is when the body is urging the pursuit of sexual gratification.

But these people have failed to notice that unspeaking animals are motivated by their nature alone and by irrational chance and that they bring nothing from their own thoughts to bear on their sexual desire. Therefore, for most animals, the time when the urge for sex emerges is fixed for them. But in humans, it is not fixed for a certain time, because often the ability to think stirs up urges because of curiosity about new pleasures or fantasies.

Now, virgins who have not been properly educated or raised to practice self-control arouse their sexual desire prematurely, so one cannot trust in sexual urges. It is a good idea to keep a girl a virgin until the time when her menstrual periods begin. This will be the sign that the uterus is now capable of performing its particular functions, one of which is conception, as we have said before.

There is a danger when the seed that has been ejaculated is conceived in a uterus that is still small in size. Because of this, the embryo is constrained by the tight space as it grows and, therefore, is either destroyed entirely or loses its features. Or, at the time of birth, there is a danger to the pregnant woman since it must pass through the narrow and underdeveloped structures around the mouth[6] of the uterus. For this reason, it also happens that some embryos fail to grow because the uterus is not yet entwined with large vessels, but only the small ones that do not provide enough blood to feed the embryo in the womb. Indeed, the first appearance of the menstrual period occurs, for the most part, around the fourteenth year. Since this is the case, it appears to be the natural time for ending her virginity. On the other hand, it is not safe to end her virginity after a number of years have passed, because the neck of the uterus remains collapsed, in the same way as the genitals of men who do not use them for sex.

And so this way, the seed is molded and finished into a living creature in the roomy fundus[7] of the uterus, but it is not able to pass easily through the narrow confines of the uterine neck[8] during childbirth and brings great agonies and dangers.

6. The mouth referred to the opening of the uterus (see fig. 21). We believe that most ancient authors had in mind what we now call the "cervix," though some might have identified the mouth as the vaginal opening.

7. The fundus referred to the bottom of the womb (see fig. 21).

8. The neck referred to the area just behind the mouth (i.e., the opening of the uterus; see fig. 21). If the author understood the mouth to be the cervix, then the neck would be the area directly behind the cervix. If the author understood the mouth to be the vaginal opening, then the neck would be the vaginal canal.

Therefore, the time discussed earlier, when the reproductive organs have been fully developed and are able to sustain conception, is the right time for ending virginity.

Book 1, Chapter 11. How to recognize women able to conceive

Most women are married for the sake of children and family succession, but not for empty pleasure, so it is completely wrong-headed to look into the quality of their pedigree and the abundance of their wealth, but not to find out if they are able to get pregnant, and if they have the right bodies for giving birth. It is therefore suitable for us to include a discussion of the matter at hand. One must recognize that women capable of becoming pregnant range in age, for the most part, from fifteen to forty years, and are not manly, husky, solid, or obese, nor overly flabby and moist. [Since] the uterus is similar in composition to the whole [body], it is unable to accept the attachment of the seed easily either because of its excessive hardness [if it even attaches in the first place], or its excessive flabbiness and lack of strength.[9]

And women who are able to conceive have a uterus that is neither too moist nor too dry, nor are they too loose or too constricted. They have regular menstrual periods, not due to some retention of fluid or pathological discharge caused by another process, but a discharge of blood, and not too much of it, nor again far too little. And they have a uterine opening that sticks out a little [into the vagina] and lies straight, because a uterine opening that is naturally out of alignment and lying farther back in the female genital tract is less suited for attracting and receiving the seed.

Also, women able to conceive digest their food easily and do not have constant watery bowel movements, and are calm in their thoughts and cheerful (because perpetual indigestion disrupts pregnancies, and diarrhea in the bowels disrupts the early pregnancy while it is undeveloped), and sadness and extreme shifts in mood dislodge the pregnancy by disrupting the breathing.

Some people, however, also say that women who [appear to] show neither joy nor grief with their eyes, and who quickly change in color, especially if the color becomes darker, are not fit for pregnancy. They say this because there is a great deal of heat in the desires of these women that is changing them and darkening them, through which the seed is boiled away in some manner. But it is a more reliable and fundamental sign, as **Diocles** says, that a woman can conceive if her loins and flanks are fleshy, broad, freckled, rosy, and if she is masculine in her face, and that women who look the opposite way are infertile. Specifically, these women are underfed, scrawny or obese, too old or too young. But he pays the most attention to an observation of vaginal suppositories involving **pessaries** of resin, rue, garlic, garden cress, and coriander. If, once inserted, their characteristics are carried up to the mouth, he says that these women are able to conceive, and if not, the opposite. **Evenor** and **Euryphon** use these substances in a **fumigation** while the women sit on a birthing chair.

9. The words in square brackets have been added by the editors of the text to make sense of the Greek. It is also likely that there are other missing words in the Greek text of this sentence.

But all this is false. Because even women who are not fleshy in the loins have gotten pregnant, and items administered as suppositories and fumigations are circulated through passages that may be observed through deduction,[10] even in someone who is not able to conceive. For **Asclepiades** says that if a waxy ointment of rue is applied to a person with ulcerated legs, the distribution of it will become noticeable to the patient. Generally speaking, one must find out what state the woman's whole body is in as well as her uterus. Because just as poor soil does not promote the growth of seeds and crops, but through its badness undoes the good qualities of both crops and seeds, so too female bodies that are not in a normal condition are incapable of taking control of the seed put into them, but due to their badness they compel the seed to sicken or even to be destroyed.

Book 1, Chapter 12. What is the best time for sex leading to conception?
Just as not every time of the year is suitable for sowing extra seeds onto the earth for the purpose of bearing fruit, so too for humans not every time is suitable for the seed ejaculated during sexual intercourse to produce conception. And so, in order that the desired end of purposeful intercourse may be achieved through good timing, it is useful to discuss that timing. The best time for sex for pregnancy is when the menstrual period is just finishing and tapering off, and urge and appetite for copulation is present, and when the body is neither hungry for something nor overly stuffed and weighed down with drink and indigestion, and after the body has been massaged, a small snack has been eaten, and a state of mental comfort with respect to everything exists.

The best time is when the menstrual period is just finishing and tapering off, for the time before the menstrual period is not suitable because then the uterus is weighed down and in an insubordinate state because of the overabundance of matter and is not able to perform two motions that are opposite to each other: expelling one type of matter, and receiving another. Just as when the stomach, weighed down by some matter to the point of heaving, is turned by nausea and is prone to vomit up that which constricts it, being averse to taking in nourishment, so too by this same principle the uterus, when it is full during the time of the menstrual period, is best able to empty itself of the blood that is inside it, but is unable to take hold of the seed and gestate it. And the time when the menstrual period is beginning must also be passed over because of the generalized contractions, as we have said, and likewise the time when the menstruation is increasing and at its peak because the seed is moist and the blood that is being pushed out washes it away with its quantity. Just as a wound does not heal when a hemorrhage is pushing it apart, and even if it is closed temporarily opens again when the hemorrhage pushes through, so too is the seed unable to be glued in place and grow into the fundus of the uterus because it is being pushed away by the bloody flow pushing forth.

And so the only suitable time is at the very end of the menstrual period, because the uterus has been unburdened and there is an appropriate proportion of warmth and moisture.

10. Soranus is here referring to invisible passages in the body that were believed to transmit odors of the substances mentioned in the previous paragraph from the vagina to the mouth.

For, again, the seed cannot be attached unless the uterus has already been made rough [or, rather,] scraped down at the fundus. And so, just as with sick people food taken during a remission and before an attack [is retained], but during the attack itself it is vomited back up, in the same way the seed that has been taken in is also safely retained at the time when the menstrual period is finishing. And even if some have conceived at another time, especially when menstruating a short while, we must not dwell on a few isolated instances, but declare the correct time for conception by drawing conclusions from scientific explanations.

We added "when urge and appetite for copulation is present." For, just as the seed is not ejaculated by the male without appetite,[11] in the same way it is not received to be conceived by the female without appetite. And just as food eaten without appetite while there is some aversion is not swallowed well and causes issues during the subsequent digestion, so too is the seed unable to be received and, even if it is captured, is unable to be carried to term unless the urge for sexual intercourse and appetite is present. And even if some women conceived under force, one can say that, in their case, the condition of appetite was surely present for them too, but was rendered imperceptible by the mind's resolve. In a similar way, the appetite for food often exists for mourning women, but it is rendered imperceptible by the grief resulting from their misfortune. Indeed later they are compelled to eat, reversing their resolve, due to overwhelming hunger.

And so the proper time is when there is appetite, so long as the body is neither weighed down nor hungry. Because it is not enough to have the urge for sexual intercourse if the state of the body is not also ready. For, just as we often have an appetite for food when the food already eaten is poorly digested and ruined, and if we should eat something, giving in to the impulse of our appetite, we also ruin this food. Similarly, the proper time is not just the time when there is an appetite for sexual intercourse, unless we observe the other factors, for in the case of women with very high libidos there is a desire for sexual intercourse all the time. Therefore, do not let the body be starved and out of shape, because it is reasonable to conclude that if the whole is weak, the parts are weak too. In this way it is likely that if the uterus is rather out of shape, it is likely unfit to perform its function, which is to conceive.

And so sexual intercourse should be undertaken neither when the body is hungry, nor again when it is weighed down, as it is during indigestion and drunkenness. First, because when the body is in a natural condition it performs its appropriate functions, but it is not in a natural condition when it is drunk and suffering from indigestion. Therefore, just as no other natural function can be performed in such a state, so too conception is impossible. Second, because the attached seed must be nourished, and takes its food from the bloody and aerated matter that is being carried to it.

But in women who are drunk or suffering from indigestion all vapor is contaminated and the **pneuma** is made cloudy. And so there is danger of the seed being degraded to a worse condition by the bad particles being pulled into it. Furthermore, being full due to drinking creates an impediment to the seed attaching in the uterus. For, just as wine causes

11. In this discussion, "appetite" refers to people's basic, animal urges for sex and food.

drunk people's wounds to resist closing up due to its spreading out in the body, it also stands to reason that the attachment of the seed is disrupted by the same cause.

What must one say about the state of the soul bringing about certain changes in the form of the fetus? For example, some women who have seen apes during sex have given birth to babies who look like apes. The tyrant of the Cyprians, because he was deformed, forced his wife to look at very beautiful statues during intercourse and became the father of attractive children. And horse breeders set well-bred horses in front of the female horses during mating.

So, in order that the child who is being conceived does not turn out to be misshapen because the soul is assaulted by strange figments of the imagination when drunk, women should be sober during intercourse. Moreover, a certain resemblance to the mother is carried over to the child not only in body, but also in soul. Therefore, it is good that the child be formed in the likeness of a soul that is in a good condition and not knocked out of balance by alcohol. It is completely ridiculous that a farmer takes a great deal of care not to sow his seeds on saturated and swampy fields, but that people assume that nature will go about creating life well when the seeds are being planted into bodies that have been saturated and blocked up due to overindulgence.

In addition to these facts, the best time, as previously mentioned, is after a massage and a small snack. Offering the snack will bring about an urgent arousal for intercourse, since the urge for mating is not diverted to a hunger for food. The massage will create a state that is more prepared for taking possession of the seed when it has been ejaculated. For just as massage encourages absorption in the digestion of food, in the same way it works toward the reception and retention of the seed, since yesterday's surplus has been cleared away, so to speak, and the cleaned-out body is in the proper state for performing its natural functions. So, just as a farmer sows only after cleaning the land and removing foreign matter from it, in the same way we advise that the body be massaged before sowing the seed of a human being.

This advice is not in conflict with what is said in *On Hygiene* that the best time for sex is before a massage, because what was said there was relevant generally to all other sorts of sex, including between men. But here, sex specifically aimed at making children is being singled out. For, however healthy it is in its own right to be massaged after the turbulence of sexual pleasure, it is equally advisable to keep still so that the seed is kept in place.

Some of the early authorities have also used external circumstances to determine the right times for conception. Thus, the time when the moon is waxing is considered suitable. For, they say, conditions on the earth are connected to conditions in the sky, and just as the creatures in the seas grow bigger when the moon is waxing, but weaken when the moon is waning, and in house mice the lobes of the liver swell when the moon is waxing, but shrink when the moon is waning, so too do the powers of seed within us and other animals increase when the moon is waxing, but decrease when it is waning.

Also, they say that the most effective time for conception to occur is the spring, because in the winter when bodies have been made more compact the seed becomes difficult to conceive, and even if it is conceived into a pregnancy, it remains stunted just like seeds tossed on the earth (for, during the winter those seeds are kept from growing, and the offspring of animals born during the winter are difficult to care for). But in the summer, they say, due to the large amount of evaporation making everything weak, the seed and the sexual organs of these creatures are also weak, in the same way that their entire bodies are.

But even without subjecting these claims to reason, there is enough evidence from observation to disprove them. We see conception occurring and being carried to term in every season of the year. And if some people are constitutionally unsuited to summer and endure heat more poorly, or others are unsuited to winter and do poorly in the cold, we will not look to the seasons for the reasons, but to the specific design of the body. This is because we define the right time generally as the time at which the body is not deprived, not weighed down, and feeling good in every respect. And as for the phases of the moon, if some change in the structure of our bodies happened, we definitely would have observed it, as is the case in mice and oysters. And if no such change in our bodies has been observed, such a claim will be believable, but also completely false.

Book 1, Chapter 13. If getting pregnant is healthy
Some people think that getting pregnant is healthy because every natural function is useful, and pregnancy is a natural function. Second, because some women who menstruate with cramping and experience pressure in the uterus are relieved of their difficulties after experiencing pregnancy.[12] In opposition to these arguments, it must be said that a menstrual period is a natural function, but is not healthy, as we have already explained previously.[13]

It just so happens that even if a function is useful, it does not follow that it is also always healthy. For instance, both menstruation and pregnancy are useful for the creation of human beings, but are not healthy for childbearing women. And even if women who have gotten pregnant are relieved of their previous uterine difficulties, it is because they have been relieved of those conditions that they go on to get pregnant.

And even supposing they have indeed been relieved through pregnancy, pregnancy becomes an aid against illnesses, and not a general measure for maintaining health, just as bloodletting does not become healthy just because it puts an end to illnesses when used as a treatment. Also, according to what was set out earlier,[14] it must be said that many burdensome conditions beset women during gestation, who are weighed down and suffering from **kissa**. Furthermore, one should know that the food needed for one organism must be split to feed and grow two organisms, and therefore there is not enough food left to nourish the pregnant woman. What is allotted to the fetus being gestated must be taken away from the woman pregnant with it. For it is impossible for her to take in more nourishment to keep up with the increasing consumption, since the process of digestion will not support the management of more food. If, therefore, she takes in as much as she is able to digest, and from that digested amount the part that is directed to the fetus being gestated is taken away from

12. Soranus may be referencing the Hippocratic treatise *On the Diseases of Virgins* for this claim.
13. Soranus, *Women's Health* 1.8.
14. Soranus, *Women's Health* 1.13.

the woman pregnant with it, then the deprivation is not healthy, and neither is pregnancy good for her health. Also, that pregnancies lead to stunted growth and lack of strength and premature aging is quite clear from the obvious evidence, and furthermore from the similarity to the earth which is so depleted that it is not able to bear fruit every year.

. . .

Book 1, Chapter 16. What is the care for pregnant women?
The care for pregnant women has three stages. Care during the first stage is directed towards the preservation of the ejaculated seed. And the care during the second stage is directed towards addressing the **sumptōmata**[15] that subsequently develop, for example the treatment of the *kissa* that develops. Care during the final stage that is already close to the birth is directed towards perfecting the embryo and an easy endurance of the birthing process. Of these three stages we will now make an overview of the first.

When pregnancy has occurred, we must guard against every excess and disturbance, both in the body and in the mind. This is because the seed is expelled due to fear, grief, sudden joy, and, generally speaking, strong disruption of the mind, and also vigorous exercise and forced holding of the breath [*pneuma*], coughs, sneezes, blows, falls, especially those affecting the hips, lifting heavy things, jumps, hard chairs, **drugs**, the application of strong-smelling substances and substances that cause sneezing, lack of food, indigestion, drunkenness, vomiting, diarrhea, a flow of blood from the nostrils and from hemorrhoids or another place, also relaxation due to a heating agent, and through high fever and shivering and cramping and, to sum it all up, everything that brings on a disturbance through which a miscarriage is produced.

And so, of these things, the items that are within our control must be prevented, and one should keep the pregnant woman resting in bed for one or two days, while she uses massage oils in a simple way to encourage her appetite and to be made ready to take in the food given to her, but she should request that there not be massaging of her belly, so that the seed that is being rooted in place not be torn away by associated motion in that area. One should massage her with newly pressed oil from unripe olives and give her grain-based food, a little less than usual. One should hold off bathing, if it is possible, for seven days; this is because bathing falls into the category of things that loosen up the entire body and will also wilt the new growth of the seed. Otherwise, one would have to believe that wounds not yet firmly closed re-open in the bath and the thickly muscled bodies of athletes are loosened up, but that seed is not melted away when it is still newly sprouted and has only just gained solid form.

For this reason, it is also appropriate to deny wine for the same number of days so that giving her food does not become violent and overpowering. For just as bones heal together at the point of fracture if they are not moved, so too is the seed implanted safely and strongly into the uterus if it is not shaken by forces capable of moving it.

15. We have left the Greek word *sumptōma* (plural: *sumptōmata*) untranslated because it lacks an exact equivalent in English. A *sumptōma* is something that happens, sometimes, but not always, with the implication that what has happened is bad or undesirable. See the word's glossary entry for more details.

That said, this therapy should not be extended too long, so that, once the body has become exhausted by going without wine and food, the uterus also will lose strength. But this therapy must be changed gradually. From the first or second day, she should use passive exercise on a stool or a large chair (the sort that happens when drawn by yoked animals must be excluded since it shakes too violently), then she should take a leisurely and gentle walk, increasing it a little bit every day accordingly. And she should eat foods of moderate character, such as fish that are not too oily and cuts of meat that are not too fatty, and vegetables that are not too biting. Indeed, she should avoid everything that is biting, for instance garlic, onions, leeks, salted meat, and foods that are very moist.[16] This is because very moist foods are easily dissolved, and biting foods cause gassiness and, besides that, are solvents and thinning, which is why we approve their use for treating chronic illnesses that require callouses to be dissolved, for instance.

But it is completely irrational not to realize that things which irritate, dry, wear down the whole physique, and dissolve calluses, that all these things are passed on through the process of distributing nourishment to parts of the uterus, will soften the seed, which has the texture of mucus that has not yet been dried into solid form, much more.

She should also be careful about sex, because it too creates motion in the whole body generally, but especially in the areas around the uterus that need to rest. For just as the stomach holds down food when it is resting, but often when it is shaken it ejects the food it has eaten by vomiting, thus also the uterus when it is not being shaken keeps control of the seed, but when it is being bumped repeatedly, it discharges the seed. She should take moderately warm baths because of both the airs and the waters, without prolonged and plentiful sweating, so as not to wear the body down and make it limp. Accordingly, she should use cold in moderation, so that no shivering sensation develops. After the massage, she should fast until her body rests and the disruption of her breathing [*pneuma*] and the sloshing of her bodily fluids has settled down. Finally, she should drink water a rather long time before her meals, but if she is used to it, also a little watered-down wine.

Let no one assume, even if a woman has violated one or all of these aforementioned rules, but a miscarriage of the pregnancy did not occur, that the pregnancy has not been injured at all. For it has been harmed in such a way that it becomes weaker and more stunted and more difficult to gestate and, in general, more prone to disruption and easily affected by harmful factors and deformed with an imperfect soul. One cannot argue with the example of house-building that if a house is built on firm foundations, it remains standing firmly for many years, and those that are built on cracked and loose foundations collapse easily and with little effort. In the case of living creatures the beginning is no different, except for the fact that they are built, as it were, on different elements and foundations

If the seed has been ejected, this will be detected from the excessive moisture of the woman's vagina, but corrective measures are available against a second failure of becoming

16. The text is uncertain here. The final item in Soranus's list here may simply be "foods that are bitter," but this seems repetitive. "Foods that are moist" is how a Latin translator interpreted what Soranus was saying here, and this seems more plausible.

pregnant. And because of this, if there is some bodily disturbance, one should remove it, and one should comfort the soul, if the worries of daily life have bothered it, and one must strengthen the parts along with the whole body, if there is a lack of strength in the uterine region. And such is the care given during the first stage of pregnancy.

. . .

Book 1, Chapter 22. What signs indicate that a natural birth is imminent?
It is useful to learn the signs that someone is about to give birth in order to prepare the things necessary to bring to a delivery. There comes upon those about to give birth around the seventh or ninth or tenth month a heaviness in the lower abdomen and in the region around the stomach, along with a burning sensation in the vulva and a pain in the groin and inner thighs and the waist radiating down to the regions lying below the uterus. Also, the uterus advances towards the vulva enough that the **obstetrician** making an examination can easily feel it, and its mouth has opened and is soft to the touch when moistened.[17] In proportion to how imminent birth is, the hips and the region around the stomach drop, and the lower belly near the groin bulges, and a continuous need to urinate develops. A viscous fluid also leaks out, then in many cases blood too, flowing out from the thin vessels being broken in the fetal membrane, and an egg-shaped bulge presses back against a finger inserted into the vulva. It has also happened that the distress was the result of inflammation, but this will be distinguished by the mouth of the uterus remaining closed and dry.

Book 2, Chapter 1. What must one prepare for a delivery?
For a delivery that is natural, one must prepare ahead of time olive oil, warm water, warm compresses, soft sea-sponges, wool, bandages, a head pillow, aromatic substances, an obstetrician's stool or chair, two beds, and a prepared room.

Olive oil is for douching and lubricating, warm water is so that the body parts can be washed, warm compresses are for relieving pains, sponges are for sponging things off, wool is so the parts of the woman are covered, bandages are so the newborn may be swaddled, a pillow is so that the infant can be placed on it below the pregnant woman while the after-birth is being dealt with, and aromatic substances (such as pennyroyal, a clod of earth, barley kernels, an apple and a quince and, if in season, a citron, a melon, and a cucumber, and everything comparable to these) for reviving the woman in labor.

And an obstetrician's stool is so that the woman giving birth can be positioned on it. It needs a crescent-shaped cavity cut out at the middle of the stool and at the point where the attendants hold her up, not so big that she is carried down through at her hips, and conversely not so narrow that the vulva is compressed. The latter problem is more difficult to compensate for, since a wider opening can be padded by the obstetrician adding folded cloth. The entire width of the whole stool should be enough to accommodate heavier women, and it should be moderate in height because a stool can be placed under the feet of very short

17. The Greek here contains what seems to be an explanation added by a later scribe who copied Soranus's text. The explanation says: "its mouth opens at a soft touch and dilates with perspiration."

women to compensate for the gap. As for the open spaces under the seat, they should be enclosed with planks, but the front and back sides should be left open for the activities of obstetricians, which will be discussed soon.

For the spaces above the seat, there should be two arms on either side in the shape of the letter Π[18] for her to press her hands upon while pushing. And behind her there should be a backrest, so that her hips and thighs will have a backstop against gradual slipping; for if they lean back against a woman stationed there, by the crooked angle they would impede the direct delivery of the fetus. Some people also include a projecting axle with cranks on each side and a knob on the lower parts of the stool, so that during the extraction of a fetus slip-knots or cables can be wrapped in loops around the arms or other parts of the fetus and, once they have tied the ends to the knob, they will perform the extraction of the fetus through traction, not knowing the general rule that the fetus extraction procedure in a difficult delivery must happen while the woman is lying down.

The stool therefore must be made according to the specifications that we just mentioned, or a chair that has been cut away at the front, or also the back, and with a hollow which often has some sort of padding attached and suspended at the back by leather straps.

And there should be two beds, one made up to be soft for her to rest on after the birth, and the other firm for reclining on while giving birth, so that a worn-out bed does not sag at the hips, as such beds tend to do . . . [and one must have her lie down][19] on her back, with her feet pulled up and together, but with her thighs spread, with something wedged below her hips so that the female genitals are angled downward . . .[20]

[. . .] First, one must sooth the pains by touching with warm hands, and next one should soak cloths with sweet and warm olive oil and apply them over the belly and labia, then keep them soaked with warm olive oil, and also one should place bladders filled with warm olive oil alongside.

When the mouth of the uterus is opening up, the obstetrician should coat her hands with warm olive oil and insert the index finger of her left hand, its nail trimmed short, encouraging the mouth open gently until the nearest portion of the fetal membrane bulges down, and with her right hand she should keep the body parts coated in olive oil, taking care not to use oil that has been used for cooking. When the bulging portion of the fetal membrane has

18. Π is the capital form of the Greek letter for "p," Pi.

19. The words in square brackets have been added by the editors of the text to make sense of the Greek.

20. There is a break in the Greek manuscripts of Soranus here. But an adapted translation of Soranus into Latin by **Caelius Aurelianus** preserves the likely sense of what is missing in the Greek: "Also, the bed should be low enough that an obstetrician in a seated position can hold the woman giving birth in place. Then the bed should also be fixed firmly in place so that it does not wobble when the fetus is being pulled out. Also, let the place in which the delivery is happening and the place where the women rest after the birth be mid-sized. This is because a small room suffocates; it is difficult to find a large room that is warm. And so let the air be kept at a moderate temperature, for cold air, due to its contrast, constricts things a bit. Likewise, high heat cuts short the strength of the woman giving birth far too much."

become about the size [of an egg] below the mouth of the uterus, if the laboring patient is weak and out of shape, she should be placed lying down for the delivery, since this way causes less tearing and it is not as frightening. But if she happens to be in good shape, she should be helped up into a sitting position on the so-called obstetrician's stool [. . .].[21] The laboring woman should be warmed thoroughly with warm olive oil [in her body parts] and given douches to keep her from becoming easily chilled. Let there also be placed on her feet as a covering . . .[22]

There should be three women standing by as assistants, capable of allaying the fear of the woman giving birth, even if they themselves do not happen to have given birth. Two of them should be on either side and one behind to hold the pregnant woman steady against slumping over during labor pains. But if there is not an obstetrician's stool available, the same posture can be achieved if she sits on a woman's lap. That woman must be in very good shape so that she can support the weight of a woman and hold her seated upright during the pains of labor. Finally, covered neatly above and below with an apron, the obstetrician should sit opposite and a little lower than the woman giving birth. For the delivery of the fetus must happen from higher areas towards lower areas. The practice of having her kneel down, as some people advise, makes it difficult for her to work and is undignified. Similarly, the practice of having her stand in a pit so that she would not be working with her hands from above, as **Hero** required, is not only inappropriate, but also impossible in a second-floor room.

Therefore, the obstetrician, with her thighs parted and leaning forward a little onto her left foot so there is good support for working with the left hand, should be seated in front of the woman who is giving birth as has been already said. I advised already that the sides of the stool's base should be covered, but that the back should be kept open for the necessary use of the attendant, because she must maintain pressure on the laboring woman's anus by pressing a small folded cloth against it to prevent it from prolapsing and splitting open while the woman is pushing. Moreover, it is a good practice for the face of the woman giving birth to be visible to the obstetrician, who should address her fear by reassuring her that the birth is proceeding without any cause for alarm.

Then, one must advise the woman to push her breath [*pneuma*][23] down into her flanks without screaming, but rather with a groan and holding her breath. For some inexperienced women, by holding their breath in the upper part of their body and not pushing their breath downwards have given themselves swollen throats. For this reason, in order to keep the flow of air unrestricted, they loosen up the woman's belt and free the entire chest from bindings, though not in order to conform to the common adage that "the feminine consents to the presence of no bindings," and because of this also loosen her hair. For the aforementioned reason, perhaps the loosening of the hair promotes the head being in good shape.

21. More of the Greek text is missing here.
22. The Greek text breaks off here.
23. In this paragraph and the next, the Greek word *pneuma* is always translated as "breath."

And so, we must encourage the women to hold their breath in and not to cringe back from the pains, but when they come, then they should especially bear down and push. The obstetrician should be careful not to hold her gaze fixed on the vulva of the woman giving birth, so as not to cause the body to freeze up in embarrassment. But the obstetrician should encourage the dilation at the mouth of the uterus with her finger in a circular motion [and] the labia . . .[24]

And the mouth of the [uterus[25]] points upwards, but sometimes it also veers downward. And then, one must slip the fingers in carefully during the interval of relaxation and pull the fetus forward, pausing when the uterus is pulling against her, but then gently pulling when it dilates. For doing this while a contraction is in progress is likely to cause inflammation or hemorrhage or downward displacement of the uterus. And the assistants standing at the sides should press downward with their hands on the bulge of the belly, straight down towards her lower parts.

Finally the obstetrician should catch the fetus herself, having first wrapped clothes around her hands or, as the obstetricians in Egypt do it, with thin coverings of papyrus in such a way that it will not slip out of her grasp or be squeezed roughly, but slide gently into place. And if the afterbirth is expelled also, it should also be dealt with immediately, but if the afterbirth is retained, while the woman giving birth is lying down the newborn should be placed nearby . . .[26]

TEXT 45. AËTIUS OF AMIDA, *FOUR-VOLUME COMPENDIUM* SELECTIONS (16.10–12, 16.22–25)

Aëtius *(sixth century CE) was a physician who seems to have served at the court of the emperor Justinian (who reigned from 527 to 565 CE) in Constantinople. Aëtius's* Four-Volume Compendium *provides a comprehensive account of how medicine was taught and practiced in his*

24. The Greek text breaks off here, and a significant section of content is missing. An adapted translation of Soranus into Latin by Caelius Aurelianus preserves the likely sense of what is missing in the Greek: "And if the sac has been ruptured not at all, it should be opened with an ointment. Or if it has broken on its own, the break should be widened [with an ointment]. Also, she should take care, if the mouth is open, that the fetus does not fall out suddenly and be broken when it slips out and cause the umbilical cord to rupture from the distention, because the flow of blood leads the patient into danger. However, once the sac has been opened sufficiently, the head of the fetus is next pushed out. For this is how it is brought out when nature's duty is performed properly. And the birth is even better if the infant's face is turned toward the mother's lower back. Then one ought to help the mouth of the uterus open with light distention so that the head can emerge more easily, but with extra caution so that it [the fetus] not develop an injury when squeezed too hard. But when the head has come out, then the mouth of the uterus should also be distended so that it does not close up back with a natural reflex and choke the infant. For it always alternates back and forth between these motions, when it now opens itself up, and then pulls itself back in. Also, when the shoulders are coming out, the fetus should be taken out by the obstetrician's hands. And it must not be coaxed out in a straight line, but rather slightly tilted at an angle, and moved along with a gentle push on both sides."

25. The missing section of text makes it unclear what word this is meant to be, but "uterus" is likely given the context.

26. The Greek text breaks off here again.

*time. Each section of the text follows a pattern of quoting from an earlier authority and then add-ing commentary drawn from Aëtius's own experiences, especially relating to **drugs** and surgeries. The selections below, which are drawn from Book 16 on pregnancy and childbirth, describe ail-ments typically experienced in pregnancy and childbirth, as well as detailed advice on abortions and embryotomies (the procedure for removing a fetus that has died from its mother's womb).*

Aëtius wrote in Greek, and large portions of his text survive in this language. But the only reli-able version of the Four-Volume Compendium *is a Latin translation made in the sixteenth cen-tury by the scholar Janus Cornarius.*

SOURCE: Translation by Lesley Bolton based on the Latin text from Janus Cornarius, *Aetii medici graeci Contractae ex ueteribus medicinae sermones XVI* (Venice: Ioan. Gryphius, 1542).

Book 16, Chapter 10. On *Pica*, according to **Galen**

About the second month of pregnancy, a particular ailment occurs in pregnant women which gets its name, *pica*, from the small bird, the magpie. Some people, though, believe this ailment is called *citta*[27] by the Greeks because of its similarity to the ivy plant, which is called *citta* in Greek. For just as ivy is in the habit of spreading and attaching itself to all manner of plants, so too women suffering from *pica* long for all manner of foodstuffs which, in turn, yield pleasure and displeasure.

The ailment generally occurs about forty days after conception. It involves an upset stom-ach accompanied by nausea and an aversion to food, resulting in the vomiting of bile and phlegm. Then, without relief, follows excess saliva, stomach-ache, and feelings of anxiety. All these things develop especially because of an excess of bloody **humor;** this is normally expelled via the vessels of the womb during the monthly periods, but it is contained by the presence of the fetus and rises upward, where it disturbs the stomach at a time when it is more sensitive than normal. Because of the varied nature of this bad humor, the women crave various and odd foods. Some crave salty food, some tart food, others crave soil, or shells, or ashes. Often this ailment lasts to around the fourth month of pregnancy. For, at the start, only a moderate amount of blood is assigned as food for the fetus. But, afterwards, with the fetus growing, more nourishment is drawn to it. Then, finally, with this bad humor purged partly through vomit, and partly by being carried off to the womb for the sake of feeding the fetus, the previously mentioned ***sumptōmata***[28] diminish.

So, for those women who retain excess blood, a moderate amount of food is adequate, and exercises that are appropriate for women can help dissipate the excess. Travel and things that tire out the body are also useful. But as for pregnant women who are not accustomed to working, they tolerate badly any sudden and arduous movements. Those whose stomach is

27. This word is also sometimes spelled *cissa*/**kissa** (see the glossary of subjects).

28. The Latin word here is *accidentia,* which translates the word *sumptōmata* in the original Greek of Aëtius's text. We have left *sumptōma* (plural: *sumptōmata*) untranslated because it lacks an exact equivalent in English. A *sumptōma* is something that happens, sometimes, but not always, with the implication that what has happened is bad or undesirable. See the word's glossary entry for more details.

pained by bitter, or tart, or salty humors will benefit from drinking lukewarm water in order to provoke vomiting that will expel the offending humor. They should abstain from sweet foods, and they should drink old, tawny, fragrant wine which is a little on the tart side. The quantity of fluids should be moderate, however, so that foods do not float about undigested in the stomach. Also, before a meal, it is advisable to serve olives preserved in brine with some soft bread, or five to seven bitter almonds, or barley meal sprinkled with the juice of quinces or pomegranates, or chicory or endive, or marsh asparagus or wild parsnip. Poultry which is neither fatty nor gamey is good. Also suitable are pigs' trotters, snouts and stomachs, and freshly caught sea-urchins. After meals, one should give raisins, pomegranates, and pears. All of these, however, should be in moderate quantity. Those who avoid eating must be enticed by the variety and delightfulness of food. This is of no use to those who eat soil, however, who should be given fresh starch in place of soil.

There are other drugs that are good for *pica,* such as extract of purslane taken with food, and peeled cucumber seeds taken in water; also, an infusion made from knotgrass or dill, or extract of rhubarb or spikenard, or juice of endive, or the plants themselves enjoyed raw as well as cooked in plentiful quantity. But if what the women vomit up is rather thick and, because of the viscous nature, can only be brought up with difficulty, they ought to eat pickled fish and radishes in honeyed vinegar, and every effort should be made to draw out the dangerous humor before pains and cramps can set in. It is also useful to apply things externally to the weakened stomach, such as **poultices** made from wine, wild grapes, the flowers and buds of the pomegranate tree, roses, myrtle, myrrh leaves, and fennel seeds; nutgall, or cumin, or wormwood can also be added. Also useful is a **plaster** made from the fleshy parts of the palm fruit that have been crushed, and soaked or cooked in wine, or a poultice of quinces, either crushed in vinegar-water or prepared with rose-oil or nard balsam, along with saffron. Or, soak unscoured wool or linen strips in wine and oil, or vinegar and oil, or rose-oil and vinegar, or nard wine and regular wine, and then apply to the stomach. For all these alleviate the pains that will vex the stomach. Furthermore, drinking warm water (not boiling hot), and slowly and regularly walking about, and covering, warming and anointing the diaphragm with soft wool, and exercising the lower parts before meals according to individual strength—all these things help the patient wonderfully regain her health.

Book 16, Chapter 11. On Swollen Feet in Pregnant Women
For swollen feet in pregnant women, massage the feet with a mix of rose-oil and vinegar, maybe add some salt. It is also useful to apply Cimolian earth in vinegar, or fissured alum in wine. It is good also to wash the feet with a decoction of lemons. Also, spread *anthylis* that has been soaked in vinegar on flattened cabbage leaves, and apply.

Book 16, Chapter 12. The Care that Ought to be Given to Pregnant Women, according to **Aspasia**
Pregnant women who have just recently conceived must be protected from fear, sadness, and every powerful disturbance of the mind. Also, travel in wheeled vehicles, strenuous exer-

cises, holding the breath,[29] and blows to the hip area must be avoided. Nor should she lift heavy weights, or jump up and down, or sit on hard chairs. Nor will we allow bitter foods, or ones that cause flatulence, or powerful enemas, or too much or too little food or drink. Also, a loss of blood brings danger to pregnant women, whether the blood comes from the nose, from hemorrhoids, or from any other place. For these reasons, then, it is best to employ a moderate amount of food that is suitable for the stomach, travel in a sedan chair, light walks, gentle massage, and exercise through wool working.

Around the eighth month, which is the most troublesome of all, the quantity of food should be restricted, and movements that are over vigorous should be limited. If the bowel movement is suppressed because of narrowing of the rectum brought on by the womb pressing upon it, foods should be given suitable for purging the stomach, such as barley juice, cooked sorrel, mallow, and lettuce. Finally, in the ninth month, frequent bathing is advisable to relax the body in readiness for the event, so that the woman who is to give birth might bravely bear the upcoming pains of labor.

. . .

Book 16, Chapter 22. Causes of Difficulty in Birthing.

Difficulty in birthing happens for various reasons: either because the woman in labor is feeble in mind or body, or both at the same time, or because of a small womb, or because the birth passage is narrow. Women who are rather short of stature because of their age generally have a womb corresponding in size to the other parts of their body. And difficulty in birthing may also happen for any of these reasons: either because of the slanted position of the neck of the womb, or because of **flesh** that has grown in the neck or mouth[30] of the womb; or, on account of inflammation or abscess or hardening in this part; or, because the fetus is not able to break through the fairly tough membrane that surrounds it; or, on account of the fluid that is collected in the womb being expelled before the appropriate time, there is no fluid near the time of birth and the parts remain dry at a time when there is special need of fluid that might provide an easy passage for the fetus; or, because the woman in labor suffers from a stone in the bladder which, if pressed on the neck of the womb, causes difficulty in birthing; or, on account of the fleshiness and plumpness of the pregnant woman. Also, pubic bones that have grown together too much cause difficulty in birthing, as they are not able to be expanded during the birth, for in women the pubic bones are not fused together as in men, rather they are held together by strong ligaments. Also, difficulty in birthing occurs because of too large a **cavity** of the loins pressing on the womb, or because of a large quantity of feces or urine retained in the rectum or bladder. Some give birth painfully because of the weakness of advanced age; others because they get distressed as soon as the birth process

29. The Latin word here is *spiritus*, which is a translation of *pneuma* in the original Greek of Aëtius's text.

30. The mouth referred to the opening of the womb (fig. 21). We believe that most ancient authors had in mind what we now call the "cervix," though some might have identified the mouth as the vaginal opening. The neck referred to the area just behind the opening, either behind the cervix or behind the vaginal opening (i.e., the vaginal canal).

begins and, because of inexperience, they do not know how to prepare their bodies appropriately beforehand; or, because of their age, they are not yet mature, nor have their bodies attained strength for they are, as yet, girls and they spend their lives childishly.

Moreover, difficult birth happens when the entire fetus, or a part of it, is exceptionally large; for sometimes the head, chest or belly develops more than normal; or, when the fetus is quite weak and is not able to assist its mother with its own leaps and turns; or, when it has two heads or three legs; or, when twins both unexpectedly enter the neck of the womb at the same time; or, when the fetus has died and offers no help to the woman in labor; or, when the dead fetus swells and lies in an unnatural position.

The natural position for the fetus in delivery is head-first with hands extended alongside each thigh. But it is contrary to nature when the head deviates to the right or left side of the womb; or, when one, or both, hands is thrust outside, and when inside the legs are spread apart. Among the remaining positions, however, the least problematic one is feet-first, especially if the fetus presents with hands extended alongside each thigh. But fetuses that present with one foot extended, the other foot being retained in the womb, or those that present doubled-up and resting on some part of the womb, require straightening, as do those that have outstretched hands. The others, that present in oblique position, are somewhat less of a problem, and it possible for this to occur in three ways, for the fetus may present from either side or from the stomach; but it is safer to present from the side, as this gives the **obstetrician** an opportunity to direct the fetus into head- or feet-first position. But those who present doubled-up are in the worst position for delivery, especially if in buttocks-first position. Doubled-up fetuses occur in three ways, for they can lie with the head and legs in the mouth of the womb, or with the belly or the buttocks in the mouth of the womb. But if the belly presents, it is advisable to press against the belly, and once it has opened, with our help, and the contents have been released, the little body settles down and changing its position becomes easy.

Birthing is also difficult if the afterbirth does not come away, either because of its thickness, or, because of its thinness, it was torn before it was time to do so.

Further, difficulty in birthing arises from external causes, such as when cold and wintry weather constricts the birth passage, and warm and summery weather loosens it.

The physician should inquire from the obstetrician about all these things regarding the ailing woman who is giving birth; nor should he rashly resort to surgery; nor should the obstetrician be allowed to tear the womb further. If, therefore, a difficult birthing occurs because of the cavity of the loins, let the woman in labor be set on an obstetric chair, leaning forward and with her knees flexed, so that the womb, slipping down, might lie in a straight line with the birth canal. Plump and fleshy women should be set up in a similar fashion.

For any narrowing, or numbness, or tightening, it is necessary to bring the aid of relaxation by means of warm sitz-baths and **fumigations,** in such a way that even the air of the house becomes warm, also infusions of oil that bring relaxation not only through their active capacity but also through their capacity of being quite warming, and also plasters and poultices of similar type. Relaxing agents should also be applied after the bath, if there is no fever or other symptoms that might prohibit this, and the woman should be carried on a litter to a warmer place. Also, strong spasms have occurred in cases such as these.

For any women who are weak through some debility, it is necessary to strengthen them for the birth with things that firm and tone and encourage sturdiness. Such things are sprays and sitz-baths of myrtle, foliage of the grape vine, pomegranates, or roses. These are scented with vinegar and oils made from wine and cold rose-oil.

If difficult birth occurs because of the unnatural position of the fetus, it must be brought to a natural position, in as far as this can be done. If the fetus extends a hand or foot, it should not be drawn out by the limb, for this causes even greater impaction, or the limb is dislocated or even broken. Instead, by applying the fingers to the shoulder or hips of the fetus, the extended part may be brought to a suitable position. But if there is impaction, and the position of the entire fetus is bad, it should first be lifted up and away from the mouth of the womb, and then redirected to the mouth of the womb again.[31] All this should be done slowly, gently, and without pressure and the parts should be regularly anointed with oil, for this way lies safety not only for the fetus but also for the laboring woman, and the womb likewise is uninjured.

If the orifice of the womb remains closed, it should be softened and relaxed with fatty drugs. But if a stone is present, we must force it out through the neck of the bladder with a catheter. If the bladder is full of urine, we must draw out the urine with that same catheter. If the rectum is full of excrement, we must cleanse it with an enema. If a woman is unable to give birth because of inflammation, abscesses, ulceration, soft or hard tumors, or anything similar, we must treat these individually according to the nature of the conditions. If difficulty in birthing occurs because a fleshy growth has formed in the neck of the womb, or because a somewhat tough membrane is present, as is the case in women who have an imperforate opening, whatever impediment there is, it must be cut away. If the membrane that surrounds the fetus is overly tough, such that the fetus cannot break it, it must be cut apart. When the fluid contained within the membranes has leaked out before the appointed time, with the result that the parts have become parched, a mixture of egg white and mallow, or cooked and strained fenugreek, or warm barley juice should be poured in. If smallness of the womb is the cause of difficulty, the parts must be anointed with some type of fat and kept warm, the mouth of the womb must be dilated by the fingers, and the fetus must be extracted with force. But if this does not succeed, the fetus must be dismembered; this must especially be done when the fetus is large or dead. We will recognize that it is dead from the fact that it is cold to the touch and it does not move. If there are twins or triplets and they are blocking the neck of the womb, the others should be pushed back into the fundus of the womb while the one which seems more ready for birth is drawn out first. If birthing is difficult because of the size of the head, or chest, or belly, it is absolutely necessary to dismember the fetus. The time for positioning the woman in labor on the obstetric chair is

31. The instruction here seems like it should also advise that the position of the fetus should be turned before it is redirected back to the mouth of the womb.

when the mouth of the womb is open and the part that is to be cut off projects and can be touched with the fingers.

Book 16, Chapter 23. On Extraction and Dismemberment of the Fetus, according to Philumenus

The physician must consider beforehand the undertaking of a dismemberment, particularly as to whether the woman will recover or not, that is, whether she can be saved or whether she is a lost cause. The physician will, indeed, accept the one capable of being saved, but reject the hopeless case. Those who are mortally afflicted are overwhelmed by a lethargic stupor and are enfeebled. They can only be revived with difficulty, and they respond to the loudest requests only weakly, and then are carried back off into stupor. Some are also seized by spasms, and tremors arise from their nerves. The pulse races vigorously, but can be detected only as faint and weak. But those who can be saved suffer nothing of this sort.

The woman should lie down on the bed on her back, with her head lower and her legs raised, and she should be held on either side by experienced and sturdy women. At first, two or three mouthfuls of bread dipped in wine should be given, to prevent a faint. During the actual procedure, the face should be continually sprinkled with wine. The surgeon should find out the cause of difficulty by spreading the vagina apart with an instrument, and seeing whether there is a growth or hard swelling, or one of the other things we have mentioned. Whatever it is, taking hold of it with a pair of tweezers, the surgeon will cut it away with a scalpel, as we will teach later on. But if a membrane obstructs the mouth of the womb, he will also cut this away, as we will describe below in the discussion of imperforate women. If the toughness of the covering surrounding the fetus is a problem, we stretch it out with a pair of tweezers, and cut it away with a sharp knife. Then we will dilate the incised area with our fingers and make it suitable for the passage of the fetus.

If the head of the fetus obstructs the opening, it is turned around to be feet-first and is drawn out in this manner. But if, in this situation, the head has become impacted and cannot, in any way, be pushed back, the extraction hook must be fixed in the eye, or mouth, or chin, and the infant drawn out in this way. The extraction instrument should be held in the right hand, but its hook should be hidden by the fingers and gently introduced by the left hand, and fixed into one of the places mentioned. Then another instrument should be inserted and affixed likewise on the opposite side, so that extraction may occur evenly, deviating to neither side. And this is safer, for with just one instrument it might, by chance, slip off during extraction, and let go of the fetus. Thus, the fetus may be pulled out evenly, not only in a straight line, but also side-to-side; and a finger smeared with some fat may be inserted between the mouth of the womb and the impacted body, and drawn around in a circular fashion. If, on the other hand, the head is very large, either by nature or by an affliction with watery hydrocephalus, and it is impacted, it must be cut open with a scalpel and thus evacuated. Once it has collapsed, then the fetus should be extracted. If it will still not come forth, it is necessary to crush the skull and to remove the bones with the fingers. If the bones are sticking out, they can be removed with dental or bone forceps. Then, finally, attach the extraction instrument and extract the fetus. If, once the head has progressed, impaction occurs around the chest, in the same way, the areas around the collar bones must be cut with a scalpel, cutting as far as the cavity so that the fluids evacuate, and the mass of the chest subsides.

If the belly is very swollen, either because the fetus is dead or because it has a condition like **dropsy**, using the same method we will open up the belly and remove the intestines.

If a hand has extended, the arm must be cut off at the shoulder. When doing this, it is necessary to wrap the hand in a linen cloth so that it will not slip and draw the arm out a little at a time, so that the shoulder joint is stretched out. Then, spreading apart the lips of the vagina, make the cut. Then insert the left hand and direct the head and so draw out the fetus. Do likewise if both hands have extended. Likewise, also, if the feet are thrust forward but the rest of the body is not following, it is necessary to cut at the groins.

If a doubled-up fetus occurs that cannot be straightened, if the head is within easy reach, we will crush the head bones without cutting the skin, and we will affix the extraction hook to some part and draw the fetus out with the legs in a straight line. If the legs are put forth more, we will make the cut at the hip joints, and pass over the hips to reach the head that is easily readied for crushing. If the doubling-up causes more of an obstruction and the feet thrust out, the head is amputated at the point where it joins the vertebrae, then, with the chest moved to the other side, the feet are drawn out. If, after the removal of other parts of the body, the head draws back and remains stuck, insert the left hand, smeared with oil, into the depths of the womb and seek the head. With the fingers, turn the head around to the mouth of the womb and affix one or two extraction hooks. As to places suitable for the instrument to be affixed: if presenting head-first, the eyes, the ear passages, and the part under the chin; if presenting chest-first, the armpits, the collar bones, the diaphragm, the breast, and the vertebral joints; and if presenting legs-first, the pubic bones and the female genital passage.

If the mouth of the womb is closed because of inflammation, nothing should be done violently, rather plentiful fatty infusions, sitz-baths, irrigations, and poultices should be used. Once the inflammation is calmed somewhat, the mouth of the womb is dilated, and the fetus is drawn out as has been previously described.

When we have reduced the entire fetus to pieces, all the parts must be collected together and we must examine them diligently, in case something is missing or has been left inside without our knowledge. Then the afterbirth must be removed quickly.

Book 16, Chapter 24. On the Removal of the Afterbirth, according to Philumenos
If the afterbirth [*secunda*], which is also called *loculus*—it is called *secunda* because it is like a second home or container after the womb, and like a covering of the fetus—if, I say, the afterbirth is retained, sometimes the mouth of the womb is closed, sometimes it is found open, and sometimes it is inflamed. Also, at times the afterbirth is found attached to the fundus of the womb, at other times it is separate.

If, therefore, the mouth of the womb is open and the afterbirth is found separate, rolled up like a ball around some part of the womb, removal is very easy. Warm and anoint the left hand with fat, insert it into the cavity, seize the afterbirth and extract it. But if it is attached to the fundus of the womb, we will insert the hand likewise and grasp the afterbirth, but we will not draw it out immediately and in a straight line, because of the fear of prolapse of the womb. Rather, gradually, and with no violence, we will first draw it gently to one side, then move it this way then that. Finally, somewhat more forcefully, will we draw it out. For in this manner it yields and is loosened from the points of attachment.

If the mouth of the womb is closed, we will apply fatty irrigations and we will gently open it with the fingers of the left hand, and we will try to dilate it gradually. If this does not succeed, it is beneficial to cover the upper abdomen with fresh barley flour kneaded with warm water and oil, and to moisten these areas afterwards and apply fatty fomentations. Also, if bodily strength is not lacking, administer substances that cause sneezing, prepared from castoreum and pepper. Given as potions, these also promote menstruation, as we will discuss later. All these things should be done on the first and second day. We will use, in addition, fumigations of aromatics, using an earthenware pot and things like cinnamon, nard, flower of scented rush, wormwood, iris, juniper, dittany, pennyroyal, and other things of this sort. The pot is placed beneath the obstetric chair, and the woman sits upon the chair with her clothes arranged around the pot on all sides. After some time, we will examine her and, if we find the mouth of the womb open, we will insert a hand and we will try to draw out the afterbirth in the manner that has been described. But if it still cannot be drawn out this way, it is not right that it should be agitated, for, within a few days, it will have putrefied and will fall out as a loosened, bloody mass. Since the foul smell fills and congests the head and upsets the stomach, appropriate sweet-smelling aromatics should be regularly burned. Tried and tested for this purpose are cardamom seed, fig, bdellium, juniper, frankincense, styrax, black jet stone, aromatic onyx, and labdanum gum. Also, one **drachma** each of castoreum and pennyroyal in honeyed water should be given to them to drink.

Suitable also for promoting lighter menstruation is a decoction of wormwood and laurel berries in honeyed wine. Also, **pessaries** inserted from below achieve this, made from myrrh and extract of cyclamen. Likewise, the afterbirth of sheep and goat, dried, ground, and drunk in wine, or applied as an ointment, or carried as an amulet. Another pessary: mix ten drachmas each of raisin pulp, cumin, resin, turpentine, and foam of soda in honey and insert. Also, they can take sitz-baths in decoctions of wormwood, laurel berries, dill, and chamomile.

Book 16, Chapter 25. Care after the Dismemberment of the Fetus, according to Aspasia
Once the afterbirth has been removed, whether immediately after the removal of the fetus or at a later time, and nothing is left in the womb that should not be there, the legs are placed together so that torn parts may come together. If the parts seem sufficiently purged, they should be washed with a decoction of mallow or fenugreek, and bathed with warm oil. The loins and pubic areas should be bathed with the same, and covered over with soft wool dipped in warm oil. Soft food should be offered, but drinking of water should be prohibited.

If the post-delivery discharges are lighter than they should be, we will prescribe sitz-baths with decoctions of fenugreek, wormwood, mallow, and pennyroyal. Likewise, we will give a decoction of pennyroyal and fenugreek as a drink. If the post-delivery discharges are heavier than they should be, moderately **astringent** irrigations and sitz-baths should be applied, the abdomen should be bound with a broad bandage, and astringent foods should be offered. If inflammation occurs, it must be remedied. If there is a copious flow of blood, it also must be treated in ways we will describe later. If none of these occur, the neck and mouth of the womb, and the pubic area, should be anointed with something fatty and kept warm.

CHILDHOOD AILMENTS AND PEDIATRIC CARE

In order to maintain stable population levels in ancient Greece and Rome, women had to give birth to five or six children on average. This was not only because of the high mortality rates in childbirth, but also because approximately one-third of all infants died during their first year, and in total up to half of all children died before they reached the age of five (see figs. 7, 66). In order to ensure demographic stability, it was imperative to keep childhood mortality rates as low as possible. Thus medical writers dedicated a good deal of attention to the care of children and to childhood ailments.

Once an **obstetrician** had successfully delivered a baby, she would cut the umbilical cord and the newborn would be bathed to clean it of uterine matter, blood, and feces. Then the infant would be swaddled in cloth blankets or strips (often made of linen), a process that many believed would mold and shape the infant's malleable body into a good form. Indeed, many sources describe the newborn child as unformed and ugly, and therefore in need of forming through the physical manipulations of swaddling (see fig. 64). Massage too helped shape and form the infant, and as we learned in chapter 10, depending on the degree of pressure applied could also tonify the infant's body, or soften and relax it.

Galen recommended sprinkling the newborn with salt prior to swaddling in order to dry infants who were thought to be wetter at a young age (Text 47). However, he warned that physicians ought to be careful to maintain the natural balance of the infant's **humors**, avoiding excessively drying treatments and favoring those that paired well with infants' natural moistness and heat. This is one of the reasons why (wet, warm) breast milk was recommended for infants, often until the age of three, a topic we will discuss in more detail shortly.

Infants were to follow a regimen particularly suited to preserve their health. This regimen was carried out by a variety of caregivers including the obstetrician, the mother, household slaves, and (if the family had the means to afford it) wet nurses. As part of this regimen, Galen prescribed frequent warm baths as a way to soothe fussy infants and to induce sleep. In fact, bathing was prescribed throughout childhood until they reached adolescence (i.e., around fourteen).

Many writers, both medical and nonmedical, addressed the question of how to nourish the newborn child. In particular, there were varying—and often strong—opinions about whether or not the infant should be handed over to a wet nurse to be breastfed by her (see fig. 63). The orator Favorinus was reported to have spoken harshly against wet nurses, emphasizing that great harm, both physical and moral, could come from handing a small child over to

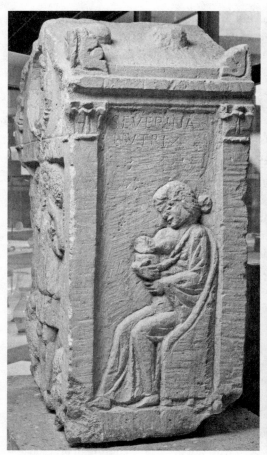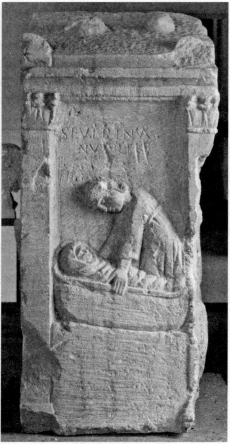

FIGURES 63 and 64 Third-century CE funerary monument of Severina, a wet nurse (*nutrix*). Various reliefs on the monument depict her engaged in her caregiving duties. In the scene on the left, Severina is pictured breastfeeding an infant. In the scene on the right, she overlooks a swaddled infant. Römisch-Germanisches Museum (inv. no. 74.414), Rheinisches Bildarchiv Köln. Photo credit: Anja Wegner.

a strange woman who might corrupt the child with her "foreign and degenerate nourishment" (Aulus Gellius, *Attic Nights* 12.1). Nonetheless, we have plenty of evidence that many elite families made use of wet nurses both for the mother's convenience and to ensure proper feeding when the mother was incapable of producing sufficient milk for her children.

Wet nurses could be household slaves or paid employees on contract. In the selection below, **Soranus** expounds on the most important qualities one is to look for when hiring a wet nurse (Text 46). Some of those requirements—especially the ability to speak Greek, an attractive appearance, and good moral character—may seem strange to modern readers. But they make sense once we appreciate the widely held belief that milk conveyed more than just nourishment (see fig. 65). Thinkers like Soranus understood breast milk also to transmit

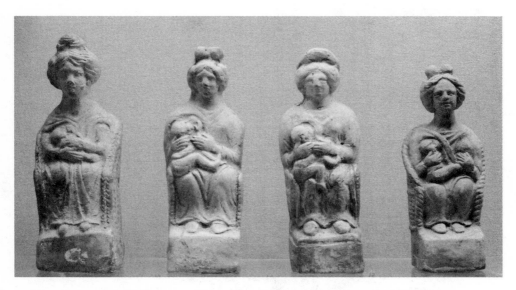

FIGURE 65 Second- to third-century CE terracotta figurines, from Roman Gaul, of women breastfeeding children of various ages. National Archaeology Museum, Saint-Germain-en-Laye. Wikimedia Commons, Creative Commons Attribution 3.0.

other substances in a woman's body, including, for instance, the semen of a man who had sex with the wet nurse, semen that made its way into the wet nurse's blood and then distilled into her milk. Moreover, the wet nurse was also thought to transmit her character to the infant (hence, Favorinus's concern about degenerate influence). Because the infant's mind (like its body) was believed to be malleable at this age (some writers describe the infant's impressionability in terms of the imprinting of a seal on wax), the infant was susceptible to receiving impressions of its parents' and caretakers' morals. Thus the character of the wet nurse who spent time with the child, and whose milk the child imbibed, was thought to be capable of either improving or ruining the health and character of the child.

We know that breastfeeding was indeed related to some childhood illnesses. We hear from Soranus that the young child could suffer from illnesses such as *aphthai* (which may be what we now call "thrush"), a yeast infection in the mouth that caused inflammations, such as canker sores. These sores could impede the child's ability to nurse and to get sufficient nourishment, which in turn weakened it and made it susceptible to other kinds of illnesses. Additionally, the time when breastfeeding ended was considered a particularly dangerous moment for the young child. Exposure to solid food meant exposure to new sources of illness (what we now identify as bacteria and parasites). Hence, weaning infants were at risk of dying from ailments that, for instance, caused diarrhea or hindered the absorption of nutrients.

Even when children were not ill with childhood afflictions, they were often fussy and prone to fits of crying. There were different views on how to deal with infants who were

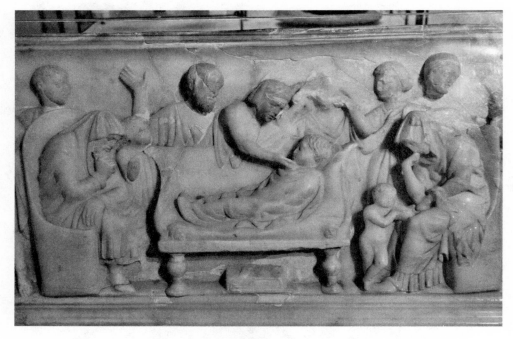

FIGURE 66 Second-century CE marble sarcophagus, from Porta Aurea at Agrigento, Sicily, depicting a mourning scene for a child. The dead or dying child is lying on the bed, surrounded by his parents at the head and foot of the bed, with heads bowed in deep sadness. Other figures express grief through raised hands or by caressing the child's face. Archaeological Museum of Agrigento. Wikimedia Commons, Creative Commons Attribution 4.0.

upset in these ways. **Plato** recommended cuddles and soothing for distressed infants, whereas **Aristotle** thought of crying as an early form of exercise. Both Galen and Soranus discussed remedies for dealing with distressed infants, and both cited breastfeeding as the favored solution. Galen also recommended soothing sounds (music) and gentle movement (rocking). Although our ancient sources do not identify a condition we today refer to as colic—frequent and prolonged episodes of crying as a result of intestinal pain—these discussions of how to soothe crying children might be evidence that colic was a problem with which mothers and wet nurses in antiquity had to contend.

If a child survived past the age of five, his or her chances of advancing into adulthood increased significantly (see fig. 7). This seems to be why medical writers tended to spend less time discussing ailments and regimen for later stages of childhood. While Galen does speak about optimal regimens for children at this stage, his focus is primarily on the development of the exemplary male child destined for a life of intellectual and political activity (Text 47, *On Hygiene* 1.12). His discussion of physical and moral character in tandem conforms to the holistic approach of ancient medicine in general. Galen does, however, recognize that individually prescribed regimens would vary according to the kind of occupation a young man might prepare for, whether civil service, manual labor, or craftsmanship. Meanwhile, as discussed in an earlier section of this chapter, regimen for young girls focused more exclusively on the preservation of chastity until marriage, and preparation for conception, pregnancy, and childbirth.

As we read the recommendations for infant and child care, we recognize that only a minority of children—namely, elite boys—would have received the idealized care described in medical sources. The majority of children would have experienced the effects of poverty and malnutrition. And we should keep in mind that many children (regardless of status) would have suffered other forms of hardship, such as physical and emotional abuse, neglect, household accidents resulting from insufficient childcare provisions, and workplace accidents linked to child labor. In a world where fathers and masters had the legal right to punish children and young slaves, sometimes severely, it is no wonder we find moralists and philosophers counseling adults on the importance of restraining emotions such as anger. Too often adults did not heed this advice, leading the children in their care to suffer as a result. Additionally, we find no warnings against bringing children to dangerous workplaces where they might sustain injuries that could affect them for the rest of their lives and sometimes even cause death (see fig. 66).

TEXT 46. SORANUS, *WOMEN'S HEALTH*[32] SELECTION (2.8)

In Women's Health, **Soranus of Ephesus** *(second century CE) is guided by two main concerns: protecting women's health and managing pregnancy and childbirth. He also discussed the ideal features of the wet nurse tasked with breastfeeding the newborn child. Soranus's advice focuses on the age and body of the wet nurse, with particular emphasis on the size and appearance of her breasts. Soranus was also concerned about the character of the wet nurse, insisting that she be a Greek woman with strong control over her emotions.*

SOURCE: Translation by Molly Jones-Lewis based on the Greek text from Paul Burguière, Danielle Gourevitch, and Yves Malinas, *Soranus d'Éphèse, Maladies des femmes, Livre 2* (Paris: Les Belles Lettres, 1990).

Book 2, Chapter 8. About the selection of a wet nurse
A wet nurse no younger than twenty nor older than forty should be chosen, one who has given birth twice or three times, who is free from sickness, in good physical condition, who has a body that is larger in size and has a healthier complexion, having mid-sized[33] breasts, spongy, soft, and unwrinkled, and nipples that are neither large nor too small and neither too firm nor too loose and spurting out milk in a gush. She should be sensible, kind, not

---

32. This text has previously been translated with the title *Gynecology*, but this traditional title may give the misleading impression that the text is only concerned with women's reproductive system, and not with women's health more generally.

33. The Greek word used here can also mean "symmetrical."

prone to anger, Greek, and with good personal hygiene. For each of these criteria the reasoning is as follows, in order.

She should be in the prime of life because those who are younger tend to be inexperienced in child rearing and they have a rather careless and childish attitude. Older women give more watery milk due to the lack of muscle tone in their body. But for those who are in the prime of life, they are in excellent shape for every bodily function. She should have given birth two or three times because first-time mothers are not yet practiced to a high standard of child rearing and have breasts whose structures are still childish and small and rather dense. But women who have given birth many times and have nursed children frequently are wrinkled and do not produce milk of the best quality. [And she should be free from sickness because healthy and nourishing milk][34] comes from a healthy body, but bad and inferior milk comes from a sickly body, just as water flowing through bad earth itself also becomes bad because it has been ruined by the quality of its source.

And she should be in good physical condition, that is plump and strong, for the same reason, but so that she does not become easily tired by her duties and her night-time monitoring, and as a result change the quality of her milk for the worse. Her body should be larger in size because, for all things being equal, milk from large bodies is more nourishing. And she should have a healthier complexion, because in such people larger vessels[35] carry material to the breasts, so that there is more milk. And she should have mid-sized breasts, because those that are small have little milk, but those that are bulky have more than is necessary, with the result that if the surplus remains after nursing, fresh milk is no longer being suckled by the newborn, but milk that is spoiled in a certain sense. But if all of it is suckled out by other children or animals, the lactating woman will become completely exhausted.

Moreover, larger breasts, when they fall onto the nursing babies, weigh them down. Some people even suggest that such breasts often have a smaller amount of milk, since the nourishment going into them is being spent on increasing **flesh** and not on the quantity of milk.

Her breasts should be spongy, soft, and unwrinkled and not riddled with visible vessels or having clotted blockages stuck in them. For breasts that are thick and hard and riddled with vessels produce little milk, but those that are shriveled and wrinkled like those found on old and skinny women produce watery milk, but those who have clotted blockages make thick and uneven milk. The nipples should be neither large nor too small because big nipples chafe the gums and make it difficult for the tongue to help with swallowing, but small

34. This phrase is not in the Greek text here; the translator has supplied it from the previous paragraph for clarity.

35. "Vessels" could refer to a number of kinds of passages in the body through which bodily fluids travel.

nipples are difficult to latch onto and they discharge milk in small quantities. As a result, newborns struggle to suckle and therefore fall prey to the so-called *aphthai*.[36]

Her breasts should also be neither too firm nor too loose and spurting out milk in a gush because breasts with narrow ducts do not release milk easily without compression. As a result, newborns are in distress in their suckling, because not as much milk is being let down as they are trying to suckle. And conversely, if they are too loose, they introduce the danger of suffocation because in suckling the milk is carried to the mouth in a gush. And the wet nurse should be "sensible" so she refrains from sexual intercourse and drunkenness and lust and other pleasure and unwholesomeness, because along with this sexual intercourse cools off the nurturing impulse towards the child being nurtured due to the distraction of the pleasure of sex. Moreover, it spoils the milk and reduces the supply or stops it entirely by stimulating the menstrual purging of the uterus or causing a pregnancy.

About the issue of drunkenness, it harms the lactating women in both soul and body, and because of this the milk is also ruined. Secondly, if she is seized by a very deep sleep she leaves the newborn uncared for or even falls down on it in a dangerous way. Thirdly, an excessive amount of wine passes its quality on into the breastmilk, and because of this, newborns become sleepy and drugged, and sometimes even have tremors and sudden paralysis and spasms, just as piglets who have been nursed by a sow fed on the dregs of wine grow lethargic and pass out.

And she should be kind and affectionate so that she will go about her duties without shirking and complaining. For some are so unfeeling towards the baby they nurse that they pay no attention to prolonged periods of crying, but do not even adjust the posture of a baby lying, allowing it to rest in one position. Often the sinews suffer damage due to compression resulting in numbness and degeneration. And she should not be prone to anger since the child being nursed naturally comes to resemble the women nursing it. Because of this, the child becomes surly from cranky nurses, and pleasant from even-tempered nurses. Moreover, angry women are frenzied and they are not able to hold on when the newborn is crying in fear, and they throw it down out of their hands or they flip it over dangerously. For this reason too the wet nurse must not be superstitious or prone to being possessed by a deity, so that she will not put the newborn in harm's way because she has been led astray by faulty logic and is sometimes trembling with madness. And the wet nurse must have good personal hygiene so that the child's stomach is not loosened up by the smell of the swaddling clothes and so that it does not lie awake because of itching or later develop any ulcers. And she should be Greek so that the child nursed by her becomes accustomed to the most beautiful of languages.

She should have had her milk for at most two or three months. This is because the earliest milk, as we have said, is rather thick and difficult to digest, but old milk is not nourishing and is thin. Some also say that it is necessary that a nurse who is going to feed a male child should have given birth to a male, and that likewise one who will nurse a female child

36. *Aphthai* likely refers to thrush, a yeast infection of the mouth.

should have given birth to a female. One should not listen to these people because they do not account for the fact that those women who have given birth to twins use one and the same milk to feed both their male and female child. And also, every type of animal feeds from the same nourishment alike, both the male and female offspring, and in no way does this practice lead to the male offspring becoming more feminine, nor the female offspring becoming more masculine.

But one must provide children with multiple lactating women in order to accomplish safe and successful child rearing, because it is risky to entrust a single child to just one wet nurse, who might then sicken and die, at which point the child is confused by the change in milk and distressed, and sometimes even refuses it entirely and dies of starvation.

TEXT 47. GALEN, *ON HYGIENE* SELECTIONS (1.7, 1.9, 1.12)

In On Hygiene, **Galen** *(c. 129–c. 216 CE) discusses how to preserve a person's "hygiene," a word that refers in this context to good health rather than cleanliness. Maintaining hygiene involved following an appropriate regimen, including diet, exercise, massage, bathing, and sexual activity. Good health would be cultivated and maintained by achieving an appropriate balance between the bodily **humors**, a concept expressed in this translation with the word **krasis**, which literally means "mixture" in Greek.* On Hygiene *includes discussion of good health at all stages of a person's life, but the selections below focus on how young children could maintain good health.*

SOURCE: Translated by Ian Johnston based on the Greek text from K. Koch, *Galeni De sanitate tuenda, De alimentorum facultatibus, De bonis malisque sucis, De victu attenuante, De ptisana,* Corpus Medicorum Graecorum 5.4.2 (Leipzig: Teubner, 1923). First published in *Galen, Hygiene,* vol. 1, Loeb Classical Library 535 (Cambridge, Mass.: Harvard University Press, 2018). Copyright ©2018 by the President and Fellows of Harvard College. Loeb Classical Library ® is a registered trademark of the President and Fellows of Harvard College.

Book 1, Chapter 7. Let us speak now about the best [constitution] in which each part is without fault in its whole substance. Certainly, such a person would be fortunate if, after the time of his birth, he came to the art of hygiene and were to have the support of this. In this way, he would also derive some benefit for the *psyche*, since a good regimen is a preparation for good habits. But even if, during one of the subsequent stages of life, he were to come to the use of the art, he would also derive the greatest benefit in this way.

What I shall say first is that, if someone were to take charge of such a person from the beginning, he would make that person healthy throughout his whole life, unless some violence were to befall him from without, for this has nothing to do with being versed in the art of hygiene. Second, I shall relate how someone would support a child, even if he were not newborn but already able to be trained; and the same with each of the other stages of life. Moreover, in the case of the newborn child who is faultless in his whole constitution, let us first wrap him in swaddling clothes, after sprinkling moderate amounts of salt over him, as a result of which the skin would be firmer and thicker than the internal parts. For when the baby is *in utero* everything is similarly soft since it is neither touched by any harder body from without nor does cold air strike it. It is due to these things that the skin becomes contracted and compressed—both harder and more dense than it was before, and more than the other parts. When it is born, the infant is inevitably going to come into contact with both cold and heat, and with many bodies harder than itself. Because of these things, it is appropriate for us to prepare its natural covering in some way, so it is best able to resist being affected [dyspathic]. In those infants who are in accord with nature, an adequate preparation is through salts alone. Those who are abnormal to some degree need to be covered over with the dried leaves of myrtle or some other such thing. However, what lies before us now is to make the discussion about those with the best constitutions. These, as I said, having been wrapped in swaddling clothes, are to be provided with milk as nourishment and baths of beneficial waters; the whole regimen needs to be moist, inasmuch as the *krasis* is more moist than in the other stages of life.

This seems to bring us immediately to the first question of what is essential for a healthy regimen. For there are those who think natures that are too moist always need to be dried, just as natures that are too cold always need to be heated, natures that are too dry to be moistened, and those that are too hot to be cooled, for each of the imbalances is increased by like things but corrected and reduced through the opposites—in short, "opposites are the cures of opposites."[37] But they must not only know and remember **Hippocrates'** statement, that "opposites are the cures of opposites," but also that in which he says, "moist regimens are beneficial to all who are febrile, particularly children, and others who are accustomed to being so treated."[38] Here he has obviously placed three things in juxtaposition—disease, stage of life, and custom. From the disease, he takes the indication of opposites while from the stage of life and custom, he takes the indication of similars. For in a fever (which is a hot and dry disease), the moist regimens are beneficial, whereas in children (for in them it is not in fact a disease but a stage of life and accords with nature), what is most similar is most helpful. It is also the same with customs, as these produce certain acquired natures in bodies for which the exhibition of opposites is very harmful. And what is right for bodies in accord with nature, is that one must preserve the proper (i.e., preexisting) state, whereas in those who are diseased, one must set in motion a change to the opposite. Therefore, each of the two is preserved by similars but changed by opposites.

One must not, then, dry children because the moistness in them is not contrary to nature, as it is in coughs, coryzas, catarrhs and **dropsies.** Rather, one must feed them with things that are moist in nature, maintaining an accord with nature by means of moist diets and baths of potable waters (for those that display any medicinal quality, such as those that are sulfurous, full of asphalt or contain sodium carbonate or alum, are all drying), and most of all provide food and drink that is particularly moist in *krasis*. And in this way too, Nature

37. Hippocrates, *Aphorisms* 2.22 and *Breaths* 1.
38. Hippocrates, *Aphorisms* 1.16.

herself gave forethought to children, preparing moist nutriment for them—that is, mother's milk. Thus mother's milk is very likely best for all infants other than those who happen to be diseased, and not least for the infant with the best *krasis*, about whom the present discussion is. Anyway, it is likely that the mother of such a child is faultless both in respect of her body as a whole and her milk.

Our nourishment, while still *in utero*, is from blood, while the genesis of milk is also from blood that has undergone the least change in the breasts. As a consequence, those children who are nourished by mother's milk make use of the most customary and fitting nutriment. So it is clear that Nature has not only prepared such a nutriment for infants, but has also provided innate powers for them, right from the beginning, for the purpose of using this nutriment. For also, when the infant has been born, if someone immediately places the nipple of the breast in its mouth, it sucks the milk and drinks it down very eagerly. And if infants should happen to be distressed and crying, the remedy for their grief is not least the breast of the nurse placed in their mouths.

There are, then, these three remedies for the distress of children discovered by nurses who have learned from experience. One is that which we have now discussed; the other two are moderate movement and a certain modulation of the voice. Those who use these things continually not only settle the infant but also put it to sleep, revealing even in this an innate predisposition toward music and exercise. Therefore, someone who is effective in using these arts well is also someone who will be best at nurturing both body and mind.

. . .

Book 1, Chapter 9. I think it is important to take the trouble to do all these things concerning the child up to the third year from birth, and in addition to these, the nurse should give no little forethought to her own food and drink, her sleep, sexual activity and exercises, so that her milk is the best in terms of *krasis*. Such a thing would occur if her blood were at its very best—that is, neither picrocholic,[39] **melancholic, phlegmatic,** whey-like, nor mixed with some other watery fluid. Such blood is produced by moderate exercises, nutriments that are *euchymous* and taken at the appropriate time and in the necessary amount, just as also by drinks that are timely and moderate. All these things will be precisely defined in the discussion that follows.

I direct women who are nursing (i.e., providing milk for) little children to abstain from sexual activity altogether. The menstrual flow is stirred up by sexual intercourse and the milk no longer remains sweet. And some women become pregnant; nothing is more harmful than this for the infant being nourished by their milk. In this case, the best of the blood is used up in the fetus, inasmuch as the origin of life is specifically contained in the blood itself and is provided for by this. Throughout, [the fetus] draws the proper nutrition as if it is rooted in the uterus and always inseparable, both night and day. Because of this, the blood of the pregnant woman becomes less suitable and of poorer quality, and also on this account,

39. Picrocholic is the condition of being affected by an excess of yellow bile; see also the glossary entries for "bilious" and "choleric."

the milk is in a bad state and little is collected in the breasts. As a consequence, I myself would recommend that, if a woman nursing an infant should become pregnant, another nurse should be found, considering and assuming her milk would be altogether better in taste, appearance and odor. And for those tasting and smelling the sweetness and looking at it, the best milk will be seen as white and uniform, and is midway between watery and thick. Poor milk is either thick and very cheesy, or watery and whey-like, livid and variable in consistency and color, and is very bitter to those tasting it. And it will give the impression of saltiness or some other unusual quality. Such milk is not sweet to the smell. Take these as your signs of bad and good milk and base your judgment on them. Whenever either pregnancy or some disease is present involving the nurse and it is necessary to go on to another nurse, make the decision and choice on this.

. . .

Book 1, Chapter 12. Since the discussion is returning again to the child of the best constitution, let me speak in detail about its stage of life from the first seven years to the second, in respect to what the *krasis* is and what kind of regimens it needs. Now the *krasis,* as I have shown in the treatises *On Mixtures,*[40] is similarly hot but not similarly moist. For always, right from the time of birth, every animal becomes drier every day but not hotter or colder in the same manner in every stage of life. But in the case of those bodies that are best constituted, the heat remains about the same up to full development, whereas in the case of those that are moister and colder than the best, their heat increases. However, the discussion is not now about those.

Let a person with the best constitution be kept to the previously mentioned regimen up to the fourteenth year, exercising neither very much nor violently, lest in some way we hold back his growth, and bathing in warm rather than cold baths, for he will not yet be able to tolerate the latter without harm. And in this stage of life, let him be molded with respect to his soul, and particularly through serious habits and studies that are especially able to make the soul well-ordered. For regarding those things that are going to be brought about concerning the body in the stage of life to follow this one, the greatest support comes from good conduct and compliance.

However, after the second seven years and up to the third, if you wish to bring the child to a peak of good health, wanting to make him either a noble soldier, or a wrestler, or strong in any other way whatsoever, you may give less forethought to the good qualities of the soul such as lead to knowledge and wisdom. For it is appropriate for those things pertaining to ethos[41] to be perfected during this time of life particularly. If, however, you prefer the parts pertaining to the body to be strengthened up to a certain point and to attain a certain healthy state and to grow, or if you hope to adorn the rational part of the soul of the boy, you will not

---

40. Galen, *On Mixtures* 1.572–645K.

41. The Greek word *ethos* can refer to the character of an individual, community, or nation. In Galen it refers to an individual's character resulting from the process of education and other kinds of training, including physical training and care.

need the same regimen in both cases. And indeed, even a third or fourth kind of life may be found at some time or other for those devoted to one of the practical arts that maintains the body either with or without exercise—such arts are farming, commerce or something else of this sort. As a result, it seems difficult to put a number on all the kinds of lives. For the profession of the art of hygiene is to give instructions regarding health to all men, which are suitable either to each person individually or to all people in common, or some of them individually and some in common. It is not possible to go over all these at the same time, but the first point is how someone, extending his life for the longest time possible, may be healthy in all respects. It is, I think, necessary for such a life to be free from all necessary activity, leaving time for the body alone. Second, in the subject under discussion, there is the issue of an art, activity, pursuit, some service (either civic or private), or some wholly necessary occupation. Otherwise our discussion would not be clear or easy to remember or accompanied by method, apart from the order spoken of just now.

GERIATRIC AILMENTS AND END OF LIFE

Given life expectancy rates in the ancient world, a smaller portion of the population of Greece and Rome would have reached old age than does today (see fig. 7). That said, if someone survived childhood, they could reasonably expect to live into their fifties or even longer. We even have stories about people who lived into their eighties and nineties—for example, the exemplary seniors Antiochus the physician and Telephus the grammarian discussed in the selection below—though such people would have been exceptionally rare.

There were many factors that affected whether or not one lived a long life. Some had to do with the activities expected of men and women: in order to live into older age, men would have had to survive injuries related to battle and risky occupations, whereas women would have had to survive multiple pregnancies and births. Other factors affecting life expectancy would have been related to socioeconomic class and wealth, such as access to proper nutrition, more sanitary living conditions, and better health care. (Though sometimes health care that involved what we now know to be dangerous procedures might have hastened death rather than forestalled it!)

Those who did reach advanced years, especially if they were men of higher status, could expect to be treated with more respect than young people. In antiquity, youth was not fetishized in the way it is today (especially in North American society); rather, older adulthood was privileged as the time that garnered more authority and respect. Yet old age was not a time of leisure. People did not retire from work in the way many today do. Rather, they stopped participating in work when they became physically or mentally incapacitated or because they died. We have reports of professional men who slowly withdrew from work life on account of waning energy in their later years. For instance, **Seneca** wrote a letter to his friend describing the discomforts of old age, while also noting how fortunate he was to have the excuse of incapacity to get out of work he no longer wanted to do: "I am grateful to old age for keeping me in my bed. And why shouldn't I be grateful for this? I can't do what I shouldn't want to do" (*Letter* 67).

Seneca's description of old age in this letter aligned with what medical writers thought of the aging process: a life stage in which the body becomes colder and drier. Seneca worried about taking baths in cold water because they exacerbated the innate chill of his body; he complained that "even in the middle of summer I can hardly unfreeze, so I spend most of my time covered in clothes" (*Letter* 67). According to **Galen**, the cold-dry bodily state of old age made people more vulnerable to certain kinds of illnesses, including chills as well as different kinds of digestive complaints because the body now lacked sufficient heat to **concoct** and digest food (Text 48, *On Hygiene*). And this undigested food, in turn, led to the buildup of morbid residues that accumulated throughout the body, causing all sorts of additional problems. Furthermore, noticing that the overall appearance of older people's bodies became thin and weakened, Galen conjectured that their inner organs were likewise becoming thin and weakened, and prone to diminished functioning. The Hippocratic text *Aphorisms* lists additional illnesses associated with older age, including catarrhal coughs, arthritis, nephritis (kidney problems), apoplexy (symptoms resulting from strokes), insomnia, failing sight, and deafness. Curiously absent from ancient sources is any mention of dementia.

Galen's regimen for older people focused on supplementing the body's waning heat and moisture (Text 48, *On Hygiene*). Galen recommended that, upon waking, his patients be massaged in order to warm the body and also to aid digestion and distribute nourishment throughout the body. He also advised older people to participate in some form of light exercise, such as walking. He recommended three light meals a day, following the Hippocratic warning that eating too much food would deplete the natural heat of the body necessary for digestion. And the patient's diet should include warming and moistening drinks and food, including wine, barley water, or gruel with honey. In order to aid digestion, and thus preserve vital heat used in the process, Galen prescribed a diuretic dish of boiled vegetables eaten with garlic and plenty of oil. And to keep the bowels moving, he recommended ripe fruits, in particular figs and plums.

Although some older people in antiquity could afford the personal care of a physician to ease the discomforts and illnesses related to aging, most people had to rely on family members for care when they became incapacitated. In these situations, the care provided to older people would have varied widely depending on the family's resources. Acknowledging this, the statesman Cicero (first century BCE) noted that old age could not be easy for those living in poverty. But few of our sources tell us much about the experiences of the elderly poor in antiquity. It was not until the development of philanthropic institutions—poorhouses and hospitals associated with the early Christian church (see chapter 2)—that older people, especially those who were poor and childless, received care.

As life came to a close, there were a number of bodily signs that announced one's impending death. The Hippocratic text *Prognosis* enumerated these signs for the express purpose of warning physicians when to withdraw care in order to preserve their reputations

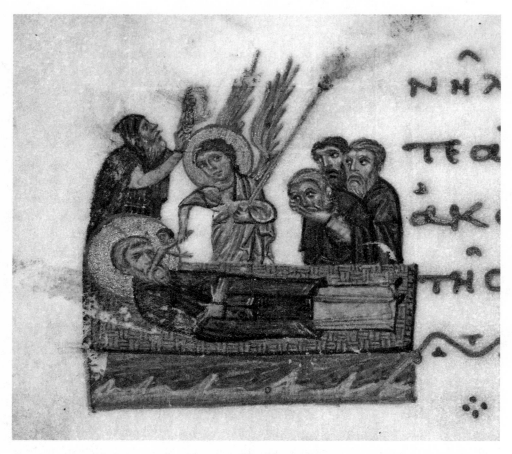

FIGURE 67 Eleventh-century manuscript illustration depicting the soul of a dying man leaving his body and delivered into the hands of an angel who will take the soul to heaven. As in many ancient representations of the moment when the soul separates from the body, the soul is depicted as a baby. From John Climacus's text, *The Heavenly Ladder* (Garrett MS.16, folio 63v). Manuscripts Division, Department of Special Collections, Princeton University. Courtesy of Princeton University Library.

and avoid blame when the patient eventually died. The signs included sunken eyes, cheeks, and temples; the nose taking on a sharp and pronounced appearance; the ears becoming cold and the earlobes drooping; the skin on the face becoming dry, stretched, and hardened; and the complexion becoming pale and dusky. Galen suggested that physicians could also discern when death was approaching by interpreting the pulse and urine. And physicians were instructed to observe the manner of the patient's sleep, whether with eyes partially opened and mouth agape, with the legs curled up, whether fitfully, and so forth. They were also warned that patients who appeared delirious and plucked at their bedclothes might be nearing the end. Finally, in accounts of dying people, we repeatedly hear about their unusual breathing pattern (what we now call a "death rattle").

TEXT 48. GALEN, *ON HYGIENE* SELECTION (5.3–4)

In On Hygiene, **Galen** *(c. 129–c. 216 CE) discusses how to preserve a person's "hygiene," a word that refers in this context to good health rather than cleanliness. Maintaining hygiene involved following an appropriate regimen, including diet, exercise, massage, bathing, and sexual activity. Good health would be cultivated and maintained by achieving an appropriate balance between the bodily* **humors,** *a concept expressed in this translation with the word* **krasis,** *which literally means "mixture" in Greek.* On Hygiene *includes discussions of good health at all stages of a person's life, but the selection below focuses on how older people could maintain good health. Galen offered specific examples of the regimens practiced by people who lived to be very old, explaining how their diet and other routines sustained them.*

SOURCE: Translation by Ian Johnston based on the Greek text from K. Koch, *Galeni De sanitate tuenda, De alimentorum facultatibus, De bonis malisque sucis, De victu attenuante, De ptisana,* Corpus Medicorum Graecorum 5.4.2 (Leipzig: Teubner, 1923). First published in *Galen, Hygiene,* vol. 2, Loeb Classical Library 536 (Cambridge, Mass.: Harvard University Press, 2018). Copyright ©2018 by the President and Fellows of Harvard College. Loeb Classical Library ® is a registered trademark of the President and Fellows of Harvard College.

Book 5, Chapter 3. What kind of body is best was stated previously. What you must know is that what departs from this does so for three reasons; that it was badly constituted from the beginning at the time of pregnancy; that after this for some reason it was brought to a condition contrary to nature; and by virtue of the stage of life (age). One must attempt to restore all these through the opposing excess. To begin with the example of old age, this is cold and dry, as was shown in the writings *On Mixtures.*[42] Correction of this occurs through moistening and heating agents. Such things are hot baths of sweet waters, drinking wine, and those nutriments that are naturally moistening and heating at the same time. Regarding exercises or massage and every movement (for it is better to begin from these since it was well said, "let exertions precede food"[43]), one must realize that what the poet said was right in part:

> when he has bathed and eaten,
> let him rest gently, for this is right for the old.[44]

But the whole matter is not so ordained. For old men need to bring the body to movement no less than young men do, since there is a danger of the innate heat being quenched in them. In the case of bodies in the prime of life, some natures discover they need rest. Concerning these, **Hippocrates** also said somewhere: "none of those who are old need complete

---

42. Galen, *On Mixtures* 2.2.
43. Hippocratic Corpus, *On Epidemics* 6.4.
44. Elsewhere in Galen's writings, he attributes this quotation to Homer.

rest, just as they do not need overly violent exercise."[45] For their heat needs to be fanned but is counteracted by violent movements. Great fires do not still need fanning but are sufficient to maintain themselves and overcome the material. Therefore, all those in the prime of life do not need to be massaged excessively in the early morning after sleep, as old men do. For certainly the objective of such massage occurring with oil is twofold: to cure the fatigue condition before it is increased to kindle a fever, and to activate a weakened distribution. I have easily restored **flesh** in a few days, in many who have been emaciated for a long time, by resorting to such massage. But what occurs to others as an incidental affection at a particular time is always in existence in the aged. Thus, in them, the whole body is cold and unable to draw the nutriment to itself, process it properly and be nourished from it.

But massage, since it stimulates their (i.e., old people) vital tone and heats moderately, makes distribution easier and nourishing more effective. Certainly, in this way too, many young men who are atrophic become enfleshed when following a regimen, while all old men are benefited. There is the one thing you should do for old people in the early morning as an exercise: after massage with oil, next get them to walk about and carry out passive exercises without becoming fatigued, taking into account the capacity of the old person. For there is no small difference between those who are exceedingly weak in movements, even if they do not yet happen to be seventy, and those who are much stronger than them who are more than eighty years old. Direct those who are weaker to passive exercises more than walking around, whereas exercise those who are stronger in both ways. You will bring both toward the second massage but not similarly; always bring the weaker quicker. Take this as one of your most general precepts: in the case of a weak capacity, nourish the body with thick and few nutriments, while in the case of a strong capacity with thin and many.

Book 5, Chapter 4. It is very easy, then, to say these and other things, but taking care of an old person and maintaining his health is one of the most difficult things, just as restoring someone to health from disease also is. This part of the art is called by younger doctors "analeptic" (restorative), while that which pertains to old people is called "geriatric." And both the conditions seem not to be in accord with the most perfect health, but to be midway between disease and health in some cases or altogether not of health in terms of a stable state, but what is called by them health in terms of an unstable state. Therefore, whether we ought to call old age a disease, or a morbid condition, or a condition between health and disease, or an unstable state of health, not giving very much consideration to any such inquiries as far as the argument of our predecessors are concerned, we must know the condition of the body of those who are old, in that it can change to disease following minor causes and must be restored to its original healthy way of life, like those recovering from disease.

45. This passage appears nowhere in the extant Hippocratic corpus. It could be a paraphrase rather than a quotation: similar subjects are discussed in Text 20, *Regimen in Health*, or from a text no longer extant.

This is why it is easy to say it is better to anoint the old person with oil after massage early in the morning, but to carry out the task properly is the most difficult thing of all. For a slightly harder massage is fatiguing, whereas that which is very soft accomplishes nothing more, just like that which is altogether brief, while a large amount of massage disperses more than it nourishes. Furthermore, if the place in which the old man's body is exposed is too cold, the massage not only accomplishes nothing useful, but also condenses and chills. If, on the other hand, the place is hotter than it needs to be, in the winter it makes the body of the old man more loose-textured than is appropriate and causes him to be easily chilled, whereas, in summer, it disperses and dissipates his capacity. Thus, in those who are healthy in terms of a stable state, none of the stronger causes change the body, whereas in old people even the smallest causes bring about great change. Moreover, it is like this in the case of the quantity and quality of the foods, for even in these, if old people overstep what is appropriate by just a little, they are harmed a lot, whereas young men are harmed very little by the largest errors.

Therefore, it is safer to give weak old people a little food three times a day, as Antiochus the doctor prescribed for himself.[46] When he was more than eighty years old, he went out every day to the place in which the council of citizens was held, and sometimes took a long route for the purpose of visiting the sick. But he walked to the Agora from his house—a distance of some three *stadia*—and in this way also saw the sick nearby. If, at any time, he was forced to be taken further, he was lifted into a chair and carried or transported in a chariot. In his house, there was a chamber heated by a fire in the winter, while in the summer this had *eukratic* air without the fire. In this above all, he spent time in the early morning, both winter and summer, obviously excreting beforehand. In his place at the Agora, around the third hour or later around the fourth hour, he used to eat bread with Attic honey. Mostly this was toasted; more rarely it was uncooked. After these things, either mingling with others in discussions or reading by himself, he continued to the seventh hour, after which he was massaged in the public baths and performed the exercises suitable for an old man—I shall speak about what kind these were a little later. Then, having bathed, he lunched moderately, first taking those things that empty the stomach and next mostly fish—those from around the rocks and those from the deep sea. Then again, at dinner, he abstained from eating fish and took what was most *euchymous* and not easily spoiled—either gruel with oxymel or a bird with a simple sauce. Looking after himself in old age in this way, Antiochus continued on until the very end, unimpaired in his senses and sound in all his limbs.

However, Telephus the grammarian reached an even greater age than Antiochus, living almost a hundred years.[47] He was in the habit of bathing twice a month in winter and four times a month in summer. In the seasons between these, he bathed three times a month.

46. The identity of this Antiochus is not certain.
47. Telephus was a famous scholar and Galen's older contemporary.

On the days he didn't bathe, he was anointed around the third hour with a brief massage. Then he used to eat gruel boiled in water mixed with raw honey of the best quality, and this alone was enough for him at the first meal. He also dined at the seventh hour or a little sooner, taking vegetables first and next tasting fish or birds. In the evening, he used to eat only bread, moistened in wine that had been mixed.

FIFTEEN

Healing Places and Spaces

Scholars in a field called "health geography" (or sometimes "medical geography") have alerted us to the important relationship between health and place. They call our attention to the spatial patterns by which illnesses spread, especially in terms of how environmental, social, cultural, and political factors mediate the spread of illness. In addition to studying the relationship between *illness* and place, health geographers are also interested in the relationship between *healing* and place. They seek to unpack how the natural and social environments in which medical treatments take place impact people's experiences of health care and even diminish or enhance health outcomes. They ask questions like the following: How are ideas and associations with natural sites mobilized in healing treatments? How do the architecture, light, sounds, symbolism, and spatial organization of healing sites contribute to patients' calmness, assurance, and optimism that they will be healed, as well as to their actual health outcomes? At times, people in antiquity spoke directly to such issues. They marked certain natural sites or regions as particularly salubrious, and they drew attention to how the organization of healing spaces impacted the experience of receiving health care, augmenting the healing process.

NATURAL AND RELIGIOUS HEALING SITES

People in the ancient Mediterranean regarded many natural and religious sites as places that possessed a special potency for healing, potency derived from highly concentrated natural resources or supernatural powers. As sick people clamored to access these resources and powers, we find that whole industries—buildings, personnel, and rituals—arose around these sites.

For example, people regarded the numerous thermal-mineral springs that dotted the Mediterranean, and regions rich with medicinal plants, as especially salubrious places. At one such site, Hierapolis (Pamukkale in modern-day Türkiye), the thermal springs gush forth from the earth, depositing a calcium-carbonate mineral that has solidified into a cascading terrace of pools. From the second century BCE onward, word spread that these springs were good for paralysis, wounds, joint pain, gout, and inflamed organs (such as inflamed bladders causing urinary tract infections or inflamed wombs causing barrenness). Thus the sick and suffering traveled here to bathe in the pools or in the bathhouses whose waters were routed from the thermal springs. Some visited thermal-mineral springs on the advice of physicians who reasoned that the temperature and quality of the water helped to restore humoral balance, or to relax constricted body parts (see a possible example of such advice in Text 8, Hippocratic Corpus, *On Epidemics* 5.9). At some sites we find nearby religious altars or temples that credited the healing powers of the natural sites to gods and goddesses, including Heracles, **Apollo, Hygieia**/Salus, and **Asclepius**.

When people visited thermal-mineral springs, they found various ways to make use of curative waters.[1] According to **Pliny the Elder,** some visitors bragged about the number of hours they soaked in the waters, while others boasted about the vast quantities they imbibed (so much that their bellies swelled). These reports suggest that ancient people thought the waters' powers intensified the more people interacted with them. Some visitors also made offerings to the gods—such as coins and anatomical votives thrown into the springs themselves, or placed at nearby altars—hoping the gods' power to heal would magnify the effectiveness of the healthful water. For those who were unable to travel to such sites, water from the springs was bottled, transported, and sold, as we see depicted in scenes from the Salus Umeritana springs in modern-day Spain (see fig. 68).

While some regions were deemed extrasalubrious for their natural springs, other regions were known for their plants and roots, which were thought to be especially effective as medicinal treatments. The Greek island of Crete, for example, had such a reputation. Pliny and **Theophrastus** reported that rare plants, such as dittany, grew only on Crete. Even for plants that were also available elsewhere, Pliny tells us that it was common knowledge that those grown on Crete were far superior. And just as the waters of natural springs were bottled and shipped, so too the medicinal plants and roots of Crete were exported; in fact they were in such high demand that they fetched high prices at markets abroad and, when imported to Rome, were set aside especially for the imperial court.[2]

In addition to natural sites, religious sites were believed to be places where healing was especially potent. Whether visiting a local shrine or sanctuary, or traveling further to seek healing at a more famous temple—such as the large Asclepian temple complexes in Epidaurus (in

---

1. At the bottom of the springs, archaeologists have discovered cups, presumably dropped by those drinking the spring water.

2. Some emperors employed botanists and root cutters on the island to avoid having to rely on traders.

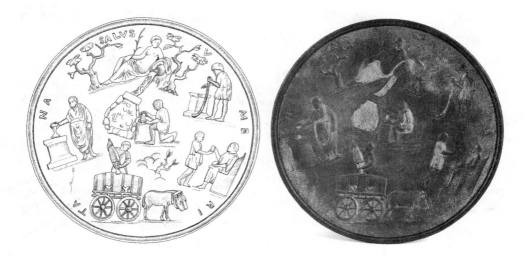

FIGURE 68 Roman period silver and gilt bowl depicting the operations at a natural hot springs in Spain. The goddess Salus—whom the Romans equated with Hygieia—is shown controlling the flow of waters into the spring (and was likely understood to be the goddess presiding over the salubrious springs). A man, likely a temple worker, scoops the water out of the spring into a cup and serves it to a visitor, while in another scene the temple worker tends to altar sacrifices. A visitor leaves an offering on the goddess's altar. Finally, a large barrel on the back of a mule-drawn cart is being filled with the healing spring water, presumably to be sold to people who could not make the trip to the site itself. Photo credit: Pátera de Otañes; 1881 © Museo Nacional de Escultura, Valladolid (Spain). Depósito en el Museo de la Biblioteca Nacional de España CER00201. Illustrator's rendering by Gina Tibbott.

mainland Greece), Cos (the Greek island homeland of **Hippocrates**), and Pergamum (in modern-day Türkiye)—ancient people endowed these sites with an aura of sacred power. Moreover, the magnificently constructed environment of temple complexes must have amplified this sense of power, boosting visitors' confidence that they would find healing there. Let's take, for example, the experience of arriving at the Asclepian complex in Epidaurus, one of the largest and best-known healing centers of the ancient Mediterranean (see fig. 49). Visitors would have entered the complex through a monumental gate and followed the pathway to the temple of Asclepius. Inside, they would have encountered a towering gold-and-ivory statue of the god, seated on a throne and holding his signature serpent staff, and they would have been surrounded by inscriptions touting the god's power and success in healing past visitors.

Beyond this awe-inspiring first impression, every other building and activity of the temple complex was coordinated to signal healing—from the *abaton,* the two-story dormitory building where the sick and suffering slept and received their dream visions or dream healings (see chapter 10) to the therapeutic sites throughout the complex where prescribed remedies were carried out—all these features must have had a cumulative impact on sick people's morale.

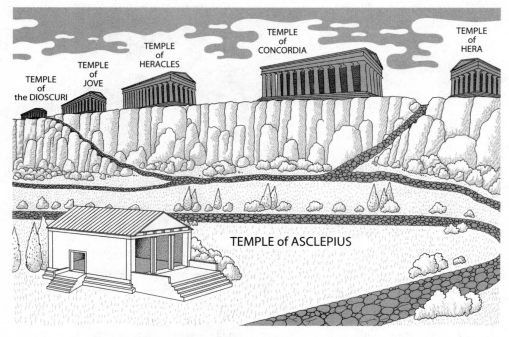

FIGURE 69 Illustrator's rendering of the Valley of the Temples in Agrigento, Sicily, with the temple of Asclepius foregrounded. Despite the fact that all of the other temples to the gods and goddesses were located on the elevated ridge, the temple of Asclepius was level with the main road, making it more possible for weak, injured, or impaired people to visit without needing to climb the hill. Created by Gina Tibbott.

And while they engaged in various treatments, visitors could be entertained by performances at the theater (which could hold 14,000 spectators!) and by athletic contests at the stadium, both within the temple complex. These leisure activities would have put them at ease, which would have further facilitated healing. The round building known as the *thumelē* or *tholos* seems to have been a place where songs and instrumental music were performed; the concentric rings of columns that encircled the building and a labyrinth of hollow spaces beneath the floor would have resonated with the songs and music for a dramatic auditory experience. All of these activities and building features made the temple complex a sensory-rich environment; and as scholars have recently shown, healing spaces with sensory input—such as sound, music, art, light, aromas, and color—foster wellness and recovery.

Some Christian churches, especially those dedicated to physician-saints, such as Cosmas and Damian or the *anargyroi* (physicians who did not charge fees), were also regarded as extrasalubrious. Visitors would pray to images of the healing saints, asking them to intercede with God on behalf of the sick. In these spaces, sick and suffering people might also engage in healing rituals. For example, the fifth-century CE bishop Augustine told stories of people with foot pain, paralysis, and hernia being healed once they were baptized, and a story of a man whose family, slaves, and even cattle were healed after they were given the Eucharist and received prayers from a church elder. In some churches, such as the church of Santa Maria Antiqua in Rome, a side chapel decorated with images of physician-saints appears to have been an incubation room, where the sick could stay overnight to receive healing dreams.

In order for the sick and suffering to tap the exceptional power of these religious sites, the sites needed to be accessible. And it seems that those who built healing temples and churches were aware of this need. The Asclepian temples in Athens and Sicily, for example, were both built below the acropolis (an elevated ridge where the temples to other gods were located), making it more possible for weak, injured, or impaired people to visit without needing to climb the hill (see fig. 69). Additionally, many healing sanctuaries provided ramps into the main buildings of temple complexes. Yet even with such attention to access, it was likely very difficult for people with serious symptoms (such as diarrhea, vomiting, weakness, and delirium) to travel too far, forcing them to visit local religious temples, shrines, or churches. And those who were bedridden and prohibited from travel altogether were forced to rely on healers who made house calls.

TREATMENT SPACES IN PATIENTS' AND PHYSICIANS' HOMES

Most people who sought the help of physicians were treated in their own living quarters.[3] Depending on the patient's status—and the expanse of their living quarters—this might mean that the patient was isolated in a room of a house, or the corner of a shared living space in an apartment (see chapter 3). Regardless, ancient medical sources explained that attention ought to be given to arranging these spaces to best facilitate recovery. For example, the Hippocratic author of *Decorum* advised physicians to calibrate the conditions—ventilation, light or dark, sounds, and smells—to the particular ailments of their patients (Text 42). Other Hippocratic and Galenic texts suggested conducting examinations, and especially surgery, in rooms that were well lit (ideally with natural light, as would come through an opening in the roof, for example) and large enough to accommodate the physician, an apprentice, and the family and friends of the patient—that is, everyone needed to assist with the procedure.

A physician's home (called *taberna medica*) also contained important spaces. We gather that many physicians grew medicinal plants in their central courtyards or back gardens, and from archaeological finds (such as mortars, pestles, scales, containers coated with plant remains and inscribed with labels that identified the plants they contained, metal boxes that held drugs after they had been mixed, and scoops and spoons to apply drugs) we surmise that many physicians used a room in their house to prepare their remedies. Some physicians' homes had a room in the front of the house that opened onto the street and served as a stall where they consulted patients and sold pharmacological remedies (see fig. 9). Other physicians treated patients in a room (often called their "workshop") within their home. In

---

3. In fact, because physicians came to patients' bedsides, their work was called "clinical" medicine, and they were called "clinicians," terms deriving from the Greek word for "bed," *klinē*.

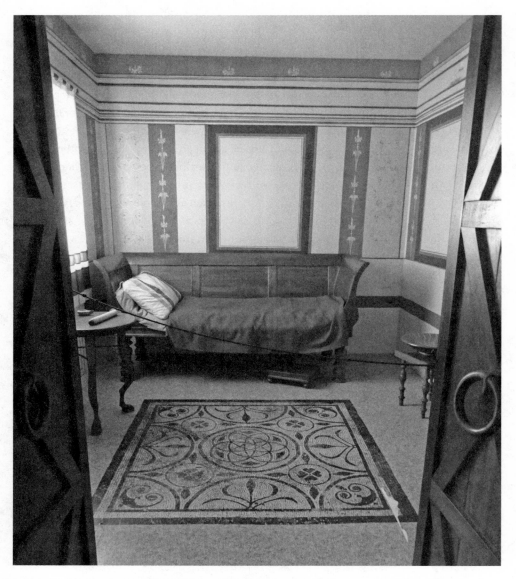

FIGURE 70 Reconstruction of a room for patients in the second-century CE residential house of a surgeon in Ariminum, Italy. This room could have been used to conduct examinations, apply treatments, perform surgery, and perhaps as a place where patients stayed overnight so they could be observed while recovering. Archaeologists found a graffito in this room, most likely scratched into the wall by a patient lying in the bed, that appears to provide the name and describe the character of the physician whose home it was: "Eutyches, good man." House of the Surgeon (*Domus Rimini*), Ariminum, Italy. Photo credit: Kristi Upson-Saia.

HOUSE of the SURGEON

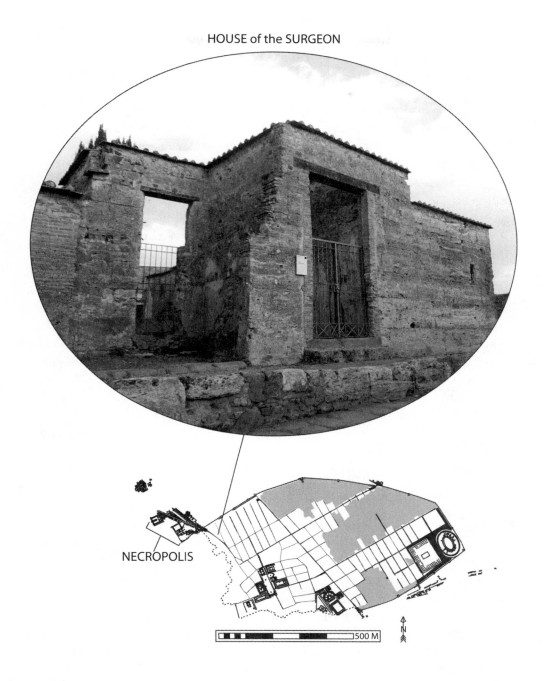

NECROPOLIS

500 M

FIGURE 71 Constructed in the mid-third century BCE, the House of the Surgeon (Regio VI Insula I, 10) in Pompeii is so named because more than forty surgical instruments, including scalpels and probes, were found there. Given the proximity of the surgeon's house to the city's necropolis, we wonder if patients and their loved ones who sought treatment there understood it to be their last resort. Photo credit: Kristi Upson-Saia. Created by Gina Tibbott.

some (seemingly rare) cases, patients might stay overnight in a physician's home. For example, **Galen** mentioned a patient with eye troubles who lived too far away from the city to be incorporated into Galen's rounds, so the patient came to live with him to receive a course of treatments.

One of the most significant of these homes is in the city of Ariminum (in northeastern Italy). In this two-story house (built in the second century CE), archaeologists have unearthed pharmacological items and the largest trove of ancient medical instruments found in one place in the Mediterranean: over 150 bronze and iron medical instruments. The cache includes basic instruments, as well as some very rare items, such as dental forceps, a lenticular (the chisel used for **trepanation**; see fig. 47), and a ceramic foot mold (similar to those depicted in fig. 41) into which patients inserted their foot for a hot- or cold-water soak. Archaeologists have also identified a set of rooms where the physician likely saw his patients: one that appears to have been his workshop, where he offered consultations, mixed drugs, and studied, and an adjoining room with a bed, where he conducted examinations, applied treatments, performed surgery, and perhaps where patients stayed overnight so they could be observed while recovering (see fig. 70).

We wonder how patients experienced these different treatment spaces. Our sources tell us that physicians' stalls were a place where neighbors congregated to catch up with one another while they waited for medical care. In contrast, we might assume that surgeons' homes might have been associated with fear and anxiety, given the risky nature of surgical treatments. In fact, in the city of Pompeii, where one surgeon's home was located on the road leading to the city's necropolis (see fig. 71), we can imagine the acute dread associated with the space. Such a location might have given the patient and their loved ones the impression that the surgical treatment they were about to receive was a last resort!

MILITARY INFIRMARIES

We are fortunate to have sources for military infirmaries (*valetudinaria*) that explain ancient reasoning on how health was related to place and space. First and foremost, when determining where to locate their encampments, Romans sought to avoid places considered unhealthy. Channeling the common medical knowledge that marshy waters are the most hazardous to health (see Text 2, *Airs, Waters, Places*)—sometimes even considered the source of toxic air that caused epidemics (see chapter 9)—the Roman military writers Onasander (first century CE) and Vegetius (fifth century CE) warned against constructing military camps on marshy sites. Additionally, within the fortification, Romans were deliberate in where they built the infirmary. Pseudo-Hyginus (first or second century CE), who wrote a detailed description of a Roman military camp, recommended that the infirmary be located at least seventy Roman feet from the animal stables and the workshop, ensuring some degree of quiet for recuperating soldiers and also distancing them from the smell of animals (and their excrement).

The layout of military infirmaries also indicates conscious attention to how the spatial configuration of the building contributed to healing. *Valetudinaria* were rectangular

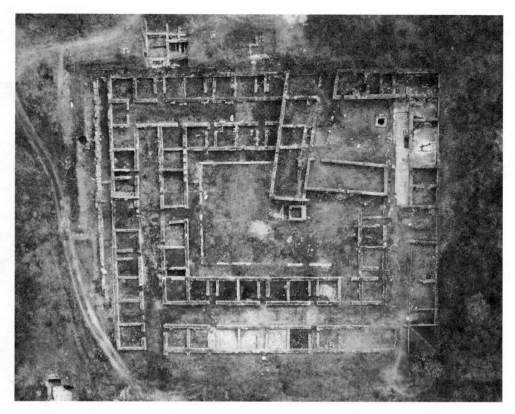

FIGURE 72 Aerial view of a Roman military infirmary (or *valetudinarium*), in Novae, Bulgaria. Like other major Roman encampments, this military base along the Danubian border had a dedicated space for the care of sick and wounded soldiers. The infirmary was organized as a set of two concentric rings of patient rooms around the perimeter, with a corridor between them. In the center was a courtyard, which was likely where medicinal plants were grown, the injured were triaged, surgery was performed, and recovering patients took recuperative walks. This image was taken during the research project on settlement structures near the Roman legionary camp at Novae (Lower Moesia) using nondestructive prospection methods, supported by the National Science Centre (no. 2011/01/D/HS3/02187), principal investigator: Agnieszka Tomas; author of the image: Michał Pisz.

buildings with two concentric rings of rooms around the perimeter, and a corridor between them (see fig. 72). This configuration would have maintained relative quiet and privacy, as the rooms that housed sick and injured soldiers were closed off to street noise outside the building, and separated from nearby rooms by the central corridor (and sometimes side hallways). Additionally, the upper-story windows would have let in light and provided ventilation to help diffuse any foul smells of the sick and injured.

In the center of the infirmary was a courtyard where a large pool of water cooled the air and absorbed bad odors. When the wounded regained enough strength to get out of bed, they could come out to the courtyard to enjoy fresh air. Or they could take a recuperative walk under the covered portico that sheltered them from the rain and wind. The courtyard environment—with gardens of medicinal plants, altars, and votive inscriptions to healing gods—must have been pleasant, boosting injured soldiers' confidence in their chances for recovery. Yet, this optimistic experience was likely tempered when the courtyard was used to triage injured soldiers or when surgeries were performed there (following the recommendations of Hippocratic texts to find natural light for surgical procedures).

Although we imagine the *valetudinarium* as the central site for healing within military fortifications, archaeologists have also discovered medical instruments in the barracks. This suggests that at times—perhaps for minor illnesses and injuries—medics treated patients at their bedside or soldiers were expected to treat one another.

CHRISTIAN "HOSPITAL" COMPLEXES

Unfortunately we have only a general sense of the layout of early Christian hospitals, and no archaeological evidence. Our literary sources describing Basil's fourth-century CE hospital complex in central Asia Minor (modern-day Türkiye) explained that it was segmented into distinct areas for the sick (where a wide variety of ailments were treated), the poor (many of whom were likely malnourished), lepers, and the dying (see fig. 6). With areas for other vulnerable populations, such as orphans and foreigners, and all of the supporting facilities (such as the kitchen, storerooms, toilet and bathhouse, workshop, stables, and housing for the monks), the complex was massive, and called by outsiders a "new city." Yet we do not know anything about the layout of the buildings, nor whether or how the monks who designed the complex thought about the relationship between spatial organization and well-being.

That said, we can imagine that Christian hospital complexes would have been sites associated with charity. These were places where sick and suffering people who could not afford to hire a physician or who had exhausted the care of relatives and friends must have been relieved to receive professional care without worrying about paying fees. Moreover, these were places where chronically or terminally ill patients—most of whom would have been turned away by physicians—could receive medical or palliative care. The ideals of care and comfort were institutionalized and must have suffused the place itself. And as we now know, health and healing are enhanced in social spaces where patients are immersed in caring and supportive relationships.

Just as the hospital spaces were meaningful social spaces for patients, they also altered the experience of those living nearby. Hospitals located in the suburbs, such as Fabiola's hospital outside of Rome and Basil's hospital outside of Caesarea, diverted many sick and suffering people from the rest of the city's population, sparing the latter from the repulsive sight of many serious illnesses. Fabiola treated individuals whose pus-discharging wounds most people "could not bear to look at" (Jerome, *Letter* 77.5), and the *leprosaria* at Basil's hospital segregated people with horrifying skin ailments, such that their neighbors reported that "there is no longer before our eyes that terrible and piteous spectacle of [lepers] who are living corpses, the greater part of whose limbs have mortified" (Gregory Nazianzen, *Oration* 43.63). This concentration of sick and suffering people—in one place and at a distance—must have shifted the everyday experience of those in nearby cities, freeing them (to a degree) from the ever-present reminder of their own vulnerability and mortality. Yet we must wonder how the segregation of the sick might also have undermined the normalization of illness and injury as the default and commonly shared bodily state, thus setting up the conditions for later ableist worldviews.

ACKNOWLEDGMENTS

Writing and organizing a book of this magnitude required considerable assistance in the form of scholarly advice and funding from many different individuals and institutions. We attempt to thank as many of them here as we can.

The following presses generously allowed us to reprint selections from their published translations: Akademie-Verlag, Brill, Hackett Publishing Company, Harvard University Press (Loeb Classical Library), Israel Academy of Sciences and Humanities, Olms, Oxford University Press, Prospect Books, and University of Chicago Press. The following institutions and individuals generously granted us permission to use objects in their collection, their photographs, or their figures: Art Resource, NY; Bibliothèque Nationale de France; British Museum; Cambridge University Press; Capitoline Superintendency of Cultural Heritage, Rome; Bent Christensen; Andrew Dunn; Ephorate of Antiquities of Chios; Folger Library; Getty Images; Cassandra Gutiérrez; Monica Hellström; Institute of Archaeology, University of Oxford; The Johns Hopkins Archaeological Museum; Matthias Kabel; George E. Koronaios; Metropolitan Museum of Art; Museo de la Biblioteca Nacional de España; National Archaeological Museum, Athens; National Museums Liverpool, World Museum; Dick Osseman; Michał Pisz; Princeton University Library; Carole Raddato; Carlo Raso; Rocky Mountain Laboratories; Römisch-Germanisches Museum, Köln; Sächsische Landesbibliothek, Staats- und Universitätsbibliothek, Dresden; Bibi Saint-Pol; Science Museum Group, London; Dr. Lisa-Marie Shillito; Staatliche Museen zu Berlin; Tahsin Firuz Soyuer; Gina Tibbott; Roger B. Ulrich; Wellcome Collection; Wikimedia Commons.

We are grateful to have been able to commission a large number of new translations for this volume and to find a group of remarkable translators who were able to bring fresh, new perspectives, while also integrating recent scholarship into their translations. Their precision and respect for our sources was matched by a concern to accurately convey the sources' meaning to modern readers. Many thanks to Brent Arehart, Lesley Bolton, Molly Jones-Lewis, Melinda Letts, Christopher Lougheed, Tara Mulder, Robert Nau, and Jessica Wright.

Carolyn Gersh served as a consultant on a number of translations, and we wish to thank her for her invaluable guidance.

Given the scope of the project, we relied heavily on colleagues who specialize in the history of ancient medicine, health, and healing, especially members of ReMeDHe (a working group for Religion, Medicine, Disability, Health, and Healing in late antiquity). Their input came to us via ReMeDHe workshops, while other help was solicited through our lively social media and listserv. ReMeDHe members have contributed, corrected, supported, inspired, and encouraged us along the way. Some individuals deserve special mention: Brent Arehart, Lesley Bolton, Sarah Bond, Clara Bosak-Schroeder, Janet Downie, Jonathan Edmondson, Kendra Eshleman, Susan Holman, Molly Jones-Lewis, Lennart Lehmhaus, Leigh Lieberman, Brenda Llewellyn Ihssen, Tara Mulder, Caroline Musgrove, Calloway Scott, Colin Webster, and Bronwen Wickkiser.

Feedback from other colleagues came through the formal peer review processes. Eight scholars reviewed our initial book proposal. Their comments served to shape the final manuscript in significant ways, and our project was greatly enhanced as a result of their suggestions. A few were willing to attach their names to their feedback, and we thank them here along with the anonymous reviewers. These include Emily Beckman, Susan Holman, Molly Jones-Lewis, Wilson Shearin, Svetla Slaveva-Griffin, and Faith Wallis. Three anonymous scholars reviewed our final manuscript, and their feedback served to further improve and enrich the project in its final stages.

We relied heavily on the exceptional scholarship of experts in the field. We list some of them in the Further Reading section, and we provide a fuller list in the instructors' guide available on the ReMeDHe website, but here we would like to give special credit to Gregory Aldrete, Patricia A. Baker, Kirsten Bos, Véronique Boudon-Millot, Lauren Caldwell, Louis Cohn-Haft, Sean Coughlin, Véronique Dasen, Lesley Dean-Jones, Estée Dvorjetski, Valerie French, Wilbert Gesler, Mark Grant, Saskia Hin, Ann Olga Koloski-Ostrow, David Leith, Orly Lewis, Lynn LiDonnici, Joel Mann, Adrienne Mayor, Kassandra Jackson Millar, Piers D. Mitchell, Steven Oberhelman, Tim Parkin, Roy Porter, Ralph M. Rosen, Christine F. Salazar, Walter Scheidel, Debby Sneed, Manuela Tecusan, Alain Touwaide, Philip J. van der Eijk, Peter van Minnen, Ingrid Wiechmann, Fikret Yegül, In-Sok Yeo, and the dozens of other scholars whose work we consulted.

We have had a number of excellent research assistants who helped us with a myriad of tasks at various stages of the project, including Heather Barkman, Cassandra Gutiérrez, Gahan Lahiri, Heather Patrick, Catherine van Reenen, and Katie Warden.

In addition to the support provided by our peers, this project was funded by numerous grants and scholarships. Funding from Occidental College—two Faculty Enrichment Research Grants, a MacArthur International Travel Grant, a Brown Humanities Grant, funding from the Department of Religious Studies Boyd fund, funding from the Center for Research & Scholarship, and funding from the Gamble Endowed Professorship—paid for travel, copyright permission fees, stipends for translation commissions, image reproduction fees, image commissions, and stipends for research assistants. Kristi Upson-Saia was a Visiting Scholar at the American Academy in Rome, which provided an intellectually enriching home base for her research trip to Italy. Funding from the University of Manitoba—the Faculty of Arts, Dean's Fund at the University of Manitoba, and a University of Manitoba Social Science and Humanities Research Council of Canada Grant—paid for research assistantships, travel, translations, and image commissions.

It has been a pleasure to work with Eric Schmidt, our editor at University of California Press. At every stage of the writing process he has offered insightful and thoughtful support. We are grateful to have had the privilege of working with such an exemplary editor and lovely human being. We also wish to thank editorial assistant LeKeisha Hughes and production editor Cindy Fulton, and the art department, for their guidance, especially in the home stretch. Marian Rogers, our copy editor, deserves special praise and gratitude for her keen eye and impeccable suggestions. Finally, many thanks to Teresa Iafolla, Chloe Wong, and Andrea Butler from the marketing team. We feel fortunate to have partnered with such an exceptional press.

TIMELINE

Included below are the major figures and historical events discussed in this volume. For short biographies of the medical figures listed here, see the glossary of people.

Date	Era	Medical Figures	Historical Events and Figures
800–700 BCE	Greek Archaic Period (800–479 BCE)		Homeric Poems (c. 800–700 BCE)
700–600 BCE			
600–500 BCE		Pythagoras (c. 570–495 BCE)	
500–400 BCE		Anaxagoras of Clazomenae (fifth century BCE)	Persian Wars (492–479 BCE)
			Socrates (c. 470–399 BCE)
			Thucydides (c. 460–395 BCE)
		Alcmaeon (early fifth century BCE)	Peloponnesian War (431–404 BCE)
			Plague of Athens (430–427 BCE)
	Greek Classical Period (479–323 BCE)	Empedocles (fifth century BCE)	
		Democritus (c. 460–380 BCE)	
		Hippocrates of Cos (c. 460–380 BCE)	
		Plato (c. 428–348/7 BCE)	
400–300 BCE		Aristotle (c. 384–c. 322 BCE)	Foundation of Plato's Academy (c. 385 BCE)
		Diocles of Carystus (fourth or third century BCE)	Alexander the Great (reigned 336–323 BCE)

Date	Era	Medical Figures	Historical Events and Figures
	Hellenistic Period (323–31 BCE)	Theophrastus (c. 372/1–287/6 BCE) Praxagoras (fourth and third century BCE) Herophilus (c. 330–c. 260 BCE) Erasistratus (fourth and third century BCE)	Foundation of Aristotle's Lyceum (c. 335 BCE)
300–200 BCE		Cato the Elder (234–149 BCE)	Foundation of Alexandrian Museum and Library (c. 300 BCE)
200–100 BCE		Agnodice (third century BCE) Nicander (late second century BCE) Asclepiades of Bithynia (c. 124–40 BCE?) Heraclides of Tarentum (first century BCE)	
100–1 BCE		Themison of Laodicea (first century BCE) Celsus (first century BCE and CE)	Development of Empiricist School of Medicine (first century BCE) Development of Methodist School of Medicine (first century BCE and first century CE) Augustus, Roman Emperor (reigned 27 BCE–14 CE)
	Roman Imperial Period (27 BCE–476 CE)		
1 CE		**Beginning of the Common Era**	
1–100 CE		Seneca (c. 4–65 CE)	Eruption of Mt. Vesuvius and Destruction of Nearby Roman Towns of Pompeii and Herculaneum (79 CE)
		Scribonius Largus (first century BCE and CE) Pliny the Elder (23 or 24–79 CE) Dioscorides of Anazarbus (second half of first century CE) Rufus of Ephesus (late first century CE)	

100–200 CE	Aretaeus of Cappadocia (second century CE)	Antoninus Pius, Roman Emperor (reigned 137–161 CE)
	Soranus of Ephesus (second century CE)	Marcus Aurelius, Roman Emperor (reigned 161–180 CE)
	Fronto (c. 95–166 CE) Aelius Aristides (117–after 181 CE) Artemidorus (middle to late second century CE) Galen of Pergamum (c. 129–c. 216 CE)	
200–300 CE		
300–400 CE	Oribasius (c. 325–400 CE)	First Hospitals Built in Roman Empire (c. 350 CE) Julian, Roman Emperor (reigned 360–363 CE)
400–500 CE	Caelius Aurelianus (fifth century CE)	Abdication of Western Emperor Romulus Augustulus to Gothic Leader Odoacer (476 CE)
500–600 CE	Aëtius of Amida (sixth century CE)	Justinian, Roman Emperor (reigned 527–544 CE)
	Procopius (c. 507–after 555 CE) Alexander of Tralles (late sixth century CE) Metrodora (between first and sixth centuries CE) Aspasia (between second and sixth centuries CE?)	Justinianic Plague (541–544 CE)
600–700 CE	Agnellus of Ravenna (c. 600 CE) Paul of Aegina (c. 625–690 CE)	

GLOSSARY OF SUBJECTS

The definitions included in this glossary focus on explaining what these terms and concepts meant within the context of ancient medical thought. The glossary also includes some ancient weights and measures that may be unfamiliar to readers. Fuller information about ancient Greek and Roman weights and measures can be found in W. F. Richardson, *Numbering and Measuring in the Classical World,* rev. ed. (Exeter: Bristol Phoenix Press, 2005).

astringent	From the Latin word *adstringere,* meaning "to bind fast," and referring to the properties of drying, condensing, thickening, and/or tightening, whether related to a substance (a drug or food) or the effect of a treatment.
bilious	A term referring to the physical and psychological conditions caused by an excess of yellow bile and to the humoral temperament of people in whom yellow bile predominates. Yellow bile was associated with hot and dry properties, the element of fire, the season of summer, and inflammatory conditions. Bilious individuals were thought to be easily angered and excitable; the term is sometimes used interchangeably with the word "**choleric.**" See figure 16.
canker	Related to the Greek word *karkinos* and the Latin word *cancer,* which both mean "crab." A canker was an erosive sore or ulcer, sometimes possibly a tumor, marked by inflammatory changes. The association of the condition with the crab may derive from the crab-like shape of some ulcers and tumors or the hardness of the surface of some ulcers and tumors that resemble a crab's shell.
cautery/cauterization	The process, usually therapeutic, of burning part of the body with hot metal instruments or chemical compounds to either stop the flow of blood, close a wound, or affect processes internal to the body through external applications

(for instance, to redirect morbid or excessive humors to a different part of the body). See figure 26.

cavity

Our preferred translation for the Greek word *koilia*, which is sometimes used to refer to a region of the body—the belly or, more literally, the hollow cavity of the abdomen—and sometimes to the parts contained therein (such as the gut, intestines, or bowel). Some ancient digestive ailments took their name from this region of the body where a person experienced distress (for example, *koiliakos* in Text 11), a custom that continues in the naming of different modern ailments that likewise affect this region of the body (such as what we now call celiac disease, though this is an ailment that is distinct from any digestive ailments described in ancient sources).

choleric

A term referring to the physical and psychological conditions caused by an excess of yellow bile and the humoral temperament of people in whom yellow bile predominates. Yellow bile was associated with the hot and dry properties, the element of fire, the season of summer, and inflammatory conditions. Choleric individuals were thought to be easily angered and excitable; a term used interchangeably with "**bilious**." See figure 16.

clyster

The process of injecting liquid, frequently containing a purgative **drug**, through the anus into the lower bowels; and the instrument—with a bulb on one end, and narrow opening on the other—used for the procedure (Greek *klustēr* means "syringe"). Also known as an enema. See figures 23 and 24.

concoct/concoction

From the Latin word *concoquere* meaning "to cook" and "to digest." Digestion was thought to use the vital heat from the body to refine raw food primarily into blood, which would then be concocted further into other homogeneous substances such as **flesh**, semen, and even vital *pneuma* (enlivening spirit or breath). The term was also used to refer to other cooking-like processes in the body, such as the heating of morbid bodily matter to produce pus.

cotyle

The basic Greek unit of measure for liquids, literally meaning "cup." One cotyle contained between 240 and 270 ml, or 8 to 9 oz.

crisis

A term referring to a turning point in an illness, the moment when the illness either begins to abate (leading to recovery) or begins to worsen (leading to death). The crisis could also be thought of as the most severe moment(s) of an illness. See also **critical days.**

critical days

Specific days in the course of an illness when a **crisis** was reached. See figure 18.

cupping	A process whereby a vacuum is created in a cup or bell-shaped device made of glass, metal (using fire), or horn (using suction) and then applied to the skin. Wet cupping was a kind of therapeutic bloodletting in which a small incision was made, and then bad blood was drawn out of the body using the cupping device. An incision was not made in dry cupping, which instead aimed to redirect toxic or morbid residues to a different part of the body or to remove them in the form of air (as opposed to liquids). See figure 48.
cyathus (plural: cyathi)	A Greek unit of measurement for liquids, literally meaning "ladle." One cyathus was equivalent to 6 **cotyles,** and contained roughly 1.5 liters or 50 oz.
denarius (plural: denarii)	Both a Roman coin and a unit of weight. One denarius weighed roughly 4.5 grams or 0.16 ounces.
drachma	Both a Greek coin and a unit of weight. One drachma weighed roughly 4.33 grams or 0.15 ounces.
dropsy	Swelling, especially of an extreme sort, resulting from water retention. It is also known as edema.
drug(s)	The Greek word *pharmakon* (plural: *pharmaka*) can mean drug as in "medicinal remedy," but it can also mean "poison," "spell," "charm," and even "scapegoat." These multiple meanings make sense, as many drugs could both heal and poison depending on application, circumstances, and quantity. Similarly, the Latin word *medicamentum* refers to a drug used as a medicinal remedy, but also to poison.
emetic	A substance, usually a drug, used to cause vomiting. Vomiting was sometimes induced in situations of poisoning, but most often emetics were used in order to purge the body of morbid or excessive humors and residues, thereby returning it to a healthful balance.
euchymous	From the Greek "well" (*eu-*) and "humor" (*chymos*). This term refers to the balanced and proportionate mixture of the four humors (blood, yellow bile, black bile, phlegm) in terms of both quality and quantity in the body. See also **eukratic** and **humor.**
eukratic	From the Greek "well" (*eu-*) and "mixture" (*krasis*). This term refers to the balanced and proportionate mixture of the four elemental qualities (hot, cold, wet, and dry). If properly blended, the body is said to be in a state of *eukrasia*.
expectorant	A substance used to induce **expectoration,** i.e., a drug used to prompt the body to bring up phlegm, blood, pus, or other substances from the chest, lungs, and throat.
expectoration	Phlegm, blood, or other substances such as pus ejected from the chest, lungs, and throat through coughing or spitting.

Expectoration was often induced using **drugs**, such as **expectorants**, as part of ancient medical therapies for chest and lung conditions.

fibula (plural: fibulae)

A metal pin, similar to a modern safety pin, used in the treatment of wounds, whether inserted into the **flesh** to hold the sides of a wound together or used to hold bandages in place.

flesh

The fatty, gluey tissues of the body, including muscles, organs, vessels, and even bones. Not to be confused with the skin, which was thought to be the surface or crust of the flesh. Some ancient medical writers believed that flesh was formed through the **concoction** of blood through a kind of congealing process. Many understood men's flesh to be tightly woven, whereas women's flesh was loosely woven, spongey, and porous, and partly to blame for some women's ailments.

fumigate/fumigation

The use of smoke—produced from both foul and pleasant-smelling substances—in medical treatments. Depending on the desired effect, smoke was mainly administered in one of two places (and sometimes both at once): the nose or the vagina. If the aim was to induce the organs (for instance, the womb) or substances (for instance, menstrual blood) to move downward in the body, repellant foul-smelling smoke was introduced to the nose and pleasant-smelling smoke to the vagina. Alternatively, attractive sweet-smelling smoke would be introduced under the woman.

humor

Bodily fluids thought by many ancient medical writers to make up human bodies in varying proportions. Humoral theory was based on four main humors: blood, yellow bile, phlegm, and black bile. Each humor was characterized by two of the four qualities (hot, cold, wet, dry) and was associated with a season and a temperament. See the entries for **bilious/choleric**, **melancholic**, **phlegmatic**, and **sanguine** for more information about individual humors. See figure 16.

kissa

Greek/Latin word that refers to unusual cravings experienced by pregnant women for unusual flavors (very tart or salty foods) or nonfood substances such as soil or ashes. Related to and sometimes called *pica* in Latin.

krasis

Greek word meaning "mixture." In medical writings it usually refers to the mixture of the four humors in the body (see also **eukratic**).

melancholic/melancholy

A term referring to both physical and psychological conditions caused by an excess of black bile, as well as the humoral temperament of people in whom black bile predominates. Black bile was associated with the cold and dry properties, the element of earth, the season of autumn, and conditions resulting from condensing, congealing, and drying. Melancholic individuals were thought to be depressive and sad. See figure 16.

miasma	Greek word connoting pollution, usually of a ritual or religious sort. Sometimes it simply referred to "bad air" or air that caused illness.
obol	Both a Greek coin and a unit of weight. One obol was worth one-sixth of a drachma, and weighed roughly 0.7 grams or 0.02 ounces.
obstetrician	Our preferred translation of the Greek word *maia* and the Latin word *obstetrix,* both of which are often rendered in English as "midwife." Ancient evidence for the activities of people given the title of *maia* or *obstetrix* suggests that they had similar education and qualities as people called "physicians" (*medici* in Latin, *iatroi* in Greek).
paroxysm	Suddenly occurring and/or pronounced symptoms in the course of an illness, such as a spike of fever, heightened delusion, increased inflammation, or sudden, violent, or heavy bodily emissions (such as bleeding, bowel movements, etc.). Sometimes called an exacerbation or attack.
pessary	A wool or linen suppository inserted into the vagina or uterus for two main purposes, either to deliver drug treatments to the womb or to provide support for a prolapsed uterus. The former were made by soaking the tampon in **drugs** mixed with congealed oil/fat; when inserted, the drugs would melt from the body's internal heat and be absorbed.
phlegmatic	A term referring to both physical and psychological conditions caused by an excess of phlegm, as well as the humoral temperament of people in whom phlegm predominates. Phlegm was associated with the cold and wet properties, the element of water, the season of winter, and conditions such as **dropsy.** Phlegmatic individuals were thought to be calm and lethargic. See figure 16.
pica	Greek/Latin word that refers to unusual cravings experienced by pregnant women for unusual flavors (very tart or salty foods) or nonfood substances such as soil or ashes. Related to and sometimes called *kissa* in Latin.
plaster	A cloth, often plant-based fibers or wool felt, soaked in oils and/or resin together with the pharmacological substances best suited to treating the ailment. The plaster would then be applied to the affected part of the body as a method by

which to administer the **drugs** (similar to **poultice**). A plaster could also be applied over a bandage to hold it in place.

pleurisy

From the Greek word *pleuron,* which meant "side" or "rib," pleurisy was generally identified by ancient medical writers as a condition associated with a pain in the side. Identification of other symptoms associated with pleurisy varied considerably, with some authors referring to some conditions more closely associated with the ribs and others more closely associated with the lungs, and some characterized by coughing up blood, rather than bile.

pneuma (plural: *pneumata*)

The Greek word *pneuma* can mean "air," "moving air or wind," "breath," "breathing," "breath of life," and "enlivening spirit"; it can sometimes even mean "flatulence." In the ancient medical context, *pneuma* usually refers to the refined substance that keeps a body alive. According to some models of the body, it arises from the concoction of blood into a more refined form that circulates throughout the body in the veins, accounting for the enlivening energy that keeps the body alive.

poultice

A paste most often made from ground-up grain (flour) and/ or macerated plants together with the pharmacological substances best suited to treating the ailment. This paste would be applied to the affected part of the body as a method by which to administer **drugs** (similar to **plaster**). Poultices were used to treat a range of maladies.

quartan fevers

Fevers characterized by a cycle of **paroxysm** and remission within a seventy-two-hour period (every fourth day, counted inclusively).

sanguine

A term referring to physical and psychological conditions caused by an excess of blood, as well as the humoral temperament of people in whom blood predominates. Blood was associated with the hot and wet properties, the element of air, the season of spring, vitality, and growth. Sanguine individuals were thought to be cheerful, optimistic, and enthusiastic. See figure 16.

stade (plural: stadia)

A Greek unit of distance that is equivalent to between 177 and 192 meters, or between 580 and 630 feet.

sumptōma (plural: *sumptōmata*)

Sumptōma is the Greek word from which the English "symptom" is derived, but there are distinct differences between the meaning of the Greek and English words (which is why we have chosen to transliterate the Greek word in our translations). The original sense of *sumptōma* is simply something that happens, sometimes, but not always, with the connotation that what has happened is bad or undesirable (e.g., getting a tan from spending too much time in the sun counted as a *sumptōma*, but so did having red skin from washing one's face too vigorously). In some medical instances, *sumptōma* carries the implication that the bad or undesirable thing is linked to an illness. But, for some Greek authors, including **Galen,** a *sumptōma* could also simply be something that was contrary to nature. By this reasoning, an illness itself qualified as a type of *sumptōma*, which differs significantly from the typical English understanding of a symptom as something that indicates the presence of an illness.

tertian fevers — Fevers characterized by a cycle of **paroxysm** and remission within a forty-eight-hour period (every third day, counted inclusively)

trepanation (trepanned) — The surgical process of drilling or scraping a hole, often down to bone, using an instrument called a **trephine.** This procedure was used in several ways, such as to bore a hole in the head to drain excess liquid collecting from a head injury, or to relieve pressure on the brain, or to manage migraines. Trepanation could also be used to make a wide opening around a foreign object (such as an arrowhead) that had become lodged in the body, so that the surgeon could have a better view when attempting to remove it and also to ensure no part of it was left in the body. See figures 47 and 48.

trephine — A cylindrical bore used to drill holes in the body, often down to the bone (see **trepanation**).

wasting ailment — An illness characterized by weakness, waning energy, and the progressive loss of weight.

GLOSSARY OF PEOPLE

We know about—or at least have the names of—thousands of physicians and philosophers from the ancient Greco-Roman world. Some were so famous that they were written about frequently, and we also have their extant writings. But we have little information about many others, both those with extant writings and those whose writings no longer survive. We might have only sporadic references to them from others who wrote about them, including hints about their area of specialization, a text they wrote, or where they were from.

We make this point to explain why some of the entries presented here are so limited, and why the dates given for their lives and career are so imprecise. Much of the information in the entries below is drawn from entries in Paul T. Keyser and Georgia L. Irby-Massie, *The Encyclopedia of Ancient Natural Scientists: The Greek Tradition and Its Many Heirs* (London and New York: Routledge, 2008).

Aelius Aristides (117–after 181 CE): Greek orator from western Asia Minor (modern-day Türkiye) who traveled extensively across the Roman Empire. Aristides was the author of a series of texts called *The Sacred Tales* that describe the many health problems he suffered, and the treatments he pursued at the recommendation of the god Asclepius in dreams. Many of Aristides's orations are still extant, including several of *The Sacred Tales*.

Aëtius of Amida (sixth century CE): Greek physician who may have served at the court of the emperor Justinian (who reigned from 527 to 565 CE) in Constantinople. Aëtius was the author of a large compendium on a wide range of medical topics. Each section of the compendium follows a pattern of quoting from an earlier authority and then adding commentary drawn from Aëtius's own experiences, especially his experience related to drugs and surgeries. This text is still extant.

Agnellus of Ravenna (c. 600 CE): Physician and teacher of medicine in northern Italy who gave lectures on the writings of earlier medical authorities, including **Galen**. Three of his lectures are still extant, and some commentaries attributed to other authors may also have been written by Agnellus.

Agnodice (third century BCE): According to a Roman writer of myths and fables, Agnodice was an Athenian woman who cross-dressed so she could learn medicine from **Herophilus** and provide medical care to women who were reluctant to have their bodies handled by male physicians. Agnodice is regularly cited as opening the door for women to become physicians, but it is unclear how much truth there is to this story, or even if Agnodice was a real person.

Alcmaeon of Croton (early fifth century BCE): Greek physician and philosopher of the Pythagorean school from southern Italy. Alcmaeon is credited with theorizing that the senses were linked to the brain, and discovering the associated anatomical structures, including the optic nerves and their connection to the brain. His writings are no longer extant.

Alexander of Tralles (late sixth century CE): Greek physician from western Asia Minor (modern-day Türkiye) who took inspiration from the writings of Galen while also displaying independence in his views on treatment. His writings on intestinal worms, fevers, and his *Twelve Books of Medicine* are extant, while his writings on several other subjects, including gynecology, are no longer extant.

Ammonius (first century BCE): Greek surgeon who lived in Alexandria. His writings are no longer extant, but several references to his treatment methods survive in other writers.

Anaxagoras of Clazomenae (fifth century BCE): Greek philosopher who lived in Athens. He proposed that matter was made up of invisible seeds, a view that allowed him to explain how food that people ate was transformed into different forms on or in their bodies. His writings are no longer extant, but many references to his ideas survive in other writers.

Andreas of Carystus (third century BCE): Greek physician who served in Alexandria at the court of the Ptolemies (the Greek rulers of Egypt). Andreas was a prolific writer on many medical topics, with his writings on pharmacology proving especially influential. His writings are no longer extant, but many references to his ideas survive in other writers. See figure 5.

Anonymus Londiniensis (sometimes spelled "Anonymus Londinensis") (late first or early second century CE): The name given to the unknown author of an incomplete but extant Greek text that has no obvious title. His text provides a valuable collection of material relating to the medical opinions of a large collection of physicians and philosophers, with sections focusing on medical terminology, the causes of illnesses, and physiology. The author does not appear to have been a member of any particular medical school. "Londiniensis" in the author's name refers to London ("Anonymus Londiniensis" literally means "Unknown Londoner"), but the author is called this only because the one extant copy of the text is now housed in London.

Anonymus Parisinus (late first century CE?): The name given to the unknown author of an extant Greek text called *On Acute and Chronic Illnesses*. The author is aware of Methodist theories but does not seem to have been a member of the Methodist school of medicine. The text includes a list of illnesses and their causes, along with suggestions for treatment. "Parisinus" in the author's name refers to Paris ("Anonymus Parisinus" literally means "Unknown Parisian"), but the author is called this only because two manuscripts of the text are now housed in Paris.

Apollo: Greek god of healing and medicine, truth, and prophecy. Apollo is the first god addressed in the Hippocratic *Oath*, and was believed to be the father of **Asclepius**.

Apollonius of Citium (early first century BCE): Greek physician of the Empiricist school who studied in Alexandria and specialized in orthopedic surgery. His commentary on the Hippocratic *On Joints* survives; his other writings are no longer extant.

Apollonius the Elder and **Apollonius the Younger** (second century BCE): Father and son physicians of the Empiricist school, both from Antioch. The son was nicknamed "bookworm." One of them may be the same person as **Apollonius of Citium.** Their writings are no longer extant.

Archigenes of Apamea (late first to mid-second century CE): Greek physician from Syria who practiced medicine in Rome and was part of the Pneumatic school. Archigenes wrote prolifically. His writings are no longer extant, but there are many references to his texts on pathology and pharmacology in other authors.

Aretaeus of Cappadocia (second century CE): Greek physician from eastern Asia Minor (modern-day Türkiye) about whom little is known. He seems not to have been part of any particular medical school, but he does display much familiarity with the Hippocratic corpus. His texts on the causes, signs, and treatment of chronic and acute illnesses are extant. His other writings are no longer extant.

Aristotle (c. 384–c. 322 BCE): Student of **Plato** and teacher of Alexander the Great, Aristotle was one of the most influential scholars and philosophers of the ancient world. His father was a physician, and an interest in medical subjects characterizes many of his texts, especially his several books about animals. Many of his writings are extant.

Artemidorus (middle to late second century CE): Greek interpreter of dreams from Ephesus (in modern-day western Türkiye) who authored an influential guidebook about the meaning and significance of dreams. Artemidorus thought it necessary for dream interpreters to have some knowledge of health and medicine, and many of the dreams that he discusses in his book relate to these subjects. His *Interpretation of Dreams* is still extant, but his other writings are no longer extant.

Asclepiades of Bithynia (c. 124–c. 40 BCE?): Greek physician from northern Asia Minor (modern-day Türkiye) who brought innovative and controversial ideas about medicine with him to Rome, favoring simple treatments involving diet and exercise more than pharmacology and surgery. His writings are no longer extant, but many references to his ideas survive in other writers.

Asclepius: Greek god of medicine. Asclepius was believed by some to have been a human physician and surgeon who, as a reward for his skill, was made a god, but by others to have been the divine son of **Apollo.** There were hundreds of temples dedicated to the god, where sick people and their families traveled to seek healing. The most famous of his sanctuaries in Greece was at Epidaurus.

Aspasia (between second and sixth century CE?): Athenian physician who specialized in obstetrics and gynecology. Her writings are no longer extant, but her ideas on childbirth and pregnancy were cited by later medical authors.

Caelius Aurelianus (fifth century CE): Roman physician from North Africa who was linked to the Methodist school of medicine. His two surviving texts, *On Acute Conditions* and *On Chronic Conditions,* were adapted Latin translations of lost texts by **Soranus.** His other writings are no longer extant.

Callimachus of Bithynia (third century BCE): Greek physician from northern Asia Minor (modern-day Türkiye) who practiced in Alexandria. He was linked with the Rationalist school of medicine and was a student of **Herophilus.** Callimachus was known for carefully examining the symptoms of patients. His writings are no longer extant.

Cato the Elder (234–149 BCE): Roman statesman and soldier who was also one of the first Roman authors to write prose in the Latin language. His extant text *On Agriculture* offers advice for the owners of estates, including suggestions about medical treatments that they might use for themselves, their family members, slaves, and animals.

Celsus (first centuries BCE and CE): Roman author of an encyclopedia that included discussions of medicine along with other topics. Only the section on medicine is now extant. Celsus must have lived in Rome, and seems to have been a follower of a Roman philosophical school that advocated vegetarianism. Scholars debate whether he was a practicing physician, but his writings offer hints of real experience, especially in matters related to surgery.

Chrysippus of Cnidus (late fourth century BCE): Greek physician who practiced in Alexandria and was the teacher of **Erasistratus.** He was known for avoiding the use of bloodletting. There were multiple physicians of this period named Chrysippus, and it is not always clear which one is which. Their writings are no longer extant.

Democritus of Abdera (c. 460–c. 380 BCE): Greek philosopher from Thrace and an advocate of atomic theories, holding that everything in the universe was made up of indivisible atoms. Some of his later reputation derived from texts on medicine and magic that were wrongly attributed to him. His writings are no longer extant, but many references to his ideas survive in other authors.

Diagoras of Cyprus (third or second century BCE?): Greek physician now known from scattered references to his recipe for an eye treatment, and his views on the use of opium. His writings are no longer extant.

Dieuches (fourth or third century BCE): Greek physician of the Rationalist school who had a reputation for the care he displayed in prescribing pharmacological treatments to patients. His writings are no longer extant, except for short quotations of his advice regarding dietary suggestions.

Diocles of Carystus (fourth or third century BCE): Greek physician who wrote on a wide range of medical topics and was known especially for his advice about regimen. Later writers associated him with the Rationalist school of medicine, but his connection to it is uncertain. His writings are no longer extant, but substantial parts of them were referenced by other authors.

Dioscorides of Anazarbus (second half of first century CE): Greek author from eastern Asia Minor (modern-day Türkiye) who wrote an influential and still extant text of pharmacology, *Medical Material.* Drawing on his own travels and experiences, Dioscorides explained the pharmacological properties and uses of more than 700 plants and other substances. See figure 5.

Empedocles of Acragas (fifth century BCE): Greek philosopher-poet and natural scientist from Sicily. His theory of four elements (earth, water, air, and fire) had a major influence on later philosophers and physicians. With the exception of a small part of Empedocles's poem *On Nature,* his writings are no longer extant.

Erasistratus of Ceos (fourth and third centuries BCE): Greek physician who practiced in Alexandria, perhaps as a colleague of **Herophilus.** His pioneering research on anatomy and physiology had a major impact on later physicians. His writings are no longer extant, but substantial parts of them were referenced by other authors.

Euelpistus (first centuries BCE and CE): Surgeon who practiced in Rome. His writings are no longer extant.

Euryphon of Cnidus (fifth century BCE): Greek physician believed in antiquity to have been a colleague of **Hippocrates**, and to have written some of the texts in the Hippocratic corpus. His medical interests included anatomy and gynecology. His writings are no longer extant.

Evenor of Argos (late fourth century BCE): Greek physician who practiced in Athens. He had interests in gynecology and also wrote a text entitled *On Therapy*. His writings are no longer extant.

Fronto (c. 95–166 CE): Roman lawyer and advocate, and the tutor of the emperor Marcus Aurelius (who reigned from 161 to 180 CE). Fronto and Marcus Aurelius exchanged a series of letters, often mentioning the health problems afflicting them and their families. A small collection of Fronto's writings is still extant.

Galen (c. 129–c. 216 CE): Prolific author and famed physician who remained independent from the medical schools of his time. Galen studied in Alexandria and later gained experience providing medical care to gladiators in Pergamum. He served as a physician to several Roman emperors. Many of his writings are extant. See figure 5.

Glaucias of Tarentum (early second century BCE): Greek physician of the Empiricist school from southern Italy. He wrote a text explaining the methods of the Empiricist school, and commentaries on the Hippocratic corpus. His writings are no longer extant.

Gorgias of Alexandria (second or first century BCE): Greek surgeon. His writings are no longer extant.

Heraclides of Tarentum (first century BCE): Greek physician of the Empiricist school who practiced medicine in Alexandria. He authored texts on pharmacology and regimen, and commentaries on the Hippocratic corpus. His writings are no longer extant, but many references to his ideas survive in other authors.

Hero (first century BCE): Greek surgeon who also seems to have had interests in eye diseases and obstetrics. His writings are no longer extant.

Herophilus of Chalcedon (c. 330–c. 260 BCE): Greek physician who practiced in Alexandria, where he made significant anatomical discoveries, including the discovery of the ovaries. Many of the terms that Herophilus coined for parts of the body are still used today. His writings are no longer extant, but many references to his ideas survive in other authors.

Hesiod (c. 750–c. 650 BCE): Early Greek poet who wrote the *Theogony*, a story about the origin of the world and birth of the gods, and *Works and Days*, a poem offering practical advice about why life is hard and how to cope with it. Some of the stories Hesiod told explain how illnesses were first inflicted on humans by the gods.

Hippocrates of Cos (c. 460–c. 370 BCE): Greek physician mentioned by both **Plato** and **Aristotle**. Biographical stories about Hippocrates were invented long after his life, emphasizing his great accomplishments as a physician, and identifying him as the founder of the Hippocratic school of medicine on the Greek island of Cos. In antiquity Hippocrates's name also became associated with the roughly sixty texts collectively called the Hippocratic corpus (corpus = a collection of written texts). But all of the texts attributed to him were most likely written by various authors across a long period of time. Even in antiquity, there was much debate about who Hippocrates really was and what he wrote. See figure 3.

Hygieia: Greek goddess who was the daughter of **Asclepius** and was worshipped in tandem with him at his temple complexes. Hygieia was the personification of health (her name literally means "health" in Greek).

Lycus of Macedon (second century CE): Greek physician likely of the Rationalist school who practiced medicine in Rome. He was a student of **Quintus** and had interests in anatomy. Lycus also wrote commentaries on the Hippocratic corpus. His writings are no longer extant.

Marcion of Smyrna (first century CE?): Greek author who wrote about drugs made from animal products. His writings are no longer extant.

Meges of Sidon (first centuries BCE and CE): Greek physician from Palestine and a student of **Themison** who practiced surgery in Rome. He was known for the treatments he developed for bladder stones and fistulas. His writings are no longer extant.

Melissus of Samos (fifth century BCE): Greek natural philosopher whose theories on existence (ontology) and mixture made him relevant for some discussion in the Hippocratic corpus. His writings are no longer extant, but many references to his ideas survive in other authors.

Metrodora (between first and sixth centuries CE): Author of a Greek text called *On the Conditions of the Womb*. We have no information about Metrodora outside of this text, which is the only known extant medical writing from the Greco-Roman world written by a woman. The name Metrodora means "gifts of the uterus" in Greek, so there is a chance this was not the author's real name but rather a moniker related to her area of expertise.

Mnesidamos (second century BCE): Figure cited by **Dioscorides** as an authority on the use of opium as a sedative. His writings are no longer extant.

Nicander (late second century BCE): Greek poet who may also have been a physician. Nicander was the author of two poems, both still extant, about poisonous substances of various sorts and antidotes to them. His other writings are no longer extant, but references to them show that Nicander wrote on a larger variety of topics, including gardening, geography, and snakes. See figure 5.

Numisianus (second century CE): Greek physician who was the student of **Quintus** and contributed to the growing interest in anatomical study in the second century CE. He also wrote commentaries on the Hippocratic corpus. His writings are no longer extant.

Ofillius (first century CE?): Greek physician of uncertain identity who discussed the use of saliva as a treatment for snake bites. His writings are no longer extant.

Oribasius (c. 325–400 CE): Prominent Greek physician and prolific author. Oribasius is best known now for his partially extant *Medical Compilations*, which collected, edited, and organized extracts from earlier medical writers, including **Galen**. Other writings of Oribasius survive in Latin translation.

Ostanes (before first century CE): Mysterious and legendary person identified by Greek and Roman authors as a Persian priest and magician. His date and identity are uncertain, and his writings are no longer extant.

Paul of Aegina (c. 625–690 CE): Greek physician who was the author of a text on pediatrics that is no longer extant. He also authored the extant *Medical Compendium,* an extremely influential treatise in seven books that covered many practical subjects and served as a reference work.

Pelops of Smyrna (second century CE): Greek physician and student of **Numisianus** who contributed to the growing interest in anatomical study in the second century CE. Pelops taught **Galen** and wrote commentaries on texts from the Hippocratic corpus. His writings are no longer extant, but references to his ideas survive in the writings of other authors.

Philoxenus of Alexandria (second or first century BCE?): Greek surgeon and pharmacologist. His writings are no longer extant, but several of his treatments and recipes are preserved in the writings of other authors.

Phylotimus (fourth and third centuries BCE): Greek Rationalist physician who was the student of **Praxagoras.** He specialized in surgery and also wrote a book about the medicinal properties of foods. His writings are no longer extant, but parts of his book on foods were summarized by other authors.

Plato (428–348/7 BCE): Athenian philosopher who was the student of **Socrates** and the teacher of **Aristotle.** Nearly all of Plato's writings were dialogues featuring his teacher **Socrates.** He was not a physician, and little relating to medicine appears in his writings, but his ideas on the creation of the universe and on human souls were of great significance for later intellectuals, including medical thinkers. Many of Plato's writings are extant.

Pleistonicus (third century BCE): Greek physician of the Rationalist school and a student of **Praxagoras.** His writings are no longer extant, but several references to his ideas on a range of medical topics are preserved in the writings of other authors.

Pliny the Elder (23 or 24–79 CE): Roman general and scholar who wrote the *Natural History,* an extensive encyclopedia that included content on medicine. For his research, Pliny drew on information from books that he and his enslaved secretaries read, as well as information he picked up during his administrative work and travels throughout the Roman Empire. Pliny's *Natural History* survives in its entirety, but the several other texts he wrote are no longer extant.

Polyides (first century BCE or earlier?): Figure known for a recipe used to treat wounds. His writings are no longer extant, but several of his treatments and recipes are preserved in the writings of other authors.

Praxagoras of Cos (fourth and third centuries BCE): Greek physician of the Rationalist school who was also the teacher of **Herophilus, Pleistonicus,** and **Phylotimus.** He had wide-ranging interests in medicine, including physiology, anatomy, and pathology. He also conducted pioneering work on the differences between veins and arteries. Praxagoras's writings are no longer extant, but many references to his ideas survive in the writings of other authors.

Procopius (c. 507–after 555 CE): Greek historian who was an eyewitness to significant events of the sixth century CE. Procopius's *History of the Wars* includes a detailed account of the plague that struck the Mediterranean world during his lifetime. Three of Procopius's writings are still extant.

Pythagoras of Samos (c. 570–495 BCE): Greek philosopher and a legendary figure in the Greek and Roman worlds whose name still lives on via the Pythagorean theorem. Most of the stories told about him are likely to be inventions. He influenced medicine through his views on natural philosophy, including ideas about the musical harmony of the universe, as well as through the vegetarian diet that his followers advocated. His writings are no longer extant, but many references to his ideas survive in the writings of other authors.

Quintus (second century CE): Physician who practiced medicine in Rome and contributed to the growing interest in anatomy in the second century CE. **Galen** praised his abilities, and also mentioned the commentaries Quintus wrote on texts of the Hippocratic corpus. It is unclear how much Quintus may have written down and published, but many references to his ideas survive in the writings of other authors.

Rufus of Ephesus (late first century CE): Greek physician and prolific author. Rufus had expertise in anatomy, physiology, and human emotions, and was a believer in the importance of questioning patients directly to assist diagnosis. Out of the more than 100 texts he wrote, four are completely extant in the original Greek, and substantial pieces are extant in translations into other languages. See figure 5.

Salpe (first century BCE or first century CE): Obstetrician about whom little is known. She was cited as an authority by **Pliny the Elder** for information about animal-based drugs. Other sources mention her recipe for removing body hair. Her writings are no longer extant.

Satyrus of Smyrna (second century CE): Greek physician and pupil of **Quintus** who followed the example of his teacher in writing commentaries on texts in the Hippocratic corpus. Satyrus taught **Galen** and contributed to the growing interest in anatomy in the second century CE. His writings are no longer extant.

Scribonius Largus (first centuries BCE and CE): Roman medical professional connected to the Roman imperial court under the emperor Claudius (who reigned from 41 to 54 CE). Scribonius wrote a major text on pharmacology that is still extant. It contains nearly 300 medicinal recipes.

Seneca (c. 4 BCE–65 CE): Roman philosopher and politician who displays considerable interest in health and medicine. His extant letters have much to say about health ailments that he himself suffered, including a condition that has often been identified by modern scholars as asthma. Many of his writings are extant.

Serapion of Alexandria (third century BCE): Greek physician associated with the Empiricist school and known for the critiques he made against other medical schools. His writings are no longer extant.

Socrates of Athens (c. 470–399 BCE): Greek philosopher who was the teacher of **Plato.** His teachings on ethics and epistemology remain influential to this day, and his "Socratic Method" of questioning bears a resemblance to the modern scientific method in inquiry. Socrates wrote nothing of his own, and is mostly known from the writings of his students.

Soranus of Ephesus (second century CE): Greek physician of the Methodist school now best known for his text on gynecology and obstetrics. Soranus practiced medicine in Rome and wrote several other texts, some of which are still extant.

Sostratus of Alexandria (first century BCE): Greek physician, surgeon, and zoologist. His writings are no longer extant.

Themison of Laodicea (first century BCE): Greek physician associated with the early development of the Methodist school and a student of **Asclepiades of Bithynia.** Originally from Syria, he practiced medicine in Rome and elsewhere in Italy. His writings are no longer extant.

Theophrastus (c. 372/1–287/6 BCE): Greek philosopher and student of **Aristotle**. Like his teacher, Theophrastus had wide-ranging interests across science and philosophy. He wrote more than 200 texts, only a few of which survive in their entirety. His two extant writings on botany have much to say about the medicinal uses of plants.

Thucydides (c. 460–395 BCE): Athenian general who wrote a history of the Peloponnesian War, fought between Athens and Sparta (431–404 BCE). Thucydides was not a physician, but he wrote a detailed account of the deadly epidemic that struck Athens in 430. This text is still extant.

FURTHER READING

Students and scholars seeking to do research on ancient medicine have a vast and ever-growing collection of sources and resources at their disposal. And many ancient medical sources are now freely and legally available online. This section offers some starting points for further reading on ancient medicine, emphasizing resources that are accessible to those who are not fluent readers of non-English languages.

ENGLISH TRANSLATIONS OF PRIMARY SOURCES

The volumes of the *Corpus Medicorum Graecorum* and the *Corpus Medicorum Latinorum* ("Collection of Greek Physicians" and "Collection of Latin Physicians") print the Greek, Latin, and Arabic texts of many ancient medical authors, often with a translation into a modern language. All the volumes of the *CMG* and *CML* are freely and legally available online at https://cmg.bbaw.de/epubl/online/editionen.html.

To find volumes in the list that include an English translation, look for the phrase *linguam Anglicam* ("English language") in the titles.

English translations of many texts by Hippocrates, Celsus, and Galen are available in the Loeb Classical Library series.

English translations of a number of other Greek and Latin medical authors are available in the following book series:

Studies in Ancient Medicine, published by Brill

Cambridge Galen Translations, published by Cambridge University Press

A collection of primary sources in the history of medicine in Europe after the Greek and Roman periods is available in this volume:

Wallis, Faith. *Medieval Medicine: A Reader.* Readings in Medieval Civilizations and Cultures 15. Toronto: University of Toronto Press, 2010.

SCHOLARLY SOURCES AND REFERENCE WORKS

With the caveat that scholarship on ancient medicine continues to be published at an impressive rate and the works listed here will quickly become outdated, we recommend this select list of important recent scholarship and reference works on the history of medicine and on important figures in ancient medicine.

Baker, Patricia A. *The Archaeology of Medicine in the Greco-Roman World*. Cambridge: Cambridge University Press, 2013.

Bliquez, Lawrence J. *The Tools of Asclepius: Surgical Instruments in Greek and Roman Times*. Studies in Ancient Medicine 43. Leiden: Brill, 2015.

Craik, Elizabeth M. *The 'Hippocratic Corpus': Content and Context*. London and New York: Routledge, 2015.

Crislip, Andrew T. *From Monastery to Hospital: Christian Monasticism and the Transformation of Health Care in Late Antiquity*. Ann Arbor: University of Michigan Press, 2005.

Cruse, Audrey. *Roman Medicine*. Stroud: Tempus, 2004.

Flemming, Rebecca. *Medicine and the Making of Roman Women: Gender, Nature, and Authority from Celsus to Galen*. Oxford: Oxford University Press, 2000.

Hardy, Gavin, and Laurence Totelin. *Ancient Botany*. London and New York: Routledge, 2016.

Israelowich, Ido. *Patients and Healers in the High Roman Empire*. Baltimore: Johns Hopkins University Press, 2015.

Jackson, Ralph. *Doctors and Diseases in the Roman World*. London: British Museum Press, 1988.

Jouanna, Jacques. *Greek Medicine from Hippocrates to Galen*. Leiden: Brill, 2021.

Jouanna, Jacques. *Hippocrates*. Trans. M. B. DeBevoise. Baltimore and London: Johns Hopkins University Press, 1999.

King, Helen. *Greek and Roman Medicine*. London: Duckworth, 2009.

King, Helen, ed. *Health in Antiquity*. London and New York: Routledge, 2009.

Laes, Christian. *Disabilities and the Disabled in the Roman World: A Social and Cultural History*. Cambridge: Cambridge University Press, 2018.

Lane Fox, Robin. *The Invention of Medicine from Homer to Hippocrates*. New York: Penguin Random House, 2020.

Longrigg, James. *Greek Rational Medicine: Philosophy and Medicine from Alcmaeon to the Alexandrians*. London and New York: Routledge Press, 1993.

Mattern, Susan P. *The Prince of Medicine: Galen in the Roman Empire*. Oxford: Oxford University Press, 2013.

Nutton, Vivian. *Ancient Medicine*. 2nd ed. Sciences of Antiquity. London and New York: Routledge, 2013.

Nutton, Vivian. *Galen: A Thinking Doctor in Imperial Rome*. London and New York: Routledge, 2020.

Petridou, Georgia, and Chiara Thumiger, eds. *Homo Patiens: Approaches to the Patient in the Ancient World.* Studies in Ancient Medicine 45. Leiden: Brill, 2015.

Riddle, John M. *Dioscorides on Pharmacy and Medicine.* Austin: University of Texas Press, 1985.

Rose, Martha L. *The Staff of Oedipus: Transforming Disability in Ancient Greece.* Ann Arbor: University of Michigan Press, 2003.

Thumiger, Chiara, and Peter N. Singer, eds. *Mental Illness in Ancient Medicine: From Celsus to Paul of Aegina.* Studies in Ancient Medicine 50. Leiden: Brill, 2018.

van der Eijk, Philip. *Medicine and Philosophy in Classical Antiquity: Doctors and Philosophers on Nature, Soul, Health, and Disease.* Cambridge: Cambridge University Press, 2005.

von Staden, Heinrich. *Herophilus: The Art of Medicine in Early Alexandria.* Cambridge: Cambridge University Press, 1989.

For helpful overviews on a wide range of topics and figures related to ancient medicine, we recommend the following handbooks:

Hankinson, R. J., ed. *The Cambridge Companion to Galen.* Cambridge: Cambridge University Press, 2008.

Irby, Georgia L., ed. *A Companion to Science, Technology, and Medicine in Ancient Greece and Rome.* Chichester: Wiley Blackwell, 2016.

Keyser, Paul T., and Georgia L. Irby-Massie, eds. *The Encyclopedia of Ancient Natural Scientists: The Greek Tradition and Its Many Heirs.* London and New York: Routledge, 2012.

Keyser, Paul T., and John Scarborough, eds. *The Oxford Handbook of Science and Medicine in the Classical World.* Oxford: Oxford University Press, 2018.

Pormann, Peter E., ed. *The Cambridge Companion to Hippocrates.* Cambridge: Cambridge University Press, 2018.

INDEX

gangrene, 98, 157, 161, 169–70
gardens, 40 fig. 9, 287, 315, 387, 392
gender. *See* gynecology; obstetricians; physicians; women's ailments
geriatrics. *See* elderly people
gladiators, 32, 92, 240, 278, 284–85
Greece, 8, 16, 20–30, 223 fig. 38, 227 fig. 42, 268 fig.49, 279 fig. 51, 286–87
gymnasia, 26, 222, 278
gynecology, 4, 133–48, 192, 287, 304–5, 339–65, 369; gendered anatomy, 4, 133, 339–40; gendered physiology, 4, 133–35, 339–40, 366–67. *See also* women's illnesses

healing sites, 6, 124, 383–93; natural sites, 383–84, 385 fig. 68; physicians' treatment rooms, 387–90; religious sites, 268 fig. 49, 384–87. *See also* Asclepian temples; hospitals; *valetudinaria*
health, 23, 54–55, 95–96, 98–99, 101; as balance, 23, 53, 55, 98–101; medical theories of, 95–106; personification of, 24, 416; religious explanations of, 17–19, 96–97
heart, 27, 29, 110, 134, 163, 204
hemorrhoids, 259
Heraclides of Tarentum, 30, 88, 415
Herophilus of Chalcedon, 29, 87, 89–90, 96, 136, 180, 238, 337, 415
Hesiod, 108, 121, 415
Hippocrates of Cos, 21–23, 87, 207 fig. 36, 415; Hippocratic question, 23
Hippocratic school, 21–24
Hippocratic corpus, 22–24, 133, 192, 338; *Airs, Waters, Places*, 55, 61–77; *Decorum*, 326, 330, 333–36, 387; *Diseases of Women*, 134, 138–42, 340; *Oath*, 2, 257, 326–27, 328 fig. 59, 330–31; *On the Art of Medicine*, 78, 80–86, 109, 312, 327; *On Epidemics*, 100, 122–31, 187, 192, 207 fig. 36, 260, 315, 344, 384; *On the Nature of Humans*, 23, 99, 101–6, 187, 208, 228; *On Regimen*, 271, 273–75; *On the Sacred Illness*, 195–205, 337; *Regimen in Health*, 228–31, 337
hospitals, 34–35, 392–93. *See also valetudinaria*
home health care, 40 fig. 9, 287, 315, 316
housing, 38–40. *See also* population density
human remains, 6–8, 38, 43, 49–50, 96, 157, 160, 209, 260–61, 285
humors, 20, 23, 53, 54 fig. 16, 102–6; humoral theory of illness, 98–99; temperaments associated with, 53, 54 fig. 16, 99. *See also* black bile; blood; phlegm; yellow bile
Hygieia, 24, 25 fig. 4, 279 fig. 51, 385 fig. 68, 416

illness, 132–218; as imbalance, 23, 54–55, 98–101, 181; bites and stings, 171–76; digestive and intestinal ailments, 148–57, 162, 164, 266–67, 377; epidemics, 51, 124, 205–18; eye conditions, 176–86, 240; fevers, 100, 186–92; medical theories of, 95–106; mental and emotional afflictions, 101, 134–35, 184–85, 187, 192–205; religious explanations of, 17–19, 96–97; respiratory ailments, 45–46; women's ailments, 4, 135–37, 141–42, 342, 351, 356–59; wounds and fractures, 157–71, 257, 262–67. *See also* pathology
incubation, 26, 36, 267–71, 387. *See also* dreams
infancy, 337–38, 365–76; ailments related to, 51, 199–201, 365, 367–68; bodily constitution of, 199, 278; infant mortality, 37, 51, 365. *See also* breastfeeding
infertility, 135, 137, 139–40, 340, 346–47
injuries. *See* fractures; occupational hazards; wounds
innate heat, 133, 148, 222, 226, 379
inscriptions, 6, 14, 19 fig. 2, 26, 173, 177 fig. 30, 267, 271–73, 288, 305–10, 312, 322–25, 385, 392
instruments. *See* medical instruments
intestines, 27, 89–90, 162, 164, 266–67; intestinal ailments, 148–57, 162, 164, 266–67

Jesus, 18, 179, 192, 179, 280 fig. 52, 281, 313

kidney, 29, 163. *See also* stones
krasis, 372, 373–75

lactation. *See* breastfeeding; breastmilk
lead, 8, 45 fig. 12, 170, 179, 264; lead pipes, 8, 44, 45 fig. 12; lead poisoning, 8, 44, 45 fig. 12
life expectancy, 37, 38 fig. 7, 376
life stages, 337–82; adolescence, 338, 339; infancy, 337–38, 365–76; old age, 337–38, 376–82; prime of life, 337–38, 379–80
lithotomy, 257
liver, 27, 109, 141–42, 148, 162–63, 193, 198
lungs, 45–46, 64, 134, 199–200, 238. *See also* respiratory ailments

well-being. *See* health

wet-nurse. *See* breastfeeding

womb, 4, 133–37, 343 fig. 62; ailments, 133–48; anatomy, 134 fig. 21, 343 fig. 62; parts of the womb: 134 fig. 21, 343 fig. 62; uterine suffocation or "wandering womb," 4, 134–37, 141–43; votives, 134 fig. 21

women. *See* gynecology; obstetricians; physicians; women's illnesses

women's illnesses, 133–48, 340, 342, 357–62; backed-up blood, 134–35, 137, 192, 226, 340; uterine suffocation or "wandering womb," 4, 134–37, 141–43, 226; treatments for, 135–48, 357–62. *See also* gynecology; womb

worms. *See* paleoparasitology; parasites

wounds, 157–71, 257, 262–64, 266–67; battle wounds, 50 fig. 15, 262–64, 266–67, 313 fig. 57, 314 fig. 58. *See also* pus; gangrene

yellow bile, 20, 23, 53, 54 fig. 16, 98, 99, 102–5, 187, 188 fig. 34; choleric, 53, 54 fig. 16, 193, 374n39, 403, 404

Zeus, 179 fig. 32, 277n54

Founded in 1893,
UNIVERSITY OF CALIFORNIA PRESS
publishes bold, progressive books and journals
on topics in the arts, humanities, social sciences,
and natural sciences—with a focus on social
justice issues—that inspire thought and action
among readers worldwide.

The UC PRESS FOUNDATION
raises funds to uphold the press's vital role
as an independent, nonprofit publisher, and
receives philanthropic support from a wide
range of individuals and institutions—and from
committed readers like you. To learn more, visit
ucpress.edu/supportus.